MW01529289

Language Function

of related interest

Assessing and Developing Communication and Thinking Skills in People with Autism and Communication Difficulties
A Toolkit for Parents and Professionals
Kate Silver
With Autism Initiatives
ISBN 978 1 84310 352 3

Incorporating Social Goals in the Classroom
A Guide for Teachers and Parents of Children with High-Functioning Autism and Asperger Syndrome
Rebecca A. Moyes
Foreword by Susan J. Moreno
ISBN 978 1 85302 967 7

Can the World Afford Autistic Spectrum Disorder?
Nonverbal Communication, Asperger Syndrome and the Interbrain
Digby Tantam
ISBN 978 1 84310 694 4

Autism and the Edges of the Known World
Sensitivities, Language and Constructed Reality
Olga Bogdashina
ISBN 978 1 84905 042 5

Language Function

An Introduction to Pragmatic Assessment and Intervention for Higher Order Thinking and Better Literacy

Ellyn Lucas Arwood

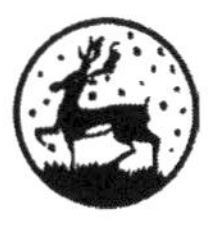

Jessica Kingsley *Publishers*
London and Philadelphia

Figures 15.1 and 15.2 reprinted with permission from Arwood, Kaakiren, & Wynne 2002

First published in 2011
by Jessica Kingsley Publishers
116 Pentonville Road
London N1 9JB, UK
and
400 Market Street, Suite 400
Philadelphia, PA 19106, USA

www.jkp.com

Library of Congress Cataloging in Publication Data
Arwood, Ellyn Lucas.
Language function : an introduction to pragmatic assessment and intervention for higher order thinking and better literacy / Ellyn Lucas Arwood.
p. cm.
Includes bibliographical references and index.
ISBN 978-1-84905-800-1 (alk. paper)
1. Language acquisition. 2. Literacy. I. Title.
P118.A74 2010
401'.93--dc22
2010025677

British Library Cataloguing in Publication Data
A CIP catalogue record for this book is available from the British Library

ISBN 978 1 84905 800 1

Printed and bound in the United States by
Thomson-Shore, 7300 Joy Road, Dexter, MI 48130

Contents

Acknowledgements

I wish to thank family members who have contributed to this work by giving up their family time, holidays, and vacations so that I may write. To Tom, thank you for the help with the technology, and to Mabel, thank you for the drawing of figures. I also want to thank my colleagues who have contributed their ideas, their students' work, their words, their drawings, and their support.

To the thousands of children and their families with whom I have worked over the many years, thank you for allowing me the opportunity. To the many families and adult learners with whom I have worked, thank you for your professional desire to help others learn. Without each and every one of you, I would not have the support to write this book nor any reason to write this book. Thank you!

Preface

The traditional approach to the study of language is structural in nature. Structural approaches examine language products: sounds, morphemes, words, sentences, vocabulary, turn taking options, and so forth. Educators develop literacy programs based on these structural units. Students learn structures and educators test for the structures. For example, educators teach students to read words and then they test the students to see how many words per minute they read as a test for reading fluency. The assumption is that the quicker children read, the better they are at reading. Educators use this approach to define reading as a measure of oral fluency. The assumption behind this approach is that a reader sees the letters and says the patterns of sound as a process of decoding. Decoding becomes the measure of effectiveness of teaching a child to read. Researchers collect data on the number of children who can decode with these methods and the oral fluency methods become the approach for teaching children to read. This reading example highlights the emphasis of teaching structures. In this case, the structures are sounds, letters, and their combinations.

This structural approach to language, and subsequently, literacy, stems from an auditory bias. The auditory bias of English "unknowingly" represents the thinking of its people. The dominant culture of English speakers uses a sound and time-based value system in school and in the workplace. Languages represent their speakers' cultures and English is an auditory language. The properties of an auditory language like English includes the following: English is alphabetic (letters and sounds), time based, and context free (words can stand alone). However, current brain research supports the author's data that the majority of English speakers (around 85%) do not learn concepts from the sound of words, and therefore do not think in sound. The properties of English do not match with the way most learners think.

Most English speakers, today, think in visual graphics like movies, pictures, printed words. Therefore, there exists a cultural and linguistic mismatch between auditory, sound-based education and the way that most people think or learn new concepts. This book will address the purpose of understanding language function as a way to deal with this cultural-linguistic mismatch, for assessing and intervening in education to promote better literacy, based on learning strengths for ultimately higher order thinking and functioning. The author defines literacy as constructing meaning for listening, speaking, reading, writing, viewing, thinking, and calculating. Therefore, the book is about all sorts of literacy programs including working on sounds for speech, teaching parts of speech for language development, teaching sounds and letters for reading and writing, and so forth. The book is also about how literacy is about thinking and viewing.

Book overview

Part I of this book will establish the basis for the difference between a structural language approach to literacy and a language function approach to thinking as a strength-based approach to literacy.

Part II will provide the reader an understanding of English, an auditory language that has its cultural roots in the way educators assume that learning to be literate must take place. This cultural auditory assumption about literacy comes from the auditory properties of English, but auditory instruction does not match the visual way that most people think. Since the majority of thinkers use a visual way of thinking, then programs for literacy (speaking, reading, writing, and so forth) will want to use a visual form of thinking.

Part III provides the reader with ways to assess how a person learns from analyzing language function and Part IV provides the reader with the way that these visual ways to approach literacy looks in the classroom.

Part I

Chapter 1 provides the structural approach to the study of language that is often the standard for developing assessment and intervention programs. But, language is more than the sum of its parts and so educators will also want to consider language functions. Language functions are a result of the acquisition of meaning so the author will describe the Neuro-Semantic Language Learning Theory in Chapter 2. This four-tier model allows the reader to understand how learning language is a process of thinking as well as using language for thinking. Chapter 3 provides an introduction to the myriad of language functions. This book is not about learning styles or preferences but about how the brain processes sensory input into patterns to form neuronal circuits for concepts of language.

Part II

Chapters 4, 5, and 6 discuss the properties of an auditory language like English compared to a visual language like Mandarin. For example, auditory languages (e.g., English, French, Russian, Spanish) displace with time whereas visual languages (e.g., American Sign Language (ASL), Chinese) displace with space. Auditory languages use the word as a referent, but visual languages use relationships for referring, and are therefore contextual or field sensitive in nature. Auditory languages allow for mobility by rearranging letters and sounds to change meanings; visual languages use the sequence of events for flexibility and productivity. These differences in language function result in differences in thinking. Typical language functions include how language displaces an event from a person such as being able to think about going into outer space but having never been in space, how language allows for learning concepts for higher order thinking (semanticity), and how language allows for global flexibility and productivity. Part II will provide an explanation for how these language functions represent thinking, learning, and the interdependence between language and literacy. Examples of application will be provided throughout this part.

Part III

Chapters 7–12 provide the reader with an understanding of the relationship between literacy and language functions versus language structures. The author will provide the reader with several examples of how to assess speakers of English for language functions at three levels of development (pre-language, language, and linguistic function). Examples of how to intervene or provide assistance in learning for these case studies will follow.

Language function becomes the tool for literacy at about seven to eight years of age when the child develops the adult grammar of structures. So, learning to become literate is a language function. Numerous examples for how learning, language, social, and cognitive development intertwine will be provided to the reader as case studies. It should be noted that the case studies are based on real examples from real children. Their names, their demographic data (age, school, gender, parent, home, and so forth), their skills, and their actual works have been modified to protect their identity and to provide the reader with the best examples of how to assess and intervene. In this way, the anonymity of the child or adult is protected while providing the best examples of assessment and intervention for the reader.

Case studies are from all levels of children and adults and from a variety of settings. Composites of studies are sometimes provided to offer the best examples to the reader. For example, a sample from an eight-year-old may be put with the picture of another eight-year-old in order to show how the writing and oral language relate. Or, the oral sample of one child may be put with the intervention strategies of another child to protect once again the identity of both children. These changes will not affect the assessment or the intervention outcomes. Case studies follow as close a description as possible without exposing the child's identity. The author has more than 40 years of effective working with clients, students, and their families and so the examples come from many places. Furthermore, she continues to refine the strategies over the years and will attempt to provide the reader with the most-up-to-date current approach to assessment and intervention based on language function.

Part IV

Intervention strategies in the book for the case studies begin in Part III for individuals and continue into Part IV, which emphasizes group use of strategies for primary, intermediate elementary, and middle school to adult levels of assessment and intervention (Chapters 13–15). Three different classroom teachers and their work will be highlighted at each of the three levels.

The individual strategies in Part III and the group strategies in Part IV utilize the theory and explanations in the first two sections as a foundation for developing effective language methods (Chapters 1–6). Because most people think with visual language function, the author has learned to use the characteristics of visual languages to develop strategies that translate auditory properties of English, an auditory language, into a visual form of acquisition and development for higher order thinking and therefore better literacy. The author refers to the methods of translating auditory English or thinking to visual methods of learning to be literate as Viconic Language Methods™.[1] Case studies (Part III) and classroom applications (Part IV) will highlight these Viconic Language Method (VLM) strategies according to

1 A trademark for Viconic Language Methods has been applied for by the author.

developmental levels as well as for those who are diagnosed with disabilities and those who are not. These methods work for a variety of disabilities that includes autism spectrum disorders (ASD), attention deficit hyperactivity disorders (ADHD), fetal alcohol syndrome (FAS), co-morbidity issues, language and learning disabilities, and so forth.

The concluding chapter of Part IV (Chapter 16) deals with the research basis for assessment and intervention methods used in this book.

Summary of the book

In summary, because language function represents thinking, learning language is both a social and cultural phenomenon. Culturally, all people in the dominant group speak the same language that represents the broad base values of that culture. But, if the majority of people think with visual cognition, it is not unusual to find that the majority of today's youth are anti-social. They cannot think about how to act in a way that matches the expected auditory cultural values. This book will address these social and cultural issues of language throughout the book. Increasing language function helps develop higher order conceptualization, the ability to be on time, and to turn in authentic homework (not plagiarized) today. Most people approach these social issues and anti-social behavioral problems of our youth as structural issues; if there is a behavior problem, work on the behavior; if there is a reading problem, work on sounds, and so on.

This book is a refreshing and a desperately needed strength-based model. Instead of working on the structures or behaviors that are found to be deficits through testing, this book explains how to examine the learning system of a person through an assessment of language function, and then use VLMs that match the thinker's learning system so as to better develop social-cognitive development.

The author realizes that many of the concepts may be new to the reader and that all learners acquire concepts (thoughts) over time and through multiple layers; so, the author provides numerous examples of new concepts in a variety of ways across the chapters for the reader to develop more depth as the reader moves through the book. The author suggests that the reader scan the text to take information off the page, rather than trying to understand each new idea the first time the author refers to it. The reader will have multiple opportunities to read about the same new concepts in multiple chapters. In this way, the reader will gain more knowledge about concepts throughout the book. The author provides the reader with an opportunity for what she believes is good conceptual learning. A Glossary is at the end of the book. Within the text, the author has emboldened and italicized the terms that can be found in the Glossary.

Note that the author is also sensitive to gender specific language so she will try to use third person whenever possible and gender specific language when the words refer to individual people such as the case studies.

The author encourages the reader to use the content of this book to develop the reader's understanding of the learning system so as to try any or all of the strategies in a variety of ways. Good luck with your applications!

PART I

LANGUAGE AND THINKING

How Do Language and Thinking Develop?

Part I introduces the reader to two different ways to think about language. First, language is a set of structures or products of the developmental systems. Second, language is a set of functions that represent the way a person thinks. Educators and researchers use these perspectives about language to establish programs, materials, and methods for teaching children and adults to become literate.

Chapter 1 provides an explanation of the structural approach to language, the standard way that most disciplines study language and the typical basis for most ways to teach literacy. Language structures include words; parts of speech; divisions of words such as letters and sounds; structural ways to look at language such as the study of sound structures (phonetics, phonology); the study of a sequence of meaningful sounds (morphology); the study of vocabulary (structural semantics); and even the structural way to analyze how two or more people talk to each other (structural pragmatics). However, language is more than the sum of its structural parts. Language is about how a person thinks; how a person learns to be literate; and how a person problem solves.

If society values thinking and problem solving, then understanding the way a person acquires both language structures and language functions is important for planning assessment and intervention programs. Chapter 2 discusses the acquisition of language structures and functions as part of a meaningful set of semantic processes; not as sounds and words but as patterns of sound and sight, and other sensory inputs, which form concepts of language. Chapter 2 introduces the reader to the Neuro-Semantic Language Learning Theory, a four-tier model that places emphasis on thinking (third tier) with language (fourth tier). Since acquisition of language is not just the result of adding structures together, but also a semantic set of processes, Chapter 3 discusses the study of language functions, an investigation of how thinking and language interact.

Speakers typically have a purpose for talking, and so their language functions to represent people's values, needs, interests, passions, and desires. For example, language allows a person to think about ideas that a speaker will never physically experience such as understanding outer space, the ancient Mayan civilization, the depths of the oceans, the government of a country, the inside of a human capillary, the concepts of respect, or the emotions of love. Language moves a thinker beyond the here-and-now of the present moment to the imaginary world of fiction. To be able to create a theme park or an animated movie requires the function of language to make the characters that no one else has ever seen, or to build the roller coaster that no one has ever ridden. Language functions improve thinking and Chapter 3 defines and explains these functions.

Even though language functions provide the purpose for learning to speak, read, write, talk, view, think, calculate, and listen (seven functions of literacy), most literacy programs emphasize the learning of language structures. This focus on language structures offers a cultural-linguistic bias that the author explains in Part II of the book as a two-tier model of sensory input and pattern processing. Most people use this model as the basis for teaching patterns of reading, writing, speaking, and so forth. However, Chapter 2 shows that if language is more than the sum of its parts or patterns, an educator will want to consider more than the assessment and intervention of patterns but also concepts and language functions. The Neuro-Semantic Language Learning Theory is a four-tier model that has rich applications for improving thinking and learning to be literate. Parts III and IV will provide the reader with assessment and intervention methods that consider language functions as part of learning to be literate as a thinker and a problem solver.

Chapter 1

DEFINING LANGUAGE

Learner objectives: Chapter 1

Upon completion of this chapter, the reader should be able to:

1. Define the term "language structures."
2. Give several examples of "language structures."
3. Define the term "language functions."
4. Give examples of what "language functions" do for a speaker.
5. Explain why language is more than the sum of its parts.
6. Explain whether most language and literacy programs emphasize structures or functions.

She knows how to play,
So she plays to know.
She learns the names.
So she knows how to learn.

A middle-aged man, Professor Smith, sits at an oversized teacher's desk studying pieces of paper with symbols on them. The ***symbols*** represent the spoken language of a group of people that is only 50 members in size. The people are from a very small, rarely visited South Pacific island. Professor Smith's colleague, Dr. Moore, an anthropologist, lived with these people for six months. During her stay, Dr. Moore video-recorded the people engaged in various everyday situations. Later, Dr. Moore transcribed the islanders' spoken ***utterances*** which Dr. Moore gave to Professor Smith to analyze. Professor Smith, a linguist, looks at the utterances that have been written in sound symbols in the hopes of finding some language patterns. For example, Professor Smith notices that most ideas begin with the sound of "eeee." This repeated sound structure is a pattern. Professor Smith is learning *about* this rare island language by finding patterns within the language. Professor Smith will then describe the language with rules he writes, for the patterns he discovers. These rules will define the grammar or elements that constitute the language. Because this island language has no written or orthographic component, Professor Smith's whole analysis will be based on Dr. Moore's data from the oral language she gathered from island speakers. Professor Smith does not know how to speak the language. He does not "know" the language. But, Professor Smith can still *study* the language by utilizing Dr. Moore's data.

The study of language structures can occur without speaking, reading, writing, or understanding the content of the language. Language can be defined by its ***structures***. These structures include the elemental patterns of sounds, words, and parts of speech used by the native speakers. This first section of this chapter provides the reader with an understanding of the structure of language. If the study of a language can occur without speaking, reading, or writing the language, then to speak, read, or write a language must be more than studying or learning structures. The latter part of this chapter will discuss language functions, the way language functions develop through ***cognition*** and with cognition.

The study of language structures

Language structures include words, sounds, sentences, parts of speech, and so forth. Language structures are observable and measurable and, on the surface, appear to define the language. To study the structures of a language, a researcher like Professor Smith observes the language. Since oral language is difficult to see, then researchers who study language structures observe them through *sampling*. ***Language sampling*** occurs by collecting a body or ***corpora*** of sentences from a ***native speaker*** just like Dr. Moore did through video-recording. The recorded spoken utterances are then transcribed and analyzed; so, the speaker's utterances can be defined, explained in units, and measured. Box 1.1 shows an example of a simple sample from an adult, native English speaker.

Box 1.1 A simple sample of an adult native speaker's language

What do you do on a typical day?

First, I walk the dog. Well, I get up, then I walk the dog. I make coffee at 7:15. I get dressed. Oh, I also get ready for work. Like sometimes I read my email. I don't always read my email. I have breakfast. I go to work. But, I also get dressed, obviously. Well, at work I do the files, take a break, have meetings, leave around 5:00. Go home. Walk the dog. Have a snack. I also have lunch. Then get ready for bed and do it again the next day.

While looking at the sample in Box 1.1, a person studying language might look for observable structures or patterns. These language structures in this type of sample include words, sentences, the way words go together or the ***grammar*** such as subject-verb agreement, and ***parts of speech*** such as nouns and verbs. Since it was a spoken sample, there is also a sound system and that sound system has structures. These observable structures or patterns fit into one of four areas of structural language study: the study of sounds, ***phonology***; the study of the smallest meaningful units, ***morphology***; the study of the word order, ***syntax***; and the study of the meanings, ***semantics***. So, the person who studies language analyzes the transcribed utterances for structures used by the native speaker which includes sounds (***phonemes***), units of meaning (***morphemes***), the way words fit together (*syntax* or word order as well as *parts of speech*), and the vocabulary (*semantics*). This means that the typical structural units of analysis are phonemes (sound units), morphemes (meaningful units like adding "s" for plural or the word dog without adding morphemes), words (vocabulary, parts of speech), sentence structures, and the general vocabulary in the language (semantics).

Activity: What are the four areas of the study of language structures? What are the four units of analysis?

Defining English structures

Look again at the sample from Box 1.1. In addition to the types of structures, what are some of the patterns of structural use? For example, most sentences begin telling about who does the ***action***. The person or noun, who does the action, is the subject of the sentence and is italicized in Box 1.2.

Box 1.2 Subjects occur at the beginning of most sentences

What do you do on a typical day?

First, *I* walk the dog. Well, *I* get up, then *I* walk the dog. *I* make coffee at 7:15. *I* get dressed. Oh, *I* also get ready for work. Like sometimes *I* read my email. *I* don't always read my email. *I* have breakfast. *I* go to work. But *I* also get dressed, obviously. Well, at work *I* do the files, take a break, have meetings, leave at around 5:00. Go home. Walk the dog. Have a snack. *I* also have lunch. Then get ready for bed and do it again the next day.

After the subject of the sentence is provided, what the subject is doing is represented by a verb or action word. Box 1.3 shows or ***marks*** the verbs (to mark a structure in language means to identify the pattern of the structure).

Box 1.3 Verbs tell what the subjects do

What do you do on a typical day?

First, I *walk* the dog. Well, I *get up*, then I *walk* the dog. I *make* coffee at 7:15. I *get dressed*. Oh, I also *get ready* for work. Like sometimes I *read* my email. I *do*n't always *read* my email. I *have* breakfast. I *go* to work. But I also *get dressed*, obviously. Well, at work I *do* the files, *take* a break, *have* meetings, *leave* at around 5:00. *Go* home. *Walk* the dog. *Have* a snack. I also *have* lunch. Then *get ready* for bed and *do* it again the next day.

So, in this sample, most of the sentences tell about the subject directly or infer the subject (noun) followed by what the subject does (verb). The action of the subject usually affects someone, some thing, or occurs some place…these are the objects of the actions. Box 1.4 shows or *marks* the objects.

Box 1.4 The object of the verb is usually a person, place, thing, or location

What do you do on a typical day?

First, I walk *the dog*. Well, I get up, then I walk *the dog*. I make *coffee* at 7:15. I get dressed. Oh, I also get ready *for work*. Like sometimes I read *my email*. I don't always read *my email*. I have *breakfast*. I go to *work*. But I also get dressed, obviously. Well, *at work* I do *the files*, take *a break*, have *meetings*, leave at around 5:00. Go *home*. Walk *the dog*. Have *a snack*. I also *have lunch*. Then get ready *for bed* and do *it* again the next day.

By observing that most of an English speaker's sentences are in a ***subject-verb-object (S-V-O)*** order, a researcher might conclude that one of the basic characteristics of English is that it consists of an S-V-O organization. *This S-V-O syntax defines the word order of English*. Not all languages use this type of structure. The islander language that Professor Smith is studying may have a different structural type.

Activity: What is the S-V-O characteristic of English language structure?

Native English speakers have learned the S-V-O pattern and therefore they are able to intuit the S-V-O order, even when they do not know the identified structures. This learned meaning of the language provides the stage for teachers and parents to want to teach subjects or nouns by labeling, followed by adding verbs or actions. The nouns and verbs are then put together to form "sentences." Some adults who learn about the structure of English conclude that because the S-V-O is the basis to English syntax, then adults should teach children who are learning English about the S-V-O structure in order for children to be good speakers or readers or writers. But, remember that Professor Smith can study *about* a language and not know how to speak, read, or write it. Chapters 2 and 3 will address how studying about the structures does not provide the basis for learning a language.

Activity: What is meant by the concept that English utilizes the S-V-O language structure?

In addition to the S-V-O word order or syntax there are also some other words, mostly time-related words that occur over and over in the sample. Box 1.5 shows or *marks* the time-based words or phrases of the sample. Again, the person who studies *about* a language grammar is looking for patterns or similarities of structure.

Box 1.5 Time-based words in the simple sample

What do you do on a typical day?

First, I walk the dog. Well, I get up, *then* I walk the dog. I make coffee *at 7:15*. I get dressed. Oh, I *also* get ready for work. Like *sometimes* I read my email.

I don't *always* read my email. I have breakfast. I go to work. But I *also* get dressed, *obviously*. Well, at work I do the files, take a break, have meetings, leave *at around 5:00*. Go home. Walk the dog. Have a snack. I *also* have lunch. Then get ready for bed and do it *again the next day.*

These ***time-based*** or ***temporal words*** or phrases are also a part of the structure of the English language. In fact, time is so important in English that the language structures show time not only in words or phrases but also in the structures of nouns and verbs. For example, in Box 1.5, there are several nouns that not only are subjects but also refer to specific events of time; e.g., breakfast, lunch, bed, break. Time is not limited to nouns; verbs show time as well; e.g., "dressed" means that the person already completed the act of dressing. In fact, the person who collected this sample asked a time-based question, "What do you do on a typical day?" since "typical" refers to "day," a temporal word. This specific question, "What do you do on a typical day?" has normative data (*Temporal Analysis of the Propositions* or *TEMPRO*: Arwood & Beggs, 1989; see also Arwood, 1991b) related to the concept that English uses time. The speaker in Box 1.5 uses a lot of English time phrases and words. *English is a time-based language. The structures consist of the S-V-O order and also time words.*

Activity: Why is English considered a time-based language?

Even though this speaker in Box 1.5 uses temporal words and temporal verbs, the speaker does not clearly let the listener know exactly what order the events occur in. In other words, this speaker has the time-based structures of English but not a complete understanding of the concepts of time. This speaker in Box 1.5 is able to use time-based words in English without understanding the cognitive meaning of time. *The cognitive meaning is the function of language, whereas the measurable surface structures make up the grammar of the language.* From studying this sample, it is apparent that English structures are time based and create an S-V-O sentence.

Activity: What are two structural characteristics of the English language?

Recognizing English structures

Even though the speaker who provided the sample is not completely clear in expressing the chronology of activity, a native speaker *listening* to this person will gain a basic idea of what happens. The speaker "gets ready" for work, which includes taking the dog for a walk, having coffee, and getting dressed. Then the person goes to work which includes some emails along with breaks and meetings. Finally, the person goes home and has dinner, goes to bed, and the routine begins again the next day. Furthermore, the syntax or word order (S-V-O) of the speaker includes all of the words that "glue" or connect the words together such as "the," "at," "to," "a," and "for." Box 1.6 *marks* these small words called ***functors***. These types of words are also structures.

Box 1.6 The functor words are marked with italics

What do you do on a typical day?

First, I walk *the* dog. Well, I get up, then I walk *the* dog. I make coffee *at* 7:15. I get dressed. *Oh*, I also get ready *for* work. Like sometimes I read *my* email. I don't always read *my* email. I have breakfast. I go *to* work. But I also get dressed, obviously. *Well*, *at* work I do *the* files, take *a* break, have meetings, leave *at around* 5:00. Go home. Walk *the* dog. Have *a* snack. I also have lunch. Then get ready *for* bed *and* do it again *the* next day.

These little words are called *functors* in English because they work or structurally function to help interpret the meaning. For example, the word "my" refers to something owned by someone or to whom something belongs. Therefore "my" is a ***possessive pronoun***. "Possessive" refers to ownership and a ***pronoun*** refers to replacing the person with a word that refers to the person. On the other hand, there are small words that *conjoin* or connect ideas such as the word "and." The word "and" is a ***conjunction*** because it conjoins two or more ideas. There are also words that *function* in the structure of an English sentence to refer to the place or location of a position of an object or person, like the word "at." The word "at" refers to the location of the person, "at work." Or the word "for" refers to the object of the action. Both "at" and "for" *prepare* the listener for what happens to the object of the sentence and are therefore called ***prepositions***. There are words that tell whether or not a noun is specific or not, such as "the ball" versus "a ball." The words "the" and "a" *function* to determine whether the noun is specific. These ***determiners*** are ***articles*** in that these words affect or determine the specificity of meaning of the noun in a phrase or sentence. Parts of English language include pronouns, conjunctions, articles, and prepositions. These structures also have a meaningful function.

Activity: What are some of the various functors in English?

These functors modify the meaning of the words, phrases, and sentences in English and therefore are part of *the study of the smallest units of meaning or morphology*. Each of these functors is one *morpheme* that consists of one meaning. But, nouns and verbs in English can be modified to have additional meaning. For example, to the word "dog," a speaker can add "-s" and therefore the listener hears "dogs" and knows that there is more than one dog. The word dog is specific and therefore the speaker is *free* to refer to the word and the listener will have an idea of what the speaker means. But, the speaker cannot use the "-s" alone so the "-s" is *bound* to another word. *Words that specify the meaning are free morphemes.* Units of meaning that are bound to specific words such as the "-s" or endings (suffixes) and beginnings of words (affixes) are *bound morphemes.*

English uses a lot of these bound morphemes to change or ***modulate*** the meanings of free morphemes. The reason that English can so easily modify the meaning of words by adding meanings through individual sounds, for example "-s," or clusters of sound such as "-ed," is because English is also ***alphabetic***. This means that the spoken words have written counterparts. An alphabetic language takes the speaker's sounds and translates them to written ***graphemes***. Each grapheme in English is a letter or letters that represent spoken

English. Sounds and letters create the alphabet. English structures are alphabetic in nature when relating spoken language to written language and the meanings of words or morphemes can easily change because of the alphabetic property of English structures.

Activity: What are morphemes? What does alphabetic mean?

So far, in this chapter, the English language is defined as including the S-V-O syntax structure, a time-based morphology, an alphabetic property, and a variety of parts of speech. When Professor Smith studies the islander language he is also taking all of the parts he knows from English and analyzing the parts. For example, the spoken words of the English language have sound. The sounds that make up the spoken English are called *phons* (pronounced phones). The sounds arranged into letters that represent the sounds are the *graphemes*. Since English does not have a one letter for one sound correspondence, a symbol system like the International Phonetic Alphabet (IPA) (e.g., Givon, 2009; Hall, 2005; Rowe & Levine, 2009) can be used to transcribe spoken language. Dr. Moore collected the videotapes of the islander speakers and gave those tapes to Professor Smith, who used the IPA to write down the islander speech. Even though Professor Smith did not know how to speak the islander language, he could use the IPA symbols to represent the sounds he heard. The sample in Box 1.7 is the same sample as the one in Boxes 1.1 through 1.6, but the IPA is used to write one symbol for each sound (note that the numbers are used as numerals but the sounds could have been written instead).

Box 1.7 Sample is written with International Phonetic Alphabet (IPA) symbols, Doulos SIL font where each sound corresponds to a letter[1]

What do you do on a typical day?

/Fɝst, ɑɪ wɔk ðə dɔg. Wɛl, ɑɪ gɪt ʌp, ðɛn ɑɪ wɔk ðə dɔg. ɑɪ mek kɔfi æt 7:15. ɑɪ gɪt drɛst. O, ɑɪ also gɪt rɛdi for wɝk. Lɑɪk sʌmtɑɪmz ɑɪ rid mɑɪ imel. ɑɪ don't alwez rid mɑɪ imel. ɑɪ hæv brɛkfɛst. ɑɪ go tu wɝk. Bʌt ɑɪ also gɪt drɛst, ɔbviʌsli. Wɛl, æt work ɑɪ du ðə fɑɪlz, tek ə brek, haev mitɪŋz, liv æt əraund 5:00. Go hom. Wɔk ðə dɔg. Hæv ə snɑɛck. ɑɪ also hæv lʌnʧ. ðen get rɛdi for bɛd ənd du ɪt əgɪn ðə nɛkst dæ./

In the sample in Box 1.7, one symbol is written for each sound; this means that the written symbol is based on the sounds made by the speaker. Until the nineteenth century, many English writers wrote the sounds of words according to their speech. All sounds were written and when a speaker read English, the speaker would pronounce all sounds. For example, in the word, "walked," the /l/ and "-ed" were pronounced.

English speakers moved across large regions of the northern hemisphere. Different people in different places would simplify the sounds or use shortcuts of pronunciation resulting in not all sounds being produced by all speakers. This simplification of English

1 For more information about the International Phonetic Alphabet, see the website: www.langsci.ucl.ac.uk/ipa.

sounds resulted in the production of fewer and less complex sounds of words. By the 1800s, the development of dictionaries of conventional spellings emerged, thus providing a conventional or expected way to write specific words, regardless of the way a word might be pronounced in different regions. With the help of a standard way to write English, the written words stayed the same but oral English continued to evolve; thus increasing the gap between oral and written language.

Finally, in the 1950s, educators developed a way to connect sounds and letters through ***phonics*** or ***phonic rules*** (Heilman, 2005/1964). A teacher might use phonic rules to show students how the letters represent different sounds. For example, a teacher might give rules like the following:

> The letter "c" produces an "s" sound when it is with the long vowel of "i" and has a silent "e" at the end of a word like "ice." But, the letter "c" sounds like "k" when it is at the beginning of a word and is followed by a short vowel as in "candy."

If these sound and letter combination rules are difficult to understand, that is typical. Rules for language structures like phonic rules describe the relationship between spoken and written English. *Language rules describe the language, not define the language.* Just like Professor Smith, the purpose of describing a language is to learn *about* the language. Learning *about* a language does not necessarily provide the tools for teaching a person to speak, read, write, think, view, listen, or calculate with the language.

Phonics was developed as a tool to describe the relationship between written and spoken language, not as a way to teach sounds and letters for reading and writing. Heilman (2005/1964), one of the original writers about phonics, very specifically indicated that describing the sound structures of English rules is based on an understanding of complete structural language. This means that phonics rules were never intended for children learning 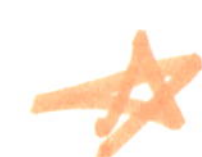 their oral language structures, nor were phonic rules intended for teaching the basic language of learning to read and write. These types of rules were described to help adults understand the translation between spoken English and written English. In other words, phonic rules help describe the language, not teach the language.

Activity: What was the intent of developing phonic rules?

Because English consists of both the spoken and written language which is alphabetic in nature, English is a language that can create new meanings quickly by rearranging the sounds. English sounds consist of combinations that are easy to arrange in as many different patterns as there are sounds. New words are created by arranging the sounds into a typical English construct. The production of English sounds is fairly easy for a human being. Speakers produce sounds by vibrating the air from the lungs up through the trachea into the mouth. As the speaker moves his or her mouth, the sounds change and so does the meaning of the word produced. For example, a native English speaker looks at a dog whose mother is a Poodle and whose father is a Schnauzer and the speaker calls the dog's new breed a Schnoodle. This new word or ***neologism*** is easily reproduced and then accepted by English native speakers because it meets the sound rules of English.

Activity: How does the rearrangement of English sounds create new words?

Describing a grammar like the Pacific Islander language or English requires finding all patterns. English has an infinite ability to combine sounds into patterns, so linguists describe the language with the rules of phonology, morphology, syntax, semantics, and pragmatics. The infinite structure of English sound patterns provides for an ***infinite grammar***. An infinite grammar like that of English provides for endless structure combinations. These combinations of English sound consist of two types of sound production. One type of sound is produced by positioning the tongue, teeth, palate, jaws, and lips and then allowing the air to flow. These types of sound are called ***consonants*** such as the sound "s." Most of the time, the "s" is produced by moving the tongue to channel the airflow into a wind tunnel right behind the front teeth. This position makes a hissing sound that can barely be heard by the speaker. Most people have difficulty hearing this "s" or hissing noise without the production of additional sound. The second or additional production of sound occurs by how open the mouth is to allow the air to flow from the vibration of the larynx through the mouth. This vibration or phonation of the air from the lungs through the larynx and into the open mouth makes ***vowel*** sounds such as "a," "e," "i," "o," and "u." So, English consists of consonants followed by vowels to form ***consonant-vowel-consonant (C-V-C)*** combinations. English consonants receive their audible "sound" or energy from the production of vowels. Without vowels, many of the consonants consist of air but little sound.

Activity: What does C-V-C combinations mean?

Once the sounds of English are combined into patterns, the speaker is consistently able to use the sound patterns to refer to something meaningful. These meaningful sound patterns are called ***words***. Words are language structures that may occur in isolation and are often considered part of a speaker's vocabulary. In other words, in English, the speaker uses these words to talk about ideas. The use of words can occur alone without any preparation for the topic. This means that English does not require much set up or ***context*** for the listener to be able to understand the meaning of a word or utterance. For example, a classroom teacher might walk into a classroom and say, "Today, we are going to study Italy." Prior to saying this sentence, the students were doing math problems. This sentence, "Today we are going to study Italy" is not related to what the class was doing before the teacher began to talk. The students are expected to be able to process and understand the teacher's words without any other preparation. This means that the words do not need context or situational cues to be understood. *English is considered a **low-context** language*. Professor Smith may discover that the Pacific Islander language does not function the same way as English (e.g., Villegas, Neugebauer, & Venegas, 2008).

Activity: What is meant by low-context language?

So far, the study of English, the language, reveals that English consists of structures or patterns. Some of these patterns include the following:

- English sounds (phonology) form into **consonant-vowel-consonant** (C-V-C) combinations.
- English **words** (semantics) in isolation convey meaning.

- English ***time*** concepts are plentiful.
- English has a written **alphabetic** sound-letter structure.
- English uses a **subject-verb-object** (S-V-O) syntax.
- English has specific types of **morphemes** (morphology).
- English is a **low-context language**.

These structural properties of English can be further described by writing rules that define the patterns. The study of language structures of rules for English or most other languages includes the following:

- How each sound is produced (**phonology**).
- How meanings are changed (**morphology**).
- How sounds relate to graphemes (**phonics**).
- How parts of speech (e.g., nouns, verbs, objects) and functors (e.g., prepositions, pronouns, articles, determiners, etc.) create the surface grammar (**syntax**).
- How words represent meaning (**semantics**).

Activity: Explain some of the structural properties of English. What are the areas of study for understanding these structural properties?

Speakers of English are able to speak to one another and understand what the other says because the speaker and listener (hearer) have rules for when people talk and what is appropriate to say. These rules for how to take turns and how to narrate or use discourse provides another area of study of language structures, ***pragmatics***. To study these structures, the researcher must write the words of the speaker and the hearer and then look for patterns between the two people's words. In the previous example, the first speaker asks the question, "What do you do on a typical day?" and the hearer of this question then changes roles and becomes the speaker. This speaker then takes a turn by saying what he does in response to the question. This shared process of rules for talking between two or more people is called pragmatics.

Activity: What is pragmatics?

English rules of structure

Comparative studies of large corpora of language transcriptions allow linguists to write the rules for the language. When Professor Smith finishes studying the patterns of the Pacific Islander language, then he will try to write rules for the patterns. For example, a researcher might want to know how all of the words relate to one another in English. So the researcher develops a tool, such as a diagram, to explain how the words relate. Figure 1.1 shows a simple diagram for words in a sentence based on the structures defined in English.

The girl walks her dog to the store.

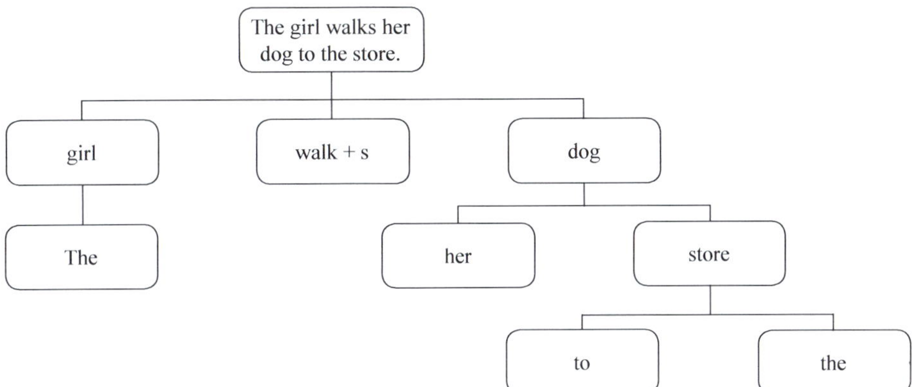

Figure 1.1 Simple diagram of a sentence

The simple diagram represents how the functor words modify words in the sentence. For example, the sentence is not about a non-specific girl; the sentence is about "the" girl; so, the first "the" adds meaning to "girl." Complex sentences result in complex diagrams. By using these types of diagrams, linguists are able to show the way words relate to one another. In this way, rules for English word structures can be written. An example of a rule might read: Articles such as "a" or "the" modify the meaning of nouns such as "girl."

Likewise, the linguist, who studies the sound rules of a language or speaker, might study the way that English sounds connect to form words and create the rules for the sound system. From this data, phonological rules may be written for a language and then each speaker of that language may exhibit variations of those rules. For example, in English there is a sound that is described as a consonantal "r" such as in the word "***r**ed.*" But English speakers also connect that sound of "r" to vowels such as in "moth***er***" or "h***er***e." Not all languages have that type of "r," and within English, the "r" varies from region to region. In the US, speakers of English sometimes even add an "r" sound to a vowel that other English speakers do not. For example, speakers in parts of the Northeast US say "idear" for "idea." Rules for how and when the "r" sound occurs with other sound patterns according to variations or dialects within the language may be written.

Rules for all the areas of language study may be written: syntactic rules, phonological rules, semantic rules, pragmatic rules, and morphological rules. These types of rules for ordering words or parts of speech or rules for creating meaning or for how English sounds are produced help define the structures of English. *Language structural rules are explanations for how to define the surface forms or patterns of the language.*

Activity: What is the purpose of language rules? What are some examples of such rules?

Development of language structures

Since children are not born with adult language structures, the question of when do children develop which structures can be addressed using the same observational methodology as the linguist, Professor Smith, uses to describe the characteristics of a language. Child development specialists audio and videotape children at various ages, observing and transcribing the development of language structures to determine what language structures develop at what ages. Table 1.1 shows the basic expectations for the development of language structures.

Activity: What are the typical stages of structural language development?

As the reader may be discerning, a child with good language development shows the production of adult language structures by the time the child is seven or eight years old. This is why some countries do not begin with reading and writing instruction until a child is seven or eight years old. By this age, the child has enough language to support reading others' works as well as enough language to write one's own ideas. Furthermore, the reader might be wondering how many US children have these adult language structures in a narrative format by seven to eight years of age (e.g., Fletcher & Garman, 1997). The answer will vary by population. For example, a colleague who teaches first grade in a Title I school[2] where 78 percent of the children are on free and reduced lunch, where there are seven or eight different ***first languages*** in each classroom, and where there is a high mobility rate, would tell you that she has only one or two children out of an average of 24 students who have age-appropriate language development when they enter her classroom. In another district, a colleague teaches fifth graders. The majority of her students do not have the solid language structures of a seven or eight-year-old when they enter her room at around ten years of age.

This author suggests that the majority of US children do not possess the language development expected of a seven or eight-year-old, even in the later grades. However, some of the research shows that children do have the language of the stages previously described at the expected ages. Most of these studies use children from college educated parents who encourage language development in the first few years. This data suggests that the adults in a child's environment play a role in the development of language structures. It is well known that children of poverty or children who lack the "right" environment for education do not show the same language development and subsequent levels of literacy (e.g., Hart & Risley, 1999; Walker, Greenwood, Hart, & Carta, 1994). Furthermore, the development of language may also affect the development of literacy (e.g., Cleave, 2005).

2 The US Department of Education provides funding to schools with at-risk populations so as to provide an equal opportunity for all children to receive a high-quality education so that they can meet academic standards. Low-income students are considered at risk, so low-income schools receive supplemental funds to assist meeting educational goals. These supplemental funds are guaranteed under titles or acts such as Title I for low-income students. Low-income students are determined by those who are enrolled in a free and reduced lunch program. For an entire school to qualify as a Title 1 school, at least 40 percent of the students must enroll in the free and reduced lunch program.

Table 1.1 The stages of language structure development

Three days after birth…differentiated cry	Different cries for different needs—mothers are able to recognize the differences.
21 days after birth…differentiated sounds	Responds to different sounds—determined by brain studies and sucking studies.
Three months…cooing	Child produces vowels like the cooing of a dove.
6–9 months…babbling	Child produces consonants with vowels such as ba-da-ga…babbling; babies can begin to imitate hand signs (American Sign Language).
9–12 months…jargon	Baby produces the C-V-C combinations like words in strings…jargon. Word patterns appear for common people, objects, and actions…Mama…da…dat.
12–24 months…***telegraphic*** utterances	Number of combined patterns increases…e.g., Mama go. Child uses the two-word utterances in a variety of ways to mean a variety of ideas…e.g., no juice can mean the child doesn't want juice, not that particular juice, the juice is gone and the child wants juice, etc.
24–36 months…simple sentences emerge	Child uses word patterns in combinations that are simple in structure…e.g., "My daddy works" or "Play toys wif me"…some of the sounds are still developing.
36–48 months…expanded structures	Child uses simple sentences and begins to ask questions…e.g., "Who plays wid dat?" or "Why are the windows dere?" "What he do?" The question forms are sometimes unique to children.
48 months…question stage	This is the question year…child asks multiple questions, sometimes the same question over and over…child refines the structure of the question, and the sounds.
Five-year-olds…storytelling stage	This is the storytelling year…children with good development of language structures are able to tell complete stories. For example, "My mom and dad took me to Granma's. Mom bought me a new dress…see? And my dad gave me shoes. Do you like my shoes? My Granma bought me a dog. I named the dog Ralph." Was it your birthday? "Yes I am five years old. I got lots of presents and I liked my dog the best." What kind of dog is it? "It is a toy dog. It is black and white and has a pink collar. I put it on my bed. When I go home, I play with my dog." The child is still developing some of the time elements and refining some of the last to develop sounds.
Six-year-olds…complex sentences	Child's language continues to increase in vocabulary, complexity of sentence structure, and sounds. "This picture is about two garbage men. They want to take out the garbage but the dog does not want them to. So, the dog bites this man on the ankle. The man tells the dog to stop so the dog leaves him alone. The men can take out the garbage. The end."
Seven to eight-year-olds…adult language structures	What do you do on a typical day? "Well, I get up and get ready for school. My mom takes me to school and then I work there for most of the day. After school, my mom picks me up and takes me to ice skating. Then, when ice skating is over, we, my mom and me, go home and have dinner. If I have homework, I do my homework or sometimes I watch some TV and then do my homework or we go do something fun like watch the ice hockey game and then go to bed. That is what we do most days."

Language structures show that the child has sufficient language for the development of literacy. Literacy may be defined as the child's psychological ability to construct meaning for and with reading, writing, speaking, viewing, thinking, listening, and calculating (Cooper, 2006). So, language structures do not develop by themselves but there must be more to development than the structures since language and literacy are interrelated.

Activity: Is there a relationship between literacy and language development? At what age are children supposed to have adult language structures?

Teaching of language structures

Linguists, like Professor Smith, who use the adult corpora of language to determine the characteristics of language, provide descriptions of languages. But using the same methodology to teach a child language is based on assumptions that may not lead to expected outcomes. For example, it is apparent that children learn the language patterns or structures of the world around them: A mother speaks Chinese and the child learns Chinese. A different mother speaks English and her child learns English. From this observation, an adult might reasonably conclude that a child learns such structures by imitation. After all, a child develops language structures in a systematic and sequential order (see Table 1.1 for an overview of such development) dependent on those around the child. But researchers discovered that there are many instances where a child produces language structures that adults never produce. For example, the two-year-old makes use of two-word utterances such as "mama go" or "me home" which the adult never produces. Or, at age four, the child might say, "Who dog that's?" for "Whose dog is that?" The order of words is not the adult order. So, imitation alone does not allow a child to develop language.

Some researchers have tried to explain these differences by suggesting that the child's language is a reduction of the adult grammar. So, the two-year-old produces only the "words" the child can produce, a reduction of the adult sentence structure. Again, the research does not support this hypothesis as children do not randomly produce words. For example, a two-year-old might say "mama go" but not "my is" of the sentence "My mama is going to the store." So, the child isn't producing only those words that the child can physically imitate. The child is learning language through processes that are greater than straight imitation. Language acquisition is not a simple additive set of structures. Chapter 2 will describe a current understanding of language acquisition. *Studying about a language and therefore teaching language structures is not the same as learning language for thinking.*

Activity: Is a child's grammar different than an adult's grammar? Does a child simply imitate the adult structures?

Underlying meaning of language structures

Children's words *mean* more than the sum of the structures (e.g., Austin, 1962; Barr & Peters, 2005; Fry, Phillips, Lobaugh, & Madole, 1996; Grice, 1989; Lucas, 1978; Robinson, 2003; Searle, 1969; Vygotsky, 1962/1934; Webster, 2008; Winkler, 2007). For example, a child might use the two-word phrase "dog go" to mean he wants the dog to come to him, he wants the dog to get a bone, he wants the dog to run, he wants to go pet the dog, and so forth. A child's meaning for the same words could vary, and different children using the same words could have different meanings. From the many studies of children's language structures, *it appears that children do imitate the patterns of the structures but they must learn the underlying meanings as part of a language acquisition process which is greater than the sum of the structures.*

Professor Smith will learn about the patterns of the observable structures of the Pacific Islander language but he will not learn about the underlying meaning of that language from studying the grammatical structures.

Language is greater than the sum of its structures, such as the parts of speech, sentence structures, or words. The human brain *functions* differently for and with language structures. For example, for a chimpanzee, the use of a tool or structure is limited in its function. After, using a stick to pull down a bunch of bananas, a chimp throws the stick down, eats the bananas, and continues on. The stick had limited use for the chimp. Even though humans possess at least 95 percent or greater of the same DNA as a chimp (Britten, 2002), a human's brain functions differently with the development of a tool. When a human uses a stick as a tool, the human finds a way to refine the stick's use, share the new found tool with others, perhaps barter the stick for the best deal, build a new and improved form of a stick, and so forth.

The stick is a structure that works as an immediate tool for the chimp. But, for the human, the stick is more than just a tool for the here-and-now. Even though both the human and the chimp can create a tool and use a tool, the human brain *functions* differently than the chimp's brain. Both the human and a chimp can learn language structures (Deacon, 1997; Shanker & King, 2002) for immediate use as a tool. But, the human brain functions with a synergy where the whole brain is greater than the parts (Arwood, 1983; Koruga, Ribar, Ratkaj, Radonjic, & Matija, 2004). The synergy of the human brain lends itself to the holistic function of the brain. Once the human uses the tool, the human brain seeks new patterns of input from the same structure. The human brain uses language as much more than an immediate tool to get something accomplished; human language functions to develop the thinking of the human. In turn, the development of the human brain allows for greater development of the meaning of language functions.

Activity: How does the human brain think differently than the chimpanzee thinks?

Summary of language structures

English, like all languages, may be studied as a set of structures—as additive parts of language defined by patterns and rules. These patterns and rules explain the surface structures of the language. English consists of an S-V-O syntax, a set of C-V-C sounds, a morphology that can easily be changed with sounds, the use of low-context words, and sound-based time elements. Such descriptions of English do not tell the whole story about the purpose of language or how language helps a person think. Furthermore, a person can learn all about the characteristics of a language like English or a Pacific Islander language without ever being able to speak, read, or write it. The meaning underlying these structures defines the acquisition of language; a process of the function of language (see Chapter 2 for a description of the acquisition of language). The learning of a language must be more than the teaching of the structures. Schools predominantly use the structures to set up curriculum. For example, Figure 1.2 shows the translation of these structures into curriculum.

Grade 4: paragraphs → essays; book reports
Grade 3: written sentences → multiple paragraphs
Grade 2: words → written sentences into paragraphs
Grade 1: letters and sounds → words to simple sentences

Figure 1.2 An example of an additive developmental product curriculum

The following section of this chapter introduces the reader to language functions, a cognitive process of learning.

The study of language functions

A three-year-old girl sits cross legged on the floor, facing the toy shelf and playing with a set of blocks. Her mom walks down the hall and peeks into the girl's bedroom and says, "Dora, put away your toys." The child hears the sound of her mother's voice. Dora quickly turns around. Mom is gone! Mom has returned to the kitchen to prepare dinner. Dora does not understand Mom's words, so she continues to play with the blocks. Mom returns in a few minutes and says, "Dora! I told you to put away your toys. It is almost dinner time."

Dora hears Mom's words as sound patterns, "wa, wa, wa, wa, wah" and recognizes the pattern "dinner." So, Dora jumps up and walks toward the kitchen. Mom stops Dora and redirects Dora back to the blocks where Mom helps Dora "put away" the blocks. Then, both Mom and Dora walk to the kitchen for dinner. Mom and Dora are engaging in a language learning lesson. Dora is learning the English language and Mom is helping to teach the language. But, because language is more than the sentence structures, the words, the meaning of the words, and the sounds of the words; Dora is also developing the cognition for language and the purpose of language. Dora is learning the ***function of language***. Language is a *function* of the ***neurobiological learning system***, specific to being human.

Activity: Why does a tool work differently for a human than a chimp?

Similarities and differences between structures and functions

The structure of language for a human is much like the chimp's use of a stick. A person can see the stick, study the stick, count the stick, and even teach another person or chimp to use the stick. Simple language structures can be seen when written down. They can be studied, counted, and even taught to a human or chimp. In this way, a person or chimp can imitate structures, repeat the patterns of structures, and even use the same structures at a later time (e.g., Fouts, Jensvold, & Fouts, 2002; Fouts & Waters, 2001). For example, children diagnosed with autism can repeat exactly what they have heard, even though they have no meaning for what they can repeat. These imitated structures are the words, the sentence structures, as well as the sounds of the words. ***Neuro-typical learners*** can also repeat structures. For example, children can repeat a rule they have been told such as "Don't touch the TV." And even though a child can repeat a rule, the child may not understand what the rule means. For example, Mom can teach Dora to say language structures such as "thank you" or "please," even though Dora may not use these words correctly.

Activity: In what way are language structures much like the use of a tool that is used in a restricted way?

The structures of language are like tools with specific, but restricted or limited use. They develop through imitation and are restricted to here-and-now usage. But, in the human brain the use of structures represents underlying thinking and learning. As the thinking develops in complexity, so do the language functions. Human language becomes the vehicle for asking, vowing, promising, creating mental constructs, planning into the future, and studying concepts that cannot be felt or touched such as Ancient Egypt. Language functions develop ideas that allow one to study or learn concepts that are far removed from the speaker without ever leaving one's home. For example, language allows the astronaut to fly into space without previously having the physical experience of being in space. Through language, the male obstetrician delivers a baby without personally being a mom. Language *functions* so that the scientist understands the mechanism of a "cell" without being able to see, touch, or physically experience the cell. Through language, the historian travels back through time without leaving the twenty-first century and the author creates a fictitious story never seen except through the mind. Through language the child who is physically unable to speak uses technology to ask for a soft drink at the basketball game, and therefore is able to fit socially with his peers. It is with language that children sit in their seats rather than run around a classroom or adults politely stay in their seats rather than interrupt a religious service. Language *functions* to develop a human's social and cognitive being! Language functions are greater than the sum of the structures!

Activity: What are some examples of what language function does for a human?

The language structures such as words, sentences, and sounds act like a tool; but, the *function of language* (not the structures of language) defines, in part, what it means to be human. The young child in the previous vignette, Dora, is learning to *function* with language. She is learning more than the words or sounds of Mom's voice; she is learning how to be a citizen. Dora is learning the social and cognitive rules of how to fit into society through the acquisition of language. As Dora learns the *functions* of language, she will be able to initiate and maintain healthy relationships, empower herself to meet her goals, and be able to plan cognitively how to work in the future. If Dora learns more than the structures of language, she will be able to use her language to learn beyond the here-and-now, to create new ideas that she can share with others, to think critically and problem solve, and to become socially competent.

On the other hand, if Dora acquires only the structures of language, then she will be dependent on what others can do to structure her world much like the chimpanzee is niche dependent. The structure of language is the here-and-now, superficial way of accomplishing a task. *The function of language is the social and cognitive path to being human, a creative being that "thinks" beyond the here-and-now.*

Activity: How is the function of language different from the structure of language?

Summary

Language consists of both structures and functions. Structures include words, sounds, morphemes, parts of speech, sentence structures, and so forth. Functions refer to the way that the learning system acquires the meaning or thoughts of cognition for social development as a human being. This human learning system functions more holistically than the simple addition of structures and the result is greater than the sum of the parts.

Linguists, like Professor Smith, study about languages for the purpose of describing its parts, its grammar, its structures. Many educators use the results from these studies to arrange programs for teaching children and adults the structures. These language structures can be easily observed and measured but by themselves do not help develop a child's cognition or a person's social being. Chapter 2 describes the way a person acquires language for more meaningful function. The study of language acquisition sheds a light on how language *functions* to help people think and to learn to think. Chapter 3 introduces the reader to the myriad of language functions that exist beyond the study of language structures.

Applications

- Examine a language literacy program and determine how much of the program emphasizes structures.
- Discuss the logic behind teaching language structures and the expected outcomes of teaching language.

Chapter 2

LANGUAGE ACQUISITION

Learning to Think

Learner objectives: Chapter 2

Upon completion of this chapter, the reader should be able to:

1. Define the four stages of the Neuro-Semantic Language Learning Theory.
2. Explain how a person learns language.
3. Explain how patterns and concepts are different.
4. Explain how concepts represent thinking.
5. Explain how learning language and thinking interconnect.
6. Give some educational applications of language acquisition to teaching.

To see is to understand
To hear is to know...
The brain writes but one poetic stanza
A full refrain of mental snow!

The author introduced the reader to Dora in Chapter 1. As a child learning language, Dora will learn to use her language to become literate. Dora's learning to be literate is not only the acquisition of language structures but also the development of the functions of language. These functions of language have a basis in brain development. As Dora's brain develops from its connection between environmental input and physical maturation, so does her language. Current, non-invasive methods are able to study brain architecture and function and therefore offer tremendous opportunities to examine the neurobiological relationship between learning and language. This chapter will provide an understanding of how language acquisition occurs as part of the development of the brain in a neuro-semantic process.

History

Language studies, during the 1950s to 1970s, explained and described language structures. Many different researchers offered models (e.g., Chomsky, 2002/1957; Katz & Fodor, 1963; McCawley, 1976) to describe the origin of language structures and their foundations. Others suggested a biological basis to language learning (e.g., Lenneberg, 1967). But, questions about how a child's brain learns language or where language physically originates remained elusive. By the 1980s, most language researchers (e.g., Lucas, 1980) limited describing language acquisition mechanisms to understanding the underlying meaning of the structures as there was little access to the organ that gave rise to language, the brain. By the early 1990s, brain research created new language studies. Using a form of qualitative research to triangulate among the literature on language (e.g., Pulvermueller, 2002; Schumann, 2004), the brain research (e.g., McEwen, 2007; Siegel, 2007; Sylwester, 1995, 2003, 2005; Trelfert & Wallace, 2007) and the concepts of literacy, a plausible theory of how the brain *learns to be literate* is available. The purpose of this chapter is to provide the reader with a brain-based theory on how a person learns language to become literate. Because the brain creates meaning as the basis to language function, the theory is ***neuro-semantic*** in nature, Arwood's Neuro-Semantic Language Learning Theory (Arwood, 1983, 1991a; Arwood & Kaakinen, 2009; Lucas, 1978, 1980).

There are four steps to the acquisition of meaning for learning language:

1. Sensory input forms meaningful patterns.
2. The sensory patterns become recognizable sets of patterns.
3. The sets of patterns form systems of patterns or concepts.
4. Language represents the concepts for greater acquisition of conceptual meaning.

This chapter will describe each of these four phases or steps in the acquisition of meaning for the development of language. The Neuro-Semantic Language Learning System[1] is responsible for the development of the language structures described in Chapter 1. Through this Neuro-Semantic Language Learning System, a child like Dora learns language for thinking so as to become literate, as well as becoming socially competent.

Activity: What different fields must connect to understand how language is acquired?

The human learning system

The human body connects to the outside world through a system of sensory ***receptors***: the ears, eyes, mouth, skin, and nose. Each receptor provides for the input of specific types of sensory input. The ears accept the particles of a sound wave. The eyes receive the particles of a light wave to enter the human body. The mouth tastes flavors of food or anything put into the mouth via the taste buds. The skin covers the body and records any pressure or movement against itself. The nose allows for smells to become part of the human physical

1 Neuro-Semantic Language Learning System refers to the neurobiological function of the acquisition of meaning whereas the Neuro-Semantic Language Learning Theory refers to Arwood's interpretation of neuroscience in developing a theory about how language is learned as a set of neuro-semantic steps.

experience. These receptor organs cover the human body and create the unity between the human body and the universe. It is through these receptors that the human being brings "all" information into the body. There appears to be no other way to bring new information from outside the person into the human body, except through the sensory receptors.

Activity: How does a child get information into his or her learning system?

Sensory input

The first step of the Neuro-Semantic Language Learning System occurs at the sensory level. ***Sensory input*** comes into the eyes, ears, nose, mouth, and skin (receptors) in the specific way that each receptor accepts information. The eye can accept only the particles of a light wave while the ear can accept only the pieces of a sound wave. Likewise, the taste buds of the mouth respond only to the flavor of items while the nose can process only smell. And, the skin accepts only touch. Two of these receptor organs, the taste buds and skin, can process only input brought to the receptor. For example, food registers a flavor when the food is actually on the taste buds, and the skin registers the pressure of touch when someone is up against the skin. Neither the skin nor the mouth will allow for information to enter from across the room or from a distance.

Infants might smell an ear or lick a mom's skin for input but older learners do not do this. They hear or see Mom at a distance. For older learners, they use the senses that allow for input from across the room or around the corner. The eyes and ears are the ***distance receptors***. The caregiver or the teacher talks to the child from a distance. The child looks at the caregivers, the chalkboard, and/or the print on the page from a distance. The distance receptors, the eyes and ears, provide the learner with the opportunity to learn language since speakers are at a "distance" from the listener who is learning language.

Activity: What are the distance senses?

What about smell? Even though the nose can pick up smells from a distance, the nose organizes these smells into a limited array of kinds of smell, e.g., pleasant, unpleasant, stinky, fragrant, etc. Because the nose creates limited types of meaning and as language refers to many different kinds of ideas than just smells, not much learning for human language occurs through the nose. The eyes and ears still remain the primary distance sources of input for language.

The bottom line is that all outside information is brought into the human body through these sensory receptors. And, not one of these receptors brings in whole products such as words, paragraphs, sentences, etc. Each of these receptors brings in only what sensory input the cellular structures can recognize. The human learning system for language literacy forms its development around these types of input.

The distance receptors of the eyes and ears connect the child to his or her mom's or dad's face and to the sound of their voices from across the room. Because the eyes and ears make this type of distance connection it is the eyes and ears that this chapter will focus on. The eyes and ears help provide the child with the meaning of what others say and do. From this meaning, the child will develop how to behave, what to say, when to be polite, how planets are different from stars, who the ancient Greeks were, how to have an acceptable work ethic, and so forth. The child will learn the functions of language such as ***critical thinking*** and problem solving through the development of this Neuro-Semantic Language Learning System. The first step of this learning system is the intake of the sensory information.

Activity: Explain how sensory input is the first step of neuro-semantic learning.

THE EARS

The ears receive sensory input from sound waves (e.g., Breedlove, Rosenzweig, & Watson, 2007).[2] The sound wave originates by compressing air and then releasing the air. For example, clap your hands together. Hear the sound? The hands did not make the sound. The clapping sound was made from pushing the air between the hands and then quickly releasing the air by moving the hands apart. This push creates a wave of compression and release. In Figure 2.1 the diagram of a sound wave shows how the air "pushes in" making a mountain top or peak and then "moves out" creating a valley.

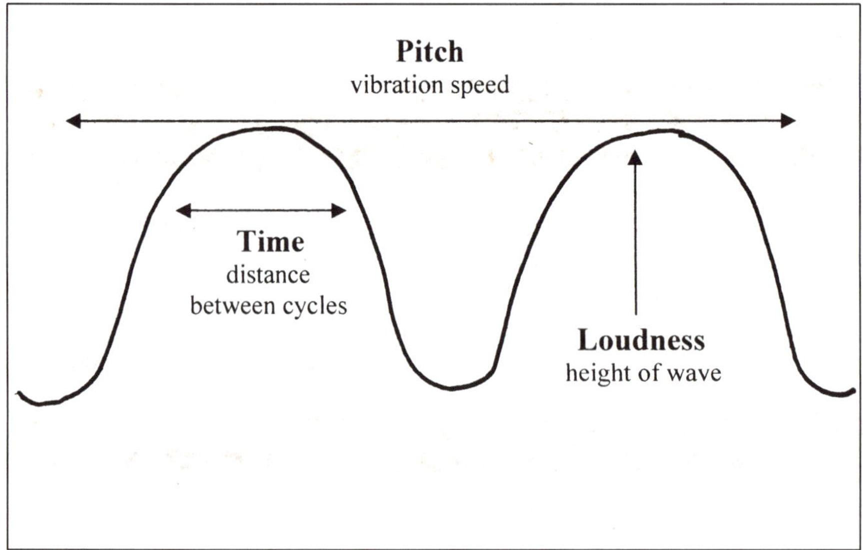

Figure 2.1 The sound wave

How fast the air moves through these cycles (cycles per second measured in hertz or Hz) of peaks and valleys determines how high or low the pitch or tone of sound. The faster these cycles move, the higher the tone or pitch. Women have thinner folds in the larynx and therefore the folds vibrate faster, producing higher voices in women. The slower the cycles move, the lower the tone or pitch. Men have thick folds on the larynx and therefore the folds vibrate slower producing lower tones of voice. Most human, male and female, speech sounds create movement around 500 to 8000 cycles per second even though the

2 There are many good sources on descriptions of the sound and the human ear. Breedlove *et al.* (2007) provide a straightforward, easy to understand option.

human ear can hear higher and lower sounds. When a parent or teacher speaks to a child, the expectation is that the child can hear the sounds of speech. But remember, the child does not physically hear the actual words. The child or baby hears the properties of the wave, the actual components of the wave such as how high or how low the sound.

Activity: How is a sound wave produced? How does the pitch change in the sound wave?

A newborn hears all sounds equally so there is a zhzhzhzhzhzhzhzh...or white noise. These sounds must become meaningful if the child is going to "understand" the parent's or educator's spoken words. To become meaningful, the child has first to be able to receive the different components of the sound wave.

The sound wave has more than just the property of how high or low the tone or "pitch." The air takes time to compress and release to create a cycle. Each cycle begins and ends over *time*. The beginning of the cycle is the "onset" of the compression and the finish of the cycle is the release or "offset" of the compression. The ear records the wave from the beginning to the end of each cycle. This recording of the beginning of the sound cycle to the end of the sound cycle allows the human body to receive the "time of sound."

As explained in Chapter 1, English is a time-based language. Therefore, the sound of a person's voice plays a major role in the properties of spoken English. The use of the time component of sound wave that comes to the human learning system through the ear allows for the development of internal time, a physical and cognitive function of English language.

Activity: In addition to pitch, what other feature of the sound wave does the ear detect?

Sound waves allow for pitch variation and time elements to become part of the human learning system. A sound wave has a third property, loudness. The harder the wave compression begins, the taller the peak or mountain of the wave becomes. Figure 2.1 shows the loudness property of the sound wave. Put your hands in front of you like you are preparing to clap. Now, think about the air that is being pushed as you bring your hands together. If you slowly bring your hands together, the clap is soft. But, if you push the air quickly then the clap is louder, the wave is taller. The height or amplitude of the wave is the loudness.

In summary, the sound wave has three components; the number or frequency of compressions and releases for the variation of tones (cps or Hz), the time of the cycles for time elements, and the height or amplitude for loudness. Similarly, the ear receives three components of sound; pitch, duration or time, and loudness.

The human ear brings all sounds into the human body as components of these sound waves. No sounds come into the human body any other way except through the wave that the ear is able to recognize. Babies as early as 21 days are able to distinguish among sound properties. Their ears have already brought in enough different wave patterns of sound that the baby is learning to distinguish sounds. Likewise, a teacher might raise or lower his or her voice and find that students attend better. The students are able to hear these tiny differences of sound. Hearing the differences between sounds or the differences in a teacher's voice does not mean that the baby or student understands what the mother or teacher is saying.

More about how this sensory input to the ear becomes meaningful patterns will come later in this chapter. *Remember that the first step of hearing sound is the ear's ability to hear the components of a sound wave.*

> ***Activity:*** What are the components of the sound wave? What is the first step of hearing sound?

THE EYES

Like the ears, the eyes connect the child with the child's learning system. The eyes receive light waves (Hubel, 1988).[3] A light wave has different properties than a sound wave and so the eye records different information than the ear. The light wave, like a sound wave, has a point of origination. In the case of a light wave, it is a source of heat or radiation such as the sun, a lamp, a flashlight, etc. Turn on a bright light and notice how many details you see… pieces of lint, flaws in surfaces, facial wrinkles, etc. Now, turn off the lights. The details disappear. In a true "black room" there is no source of light. A person in this type of room "sees" nothing even though the objects and people have not left the room. People see objects and other people because particles of the light wave reflect off surfaces, literally lighting up the objects and people in one's environment. Figure 2.2 shows the shapes of an object lit up by a light source.

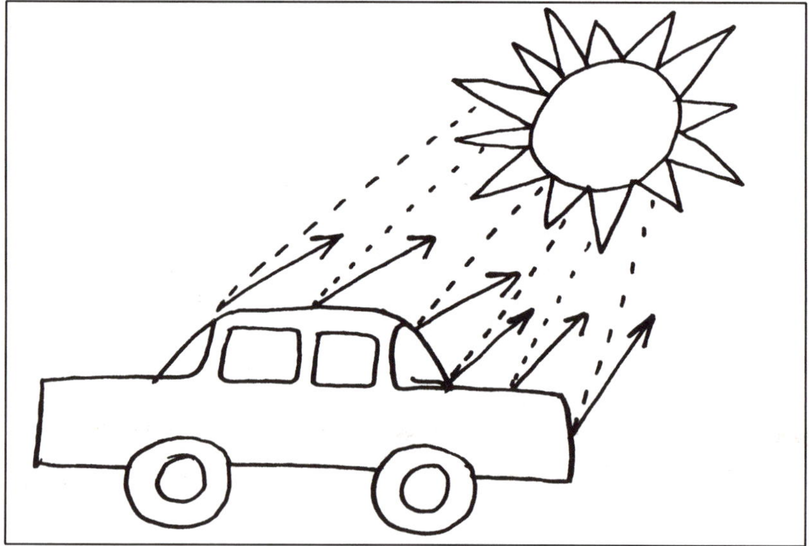

Figure. 2.2 The light wave

Sources of the light wave, such as the sun, emit the radiation particles that gather, spin out, and move together in the form of waves away from the radiation source. As the waves of energy travel further from the source, more energy spins away. Therefore, the closer one is to the source of radiation, the more energy or heat and light. Further away from the source

3 There are many good sources on the eye. One of the classic references is David H. Hubel's (1988) *Eye, brain, and vision.*

the eye perceives darkness and the skin perceives cold. For example, the sun is a very hot and powerful source of light while a penlight is a very small, cool source of light. The eye accepts and processes the radiation particles or photons that reach the eye.

The shape of the eye is crucial to the processing of light particles. Notice in Figure 2.3 that the eye forms a curved surface.

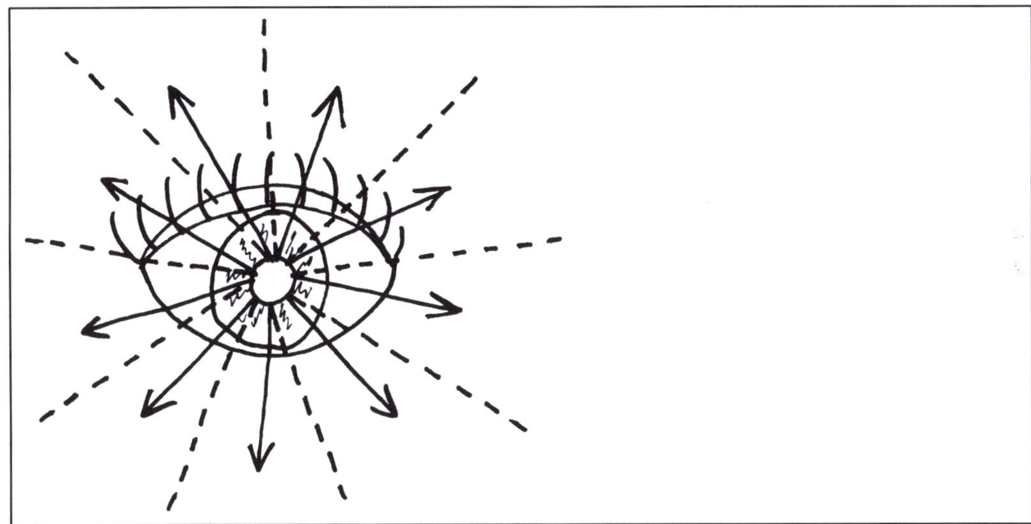

Figure 2.3 The shape of light

The curved surface allows for greater reflection of light or photons. The light is able to reflect off the interior surface of the eye. Each point of reflection creates a pinpoint of light. These pinpoints of light fall along the edges of objects, people, things, etc. In this way, the eye literally records the points of light off a surface as shapes. These points of light on the surfaces will gather over time in a way that outlines the shape of what a person sees. In the meantime, the newborn infant sees no people or objects only light, light that appears so bright to the baby that the baby cannot focus attention. These light points on surfaces of objects eventually will create the shapes of people, objects, anything visible as the eye records more and more input of various objects and people across time.

Activity: How do the eyes work to bring in information?

In the same way that a newborn hears the zhzhzhzhzhzhzhzh of sound, not words or paragraphs, a newborn does not see people or objects. The eyes do not see people or objects, just the points of light that outline the edges or shapes of people and things. In order to increase the points of light, the eyes move. Because the eyes are able to move, the eyes scan the edges or surfaces of people and objects. This scanning becomes a form of ocular tracking which allows the moving eyes to see more of the surface images of light points. The human head also moves which allows the eyes to see more surfaces within a given space. All points of light fill the surface of a plane so that by moving the eyes or head, a person begins to recognize the surfaces of all objects as two-dimensional (2D) planes. These two-dimensional planes consist of the points of light falling on the surfaces of objects, people, etc. The eye sees only in two dimensions, the points of light on the surface of horizontal and vertical planes. Figure 2.4 shows the two-dimensional flat planes of light that the eye sees and records. These points of light create two-dimensional shapes or patterns. More about the light patterns may be found later in this chapter. Also, later, the reader will learn that if the reader thinks he or she is seeing in three dimensions, it is because functional language is filling in the information. Remember that the eye sees only in two dimensions.

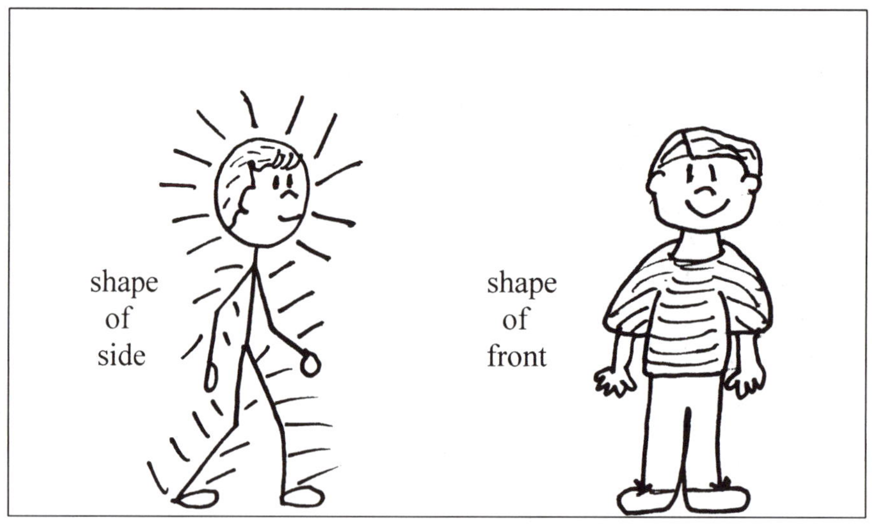

Figure 2.4 The eye sees two dimensions

Activity: What does the eye see?

THE NOSE, THE MOUTH, AND THE SKIN

The nose, mouth, and skin are all specific sensory receptors that record incoming ***sensation***. But, as previously mentioned, these sensory receptors do not bring information into the body from a distant source such as a person speaking or a printed page. Since the nose, mouth, and skin do not record distant sensory input, they also do not form widely used languages. One of the functions of language is to communicate about people and objects that are at a distance. Therefore, it should not be surprising to find out that these receptors are not a significant part of the Neuro-Semantic Language Learning System. Even though it is important to understand what these sensory receptors do, they do not form language. Since language is universal to literacy, little time will be spent on describing the nose, mouth, and skin receptors in this book.

These non-distant or sometimes referred to as immediate sensory sources (nose, taste, and touch) of input receive information in very specific ways. The nose has cells that record the various chemical changes in the air that people call smells. The nose or olfactory system is one of the oldest sensory systems with cellular structures carrying information to the brain where the brain connects the meaning to other forms of input. For example, a person sees a picture of a skunk and immediately remembers the smell of a skunk. The smell is part of the meaning of the idea of a skunk. The smell cannot create the meaning of the concept "skunk" but it can attach meaning, a specific odor, to the word or concept "skunk." Or, for example, a person might say, "Think of fresh baked bread." Immediately, a person who remembers putting a positive meaning to the odor of bread baking will "think" he or she smells the fresh baked bread, even when the bread is only a memory. The olfactory system creates a powerful link between the meaning given to something and the memory of the meaningful concept. If concept-based meaning is *not* given to the odor through the language learning system, there is no olfactory semantic memory. It should be noted that there may exist a physical memory in the brain but not a semantic memory that can be recalled.

Babies do not know the names for the odor differences, only that some odors occur more often than other odors. For example, the smell of baby powder occurs more often than Aunt Suzie's perfume. In other words, the olfactory system records changes in odor. And the brain, not the nose, interprets these changes with meaning from other distant senses. These interpretations of meaning that occur at the brain are part of higher levels of the Neuro-Semantic Language Learning System. Remember: The lowest level of meaning is the receptor level of incoming sensory input.

Activity: How does the nose record information?

The mouth has a number of bundles of cells on the surface of the tongue that will record specific flavors that the mouth tastes. These tastes will not form concepts as part of a language but help differentiate among pleasant and unpleasant items, for example, sugar and dirt. This information will connect with the olfactory system as well as with the distant senses. The taste buds cannot create language learning but will bring information into the human being that the eyes and ears or distant senses can use as part of the language learning system. Babies taste only the differences, not the substance. They taste that bitter is not sweet but they do not know it is spinach versus sugar.

Activity: How does the tongue record information?

The skin covers the entire body. The skin serves as a semi-permeable barrier to protect the inside organs, muscles, tissues from direct contact with germs, undesirable chemicals, and temperature changes. As a receptor organ, the skin serves to accept pressure. When a person touches the skin, the cells of the skin recognize the amount of pressure by chemically changing. The pressure increases with harder touches. Likewise, a gentle touch is a light amount of pressure. Babies only feel pressure; any names or interpretations for the amount of pressure such as "hurt" or "pain" have to be learned by the brain, not the skin.

Activity: How does skin record information? Why are the mouth, nose, and skin senses not as important as the eyes and ears for learning language?

Receiving the sights, sounds, tastes, touches, and smells into the human body is the first step in the Neuro-Semantic Language Learning System. It is a meaningful step at the receptor organ level. Each receptor organ recognizes those pieces of input that the cells of that organ are capable of accepting. *At this receptor level of raw data, there is no interpretation of what the sights, sounds, tastes, touches, or smells mean.* The only meaning or semantic piece is that the sensory organ receives or doesn't receive the input. The educational application at this first level of the Neuro-Semantic Language Learning System has to do with whether or not a child has normal sensory reception which is determined as a sensory impairment or deafness and/or blindness. If there is impairment at this level, then the sensory input difference will create a difference in the rest of the language learning system.

Activity: What is the first level of the Neuro-Semantic Language Learning System? Why do newborn babies not see or hear people?

Perceptual patterns

Once the sensory receptors accept the input, *the second step of the Neuro-Semantic Language Learning System begins to sort the sensory input into* ***perceptual patterns***. The ears and eyes filter and, therefore, begin to process the features of the sound and light waves. Likewise, there is also information coming into the learning system through the non-distance sensory receptors of the nose, mouth, and skin. The human learning system must organize all of this sensory input in a way that the body can utilize. Bringing information in as raw data is the first step; sorting this information and then organizing it becomes a second step. Because language learning requires the use of distance input, emphasis in this part of the chapter will be on the data brought in from a distance, the eyes and ears.

The simultaneous input of sensory input from the various sensory organs creates ***patterns***. These patterns consist of specific sets of acoustic and visual data or features. The immediate task for the learning system is to figure out a way to organize all of this data. For example, if the reader receives 100 reports from colleagues every day, the reader must organize these incoming reports or the reader will eventually be physically covered by stacks of reports. Feeling overwhelmed by the volume of reports, the reader begins to decline in the ability to function. Instead of allowing the reports to stack up, the reader develops a way to sort and organize this incoming volume of reports. So, some reports are filed away, some are discarded, some are sent on to other people, etc. The human body does a similar sorting and organizing of the incoming sensory input from the eyes, ears, and other sensory systems.

Activity: What is the second step of the Neuro-Semantic Language Learning System?

PATTERN RECOGNITION

As the sensory information comes into the receptor organ, the organ processes as much of the information as it can *recognize*. The eyes and ears will recognize those parts of the sound wave and light wave that the human body is able to process. As soon as the features of light and sound enter the receptor, the receptor begins to send the input to the next body of cells. The cells of the receptor organs convert the physical properties of the sound and light waves into chemical changes of the receptor cells. These chemical changes in the cells become messages. Each message moves from one cell to another as a wave of chemical change. From the outer receptor organs toward the brain, the chemical changes move. The primary pathway from the eyes and ears begins in the cranial nerves (e.g., Greenfield, 1997; Howard, 2006). The cranial nerves occur in pairs as part of the central nervous system (CNS) responsible for moving information from the receptors to the brain (Figure 2.5).

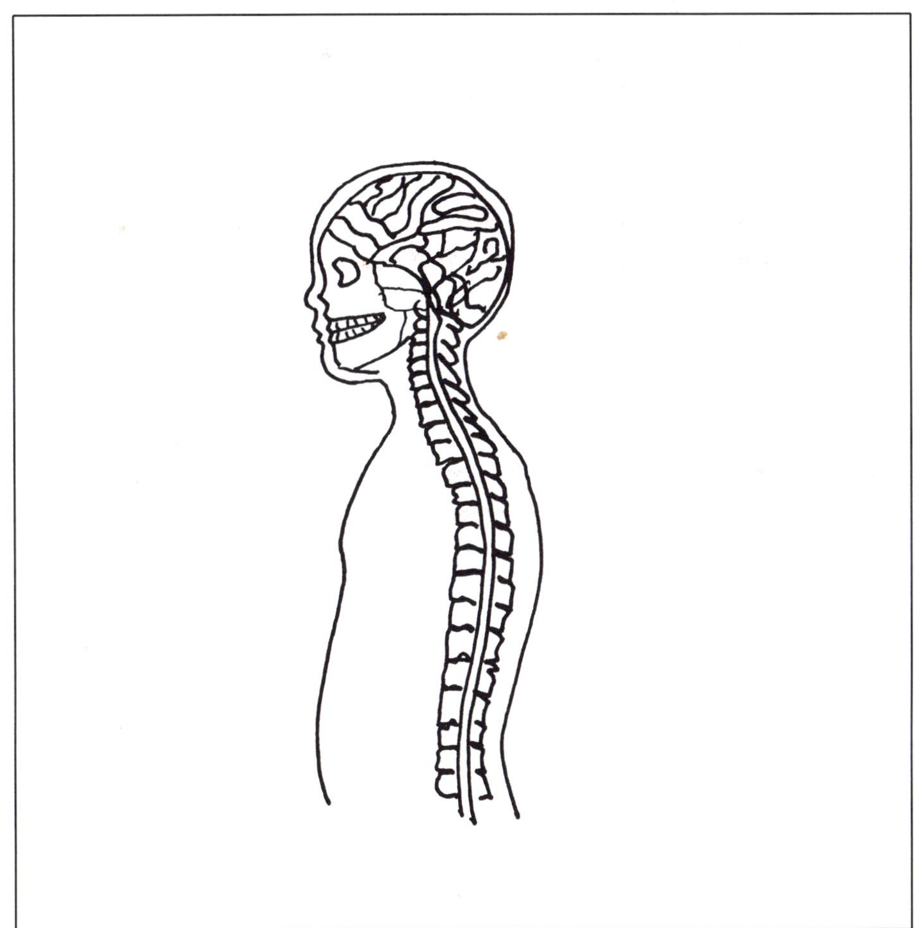

Figure 2.5 Central nervous system

In order for the sensory information to change systematically into chemical messages, the features of the sensory input begin to integrate as the cranial nerves enter the brain stem. The cells move the messages along by bundling them at different stations along the pathway. These bundles of messages move into the brain stem and then on into the midbrain. The bundling of the messages creates structures that are specific to tracking and relaying the messages. This is the second step of the Neuro-Semantic Language Learning System in that the structures of these cells allow for ***pattern recognition***. The cellular structures are recognizing patterns of past and present sensory input.

Activity: What happens first to the sensory patterns?

PATTERN ORGANIZATION

There are several characteristics about how these sensory patterns organize themselves that apply to language learning. *First, these patterns of sensory organization are unique to each and every person.* Even when the input appears to be the same for two different people, the processing of what input is important is unique to each person. This uniqueness occurs because the input for each person is different and because each person's experiences are different. Whether the cells recognize the sensory input as old or new information is dependent on whether the input consists of past sensory features or new sensory features, for that particular person at that particular time. Because each person has unique experiences, then the cells recognize the uniqueness of each person's past experiences as unique input.

Second, because the brain seeks out new patterns, new input takes priority over repeated input. New patterns create more chemical changes in the brain. Chemical changes in the brain "wake up" or activate areas of the brain (e.g., Bookheimer, 2004). In other words, the brain is "hungry" for the new input. And when the new input activates the brain, the brain uses the oxygen, glucose, and other nutrients for metabolism. The brain gets "high" on new activity.

Third, not all input forms patterns that will eventually develop into language. The immediate development of patterns appears to be an easy, brain task. But some types of patterns do not create the bundling of messages that will later be used by the human brain for language. For example, birds can mimic acoustic patterns. But, these acoustic patterns are imitated sound structures without language function. Because acoustic bundled acoustic patterns will not form language, there are no *complex* acoustic languages in the world that use only sound. There are a couple of restricted or rudimentary forms of acoustic communication, the rare clicks or whistles of tribes. These forms of communication are limited in form and function and lack the properties of the higher language functions of English (see Chapters 4–6 for more explanation of language properties and language functions).

Activity: What are three important principles of pattern organization?

PERCEPTION

The second step of the Neuro-Semantic Language Learning System is meaningful in the way that the patterns organize themselves. Such meaningful organization is ***perception***. These patterns come from the complex sensory input of the eyes and ears. For example, ***acoustic patterns*** will ***overlap*** with ***visual patterns*** to produce ideas that include both the sound and sight, like a movie or a spoken narration of a place visited on vacation. When acoustic patterns are the only input that a human processes, then echoic (e.g., ***echolalia***) utterances or imitated regurgitations of what others say occur. These imitations are the structures of language without the language function. In other words, a person can produce these acoustic patterns like a bird does, but there is limited, if any, conceptual meaning. Acoustic patterns alone will not create the necessary patterns for thinking. When patterns overlap to form meaningful connections with concepts, then perception occurs. In the case of acoustic patterns, the imitation of such patterns does not result in meaningful perception, and therefore no conceptual meaning.

Visual patterns, however, can create meaning like seeing a mental image of a picture. These pictures can be elaborate just like replaying a movie. The sorting and organizing of visual patterns creates mental images which will create visual concepts at the next stage. So, thinking can occur with visual patterns forming concepts. However, at the perception level, there are no concepts.

Activity: After the brain recognizes patterns, explain how these patterns overlap.

The pattern sets or messages of the brain stem and midbrain structures create an internal stimulation to which the human being can physically respond. The human being uses the motor system—hands, feet, arms, legs (large muscle groups), and fingers or mouth (small muscle groups) to respond to the sensory sets of patterns. For example, a child sees an object (pattern organization of visual input) and so the child reaches for the object. At this second step of learning language, the child may not know what the name of the object or what the object is for, but the child can see it. And, because the child has sufficient organization of past patterns with the new patterns, the child is able to begin to recognize the shape of the object. This cycle between what the child's brain recognizes and how the child responds by reaching, smiling, kicking, or any motor act establishes a feedback system. The child's learning system recognizes a set of patterns, and so the child *perceives* the object, the person, the action, and so forth. The child is learning the prerequisites to thinking. But, patterns do not mean that the child is thinking about what the child sees or hears.

The educational implications of understanding this second stage of learning patterns are many:

- *Each person's patterns are unique*. Each child's experience is unique. The uniqueness of perceptions is brain based. Each child's own patterns represent what each child, not teacher, understands or processes. Because each child processes the patterns of input in the classroom uniquely, the same presentation within a classroom has unique meaning to each child. This supports the notion that all perceptions of the world are valid.
- *Patterns of sensory input will organize into systems of patterns.* The human body recognizes these patterns based on past and present organization. So, new input connects to old input suggesting that we learn new information when we connect the input to something we already know. This notion of connecting new information to old information for better learning has been part of the educational literature for some time, but the reason behind the rationale for why this works rests with how the brain functions for learning.
- *Pattern sets occur as a result of sensory input.* This is only the second level of learning and is at a low level of processing in the brain. A person can easily imitate patterns. Pattern learning is a *low level* of brain function; a low level of learning. Many, many activities in education consist of pattern recognition, imitation, and regurgitation such as copying letters, spelling words, matching questions at the end of the chapter to sentences in the chapter, worksheets consisting of filling in the patterns or blanks, many multiple choice tests, word calling for reading fluency, practicing sounds, working on sentence structures, vocabulary matching, role

modeling, giving back the professor's words, and so forth. Therefore activities that emphasize patterns are not asking for higher order thinking (see more about applications in Parts III and IV). Remember that animals like dogs, cats, and birds are able to learn patterns. The human brain processes patterns. Higher order thinking requires more processing than imitating and matching or copying patterns. Learning patterns will not allow for higher order thinking or problem solving.

- *A person can learn to imitate or copy patterns because the brain processes these patterns; therefore teaching patterns is easy.* For example, Merzenich and his colleagues (Merzenich, Tallal, Peterson, Miller, & Jenkins, 1998; Merzenich, Saunders, Jenkins, Miller, Peterson, & Tallal, 1999) have been able to develop computerized programs for developing skills of pattern recognition of the sound patterns for teaching alphabetic reading. Brain scans of these trained learning systems show recognition of the patterns. Patterns can be taught! Pattern recognition is the second level of neuro-semantic development.
- *Patterns sometimes form concepts, but not all patterns will form concepts*. Learning the patterns of a skill or task may not develop a higher conceptual understanding. For example, a child can fluently word call the printed messages by learning the sound to letter patterns of English, but not understand the meaning of the print. Sometimes, this is referred to as word calling. Assessing a child's learning system for thinking will need to be present to be able to provide the patterns necessary for a particular child to learn conceptually. More about assessment and intervention will be provided in Parts III and IV.

Activity: What does the information about pattern recognition and organization tell us with regards to educational application? Do patterns always create meaningful concepts? How high a level of brain functioning is pattern recognition?

EDUCATIONAL USE OF PATTERNS

Once pattern recognition occurs, the patterns overlap to form pattern organization. Pattern organization results in motor responses. These motor responses are easy to see by others, so teachers and parents create many opportunities for their students and children to produce responses to the patterns. In this way, teachers and parents are able to count these motor productions as evidence of pattern organization. These opportunities include imitating what someone says, copying the letters of one's name, counting to 10, singing rhymes, saying the alphabet, writing a definition for a vocabulary word 10 times, reciting the multiplication tables, using flash cards, improving oral reading fluency with sounds and letters, matching someone else's words to the exact words on a test or essay, and so forth. The learning of patterns is only the second level of neuro-semantic processing.

Current brain researchers (Bookheimer, 2004) show that the rehearsal or practice of patterns results in the brain disengaging. In other words, practicing without feedback provides no new input for the brain. When the brain does not have the new patterns, the brain becomes disengaged. For example, practice may perfect the muscle memory of writing, but not the cognitive understanding of what the movements of the hand mean. For pattern "practice" to have value, there must be conceptual meaning or an interpretation of meaning through language added to the practice activity (stages three and four of the Neuro-Semantic Language Learning Theory). There must be more than pattern recognition or simple pattern organization to create a higher, conceptual, level of learning.

Activity: What are the first two levels of the Neuro-Semantic Language Learning Theory? What are some educational types of activities that represent the second level of pattern learning?

PERCEPTUAL FEEDBACK SYSTEM

The feedback system (e.g., Hood, 1998) provides two important functions: First, the feedback system helps the cells to recognize whether the input is old or not, so that old patterns can move forward and connect to new information for higher order thinking (see section on concepts). This function is known as neurological ***integration***. Second, the feedback system prevents old patterns from moving on if there isn't anything to connect them to or make them meaningful (recognizable). This function is known as ***inhibition***. Inhibition is needed for integration at a higher level to occur. Higher order thinking requires both a sufficient amount of inhibition as well as integration.

A feedback system is necessary in order to create larger bundles of meaningful messages to reach the higher levels of the brain. Patterns sort and integrate in the brain stem and midbrain to form larger messages. These messages or chemical changes move through the cerebrum to the cortex or surface of the brain. The sorting or integrating of patterns systematically occurs if the brain actively responds to the input as important or new. This feedback system consists of many, many more cellular structures coming back down from higher structures, as many as five times the number of fibers coming down than what goes into the brain from the receptors. But, this feedback system does not develop unless there is sufficient information that can leave the midbrain structures for movement to the cortex. Activation of the cellular systems depends on integrated input (e.g., Sparks, Friedman, Shaw, Aylward, Echelard, Artru, Marawilla, *et al.*, 2002). In other words, the feedback system is built partially from what the system is able to integrate from the sensory patterns of input.

Whether or not a child is able to use patterns for a higher order of meaning depends on several factors:

- Whether or not a feedback system adequately develops to allow the patterns not only to be recognized, but to overlap onto past patterns to create new circuits of meaning (*inhibition*).
- Whether or not the sensory input integrates to allow for more conceptual meaning (*integration*).
- Whether or not the learner's neurological system recognizes the overlap of specific perceptual patterns to allow for the development of neuronal circuits for concepts to occur (*neuronal circuits*).

For the learning system to recognize the pattern sets as important or new there must be sufficient organization at the midbrain level. The midbrain structures compete (e.g., see Honda, 2003) to sort and organize the input. The more patterns that go into the midbrain structures, the more the system must recognize whether the patterns are new or old. Messages of the cells send out new connections (e.g., dendrites) to create a feedback system. As the patterns of cells become larger, more of the brain cells become active in the cortex (e.g., Begley, 2007; Gazzaniga, 1999, 2005; Goldberg, 2001; Goldblum, 2001; Hampson, Pons, Stanford, & Deadwyler, 2004) necessitating more feedback to lower structures.

This feedback system is much like a sophisticated watering system. The water flows into the field. As soon as an area has sufficient water, there is a moisture sensor that sends a message to the watering system to close the duct and divert the water to another part of the field. In this way, all of the areas of the field receive sufficient water.

Like the sophisticated watering system, the midbrain of the human cerebrum must have sufficient *recognizable* input for the feedback system to develop and work efficiently. Otherwise, the patterns continue to enter and enter and enter (Arwood & Kaulitz, 2007) which results in ***perseverative*** or repetitive types of behavior often observed in children with language learning problems such as those diagnosed with an autism spectrum disorder (ASD). These problems demonstrate a difficulty with converting the incoming patterns into a higher, conceptual, form of learning. The connection between the patterns and other functions of learning also occur in other disabilities. For example, children diagnosed with ADHD have difficulty sorting the input at the pre-frontal cortex in a way that allows for attention to details. Any type of perceptual pattern problem, such as sorting, recognizing, or providing feedback for the patterns, will result in differences in language function or thinking.

Activity: What is the importance of pattern recognition, organization, and feedback?

The learning systems of some children with specific learning differences have been known to have deficiencies or smaller bundles of cells for specific structures of the midbrain or structural anomalies. For example, *some* children diagnosed with an ASD show deficiencies in the size or existence of the amygdala (Shanker & King, 2002; see D. B. Webster, 1999 for neuroanatomy), a structure used to track the cellular messages important to memory. Some individuals diagnosed with ADHD (Lou, Henriksen, Bruhn, Børner, & Bieber Nielsen, 1989) show deficient blood flow in the frontal lobe which also means lower metabolism (oxygen and glucose uptake) for better transport of messages to the language parts (cortex) of the brain. The frontal lobe provides feedback to the tracking and organization of the midbrain (memory, focus, attention) via other lobes of the cortex.

With children diagnosed with ASD, their learning systems are very good at pattern development and pattern recognition, but their learning systems have difficulty moving the chemical patterns of the messages into the cortex of the cerebrum where concepts develop. For example, children with autism often have difficulty with assigning conceptual meaning to faces (requires a higher order interpretation of meaning), understanding inferred meanings, or understanding the concepts of time. These children actively seek patterns by self-stimulation or repetition of acts. Children with ADHD have difficulty with temporal concepts for organization, focus, and often impulsivity or hyperactivity. This lack of organization, focus, impulsivity, and hyperactivity demonstrates a lack of feedback from the higher structures (e.g., frontal, parietal, temporal lobes of cortex) to the midbrain where the patterns become organized. Both children with ASD and children with ADHD are very good at pattern development.

Activity: The brain uses patterns in many different ways. What are some effects of brain differences in how individuals with ASD or ADHD may function?

In developing literacy, teaching children diagnosed with ASD or ADHD the rules for their behavior through visual-motor cartoons or learning to read with the visual-motor shape of an idea (instead of sounds and letters) (see Parts III and IV for applications) actually helps decrease pattern repetition because their learning systems are able to recognize the visual-motor patterns as meaningful. The meaningful bundles of patterns develop an increase in the meaning for better focus, attention, and ***conceptualization***. When the sensory input matches the way children are able to recognize, organize, and perceive patterns, then they are able to think at the next level of learning. Children diagnosed with ASD and ADHD do not use sound patterns (acoustic or auditory) well, but they do use visual-motor types of patterns. Therefore, giving the rules of the world in a form of visual-motor patterns actually positively affects the organization or meaning of the patterns, because more of the patterns reach the cortex for better feedback and higher order meaning. *Therefore, when the learner receives patterns that work within his or her learning system to form concepts, there exists a better feedback system.* More about this type of intervention may be found in later chapters.

Activity: Why does pattern organization into larger circuits affect the acquisition of meaning?

Concepts

The third phase of the Neuro-Semantic Language Learning System is the change of recognizable or meaningful patterns into concepts. The sensory receptors accept the various forms of input, light, sound, taste, touch, and smell at the first phase of learning. Then, these sensory forms change into chemical messages that integrate and become recognizable patterns. These perceptual patterns continue through the structures of the midbrain where patterns integrate and higher structures provide feedback or inhibit old patterns (e.g., see Lakatos, Shah, Knuth, Ulbert, Karmos, & Schroeder, 2005). These old patterns move to the next phase or step of learning when there is new information to connect. Because the chunks of old patterns become greater and greater, the size of messages also becomes larger. These large chunks of information require more "brain real estate" (Begley, 2007) to process.

In a Neuro-Semantic Language Learning System, these larger, cortical messages are systems of concepts. Concepts consist of three important components: First, they represent the underlying meaningful patterns or semantic relationships; second, they build over time by connecting old patterns with new patterns for larger or more abstract concepts or ideas; and third, their sum is greater than their parts (C. S. Peirce (2000) coined the term ***pragmaticism***: see Arwood, 1983). It is at this third phase of neuro-semantic development that the learning becomes a part of the mind, and not just the brain (e.g., Greenough, Black, & Wallace, 1987). This is where thinking, as a human thinks, begins!

Activity: What is the third level of the Neuro-Semantic Language Learning Theory?

Thinking occurs when the cells of the outermost part of the cerebrum known as the surface or cortex become active. Within this system there are over 1 trillion cells in an adult human brain (100 billion neurons plus other types of recognition and transport cells such as glial and mirror cells; e.g., see Hirsch & Kramer, 1999). These cells are busy sending messages, recognizing messages, and integrating the patterns of old input with new patterns into new messages. These larger sets of patterns are concepts, the part of the brain known as cognition or thinking. At the cerebral cortex level of cellular activity, the brain completes the dynamic learning of concepts, socially (e.g., see Gallese, 1999) and cognitively. This closed circuit creates a product greater than the sum of the parts; see Figure 2.6.

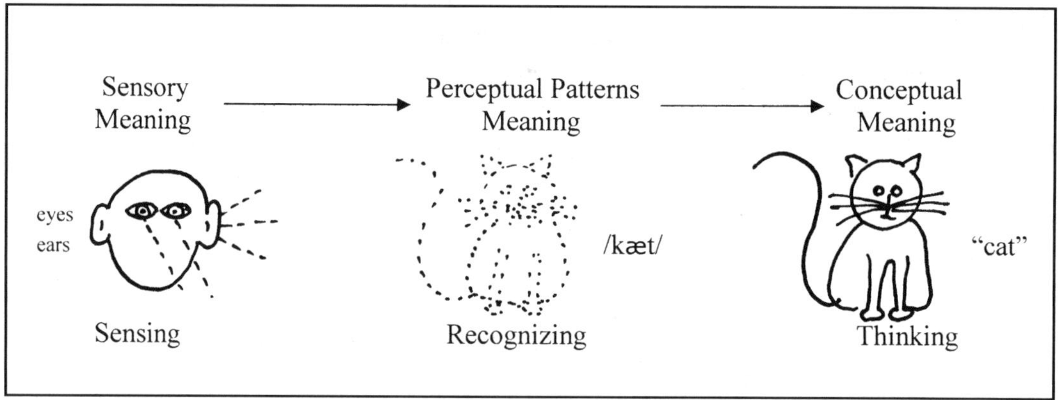

Figure 2.6 Neuro-Semantic Language Learning

At each level, there is more complexity of the system resulting in more feedback along with more complex functions (e.g., see Buccino, Vogt, Ritzl, Fink, Zilles, Freund, & Rizzolatti, 2009, regarding neuronal circuits and hand movements for music; or Monchi, Petrides, Petre, Worsley, & Dagher, 2001). As cell circuits interconnect with a variety of cellular structures in the cerebrum, the patterns become concepts (e.g., Arwood, 1983, 1991a; Gallese & Lakoff, 2005). Although the exact neuro-anatomical mechanisms are still be ascertained, it is certain that at some point the neuronal complexity yields human thinking. Thinking is the third stage of the neuro-semantic level of development and is typically referred to as cognition.

Activity: How does thinking come about?

EDUCATIONAL UNDERSTANDING OF CONCEPTUAL LEARNING

The typical cultural and educational assumption is that if a person can see and hear then that person can *understand* what they see and what they hear. But, remember all input is unique and so is the ability of individuals to organize the patterns into concepts. In fact, not all people are able to create concepts from the same input or recognition of patterns. For example, some people hear the sound of another person's voice but the sound holds little conceptual meaning. And, yet, there are others who not only hear the sound of others' voices but also are able to understand what is said without additional input from other sources such as a speaker's face.

It should be noted that the author is *not* referring to learning styles which are educational or personal preferences, but to how the learning system processes patterns to form concepts. Educationally, if a learner's input does not match the way a learner is able to form concepts from patterns, then the learner will not develop concepts efficiently. In other words, knowing how students learn concepts is important to helping a student understand content, problem solve, critically think, and conceptually learn.

Activity: Why must a learner receive patterns in the way that the learner acquires meaning for concepts? What is the difference between a learning system and a learning style?

CONCEPT DEVELOPMENT

Human receptors have very specific ways to receive input. And, the sensory data for the most complex concepts involves the eyes and ears; so there are only those types of data available to form patterns that yield concepts: the overlap of acoustic data; the overlap of visual data; and the overlap of acoustic and visual data or ***cross-modal*** integration. As mentioned earlier, the overlap of acoustic data allows for the imitation and regurgitation of patterns as in parroting and echoing, but acoustic patterns alone will not form concepts. So, this leaves the overlap of visual data or the overlap of acoustic and visual data to develop concepts.

Visual overlap of concepts will form visual constructs like mental pictures or mental movies or visual characters like in Mandarin Chinese; and, the overlap of visual movements will form shapes, like hand-in-hand signing. For example, Braille (e.g., see Sadato, Pascual-Leone, Grafman, Ibanez, Deiber, Dold, & Hallett, 1996) will form mental shapes within the visual cortex, even for those who are blind. Visual overlap of patterns will form visual concepts for language learning.

The simultaneous integration of acoustic and visual patterns will form ***auditory*** concepts. For a thinker to be able to use the simultaneous bundling of acoustic and visual patterns for auditory tasks, the thinker must be able to learn auditory concepts. For example, phonics, spelling, memorizing the multiplication tables with self-spoken repetition are auditory tasks. All of these tasks require auditory processing such as the use of visual (letters) input with the sounds (acoustic) that go with those letters.

Chapters 4 through 6 will provide the reader with more information about the different ways that patterns form concepts. *Concept development is the third stage of the Neuro-Semantic Language Learning System.*

Activity: What are the three ways to connect sensory patterns (perception) into complex concepts?

Language

The acquisition of language is the fourth and final stage of the Neuro-Semantic Language Learning System. Language represents the underlying development of concepts. Natural language functions (Chapters 3 and 4) parallel the development of the underlying concepts. The higher the conceptualization emerges, the better the language usage. The complexity of the human Neuro-Semantic Language Learning System relates to how well patterns overlap to create concepts and then how well language functions to represent the concepts. For example, the child sees the patterns of the surface of a person's body. The patterns of the outline of a body overlaps with the spoken pattern "mama" which several people say over and over in various combinations. The spoken pattern of "mama" is an acoustic pattern or tag to the outline of the physically seen features of a person. Integrated into these two patterns is the overlap of the smell of perfume, the sound of a familial voice, etc. The child responds to this set of overlapping patterns by reaching for "mama" or "smiling" in response to the pattern of mama's smile, etc. The overlapping patterns create feedback which adds a dimension of complexity for more concepts to develop. This complexity creates a relationship between cognition or thought and language (Vygotsky, 1962/1934) that is truly synergistic, parallel to the feedback of the central nervous system.

As people in the child's world assign meaning through more patterns, the child picks up the larger messages or concepts. "Mama" gives food, gives milk, picks the child up, etc. These interpretations create more overlapping patterns matched to perceptual patterns the child develops. When the child physically responds to the perceptual patterns, then the child's actions provide more feedback to the child's learning system. The child begins to develop the spoken patterns of those around him or her. In this way, those who speak English pass the English patterns on to their children while those who speak Farsi pass the patterns of Farsi on to their children. The language structure differs according to the patterns used to indicate the meaning of the concepts (see Chapters 4–6).

***Language** represents the thinker's underlying ideas or concepts*: The greater the use of language(s) the greater the conceptual development. Language is an ultimate product of the neurobiological system. Because language represents cognition, then language function represents how well a person thinks and therefore acts. Language structures, on the other hand, represent only the surface interpretation of the observable products of the learning system. Language structures are patterns while language functions are concepts and the use of language to represent those concepts.

Activity: What is the fourth stage of the Neuro-Semantic Language Learning Theory? How is language function different than language structure?

Summary

The Neuro-Semantic Language Learning Theory consists of four stages: sensory input, perceptual patterns, concepts, and language. Language represents the concepts that are made from the integration and inhibition (feedback) of large sets of perceptual patterns formed from the sensory input. There are some language properties that are crucial to understand in the development of all literacy programs.

- *The properties of languages mirror the properties of thinking*. Therefore, an educator is able to assess a student's thinking through examining the student's language. Chapters 7–12 will show the reader how to assess thinking and language at different stages of development.

- *Examining the function of language is critical in understanding whether a person is learning the conceptual level of knowledge or is just repeating borrowed patterns as language structures*. The function of language parallels the level of cognitive functioning but the language structures can be borrowed, taught as patterns, or imitated as patterns.
- *Teaching structures or patterns will not result in conceptual learning unless the learner puts his or her own language to the patterns or structures*. Therefore, language functions have to be the focus of conceptual learning.
- *Natural development of concepts comes from the sensory input matching the way a person thinks or creates concepts, not from teaching the patterns.* This means that parents and educators may want to provide a plethora of opportunities for children to use their thinking rather than regurgitating the words, sounds, sentences of others.
- *Once concepts begin to develop, the thinker can begin to assign meaning through language to his or her concepts*. Language becomes a tool for higher conceptualization of ideas that cannot be touched, tasted, smelled, heard or seen, such as ideas about liberty, freedom, respect, loyalty, consideration, collaboration, and so forth.
- *Language assigns meaning to underlying concepts and therefore creates a meaningful lasting memory.* Semantic memory requires the most tracking of the patterns within the midbrain and therefore is the most permanent type of learning. Re-teaching occurs when patterns do not form concepts that are assigned meaning with language. Semantic memory is long term memory.
- *Learning of concepts requires an increase of pattern development through the learner's own Neuro-Semantic Language Learning System.* By assigning meaning with language to one's own concepts, the learner increases the likelihood of the patterns becoming part of semantic memory.
- *In order for a learner to retrieve concepts at a later time, the learner must use language (semantic memory)*. Education without conceptual meaning (through language) results in temporary rehearsal of patterns. This type of short memory of rehearsed patterns can last for as long as six weeks or as short as a few seconds. When a person connects language to the concepts, then the meaning becomes part of a long term memory, semantic memory.

Activity: Explain the four steps of the Neuro-Semantic Language Learning Theory. What are some of the educational implications?

The purpose of this chapter was to explain how the language learning system is neuro-semantic in nature: All language has a semantic basis that rests in the ability of the learner to make meaning from the input to form concepts that language will represent. Dora, in Chapter 1, learns the meaning of her world from what the parents and others assign with language. Because her learning system is neuro-typical, she is able to process what others do and say and therefore she learns not only the structures of what she hears and sees but also the underlying meaning. Chapter 3 will provide the reader with an understanding of how the language learning process provides opportunities to think and understand in all forms of literacy—reading, writing, thinking, viewing, listening, calculating, and speaking.

To summarize this circuit of learning, the sensory input comes into the human body through the sensory receptors. The sensory input moves as chemical messages through the CNS pathways to the midbrain where structures compete for recognition of the input. When the cellular bundles or structures recognize the input, then they move the message through tracks that eventually arrive at the cortical level. This type of recognition also allows the input to become more organized. All along this system, there is feedback to the previous level. Figure 2.7 shows the neuro-semantic language system.

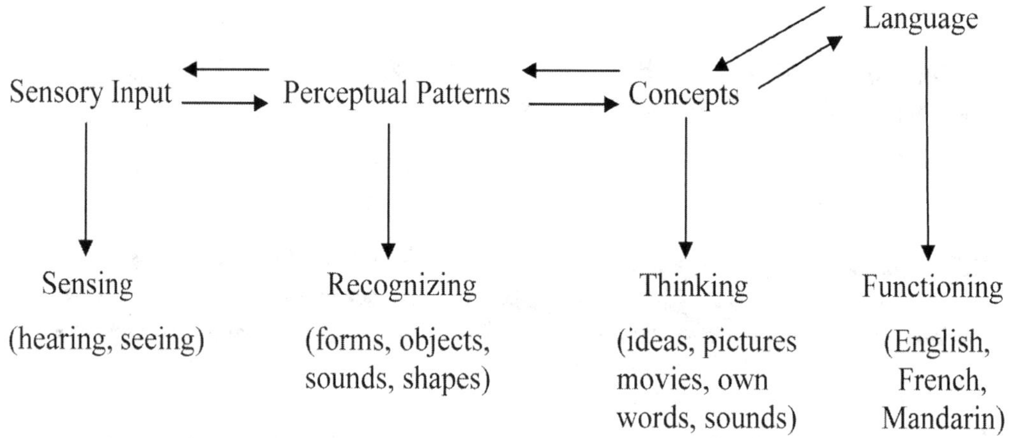

Figure 2.7 Neuro-Semantic Language Learning Theory

After the patterns overlap from integration and inhibition of new and old patterns, concepts or neuronal circuits of meaning develop. These concepts are recognized through the use of language that assigns meaning as well as assists to develop more meaning. Chapters 3–6 will provide what the conceptual language function is like for English.

Applications

- Examine some educational materials and determine what level of learning the materials expect from the learners.
- Observe a classroom teacher and determine what type of input the teacher assumes that the learners are able to process.

Chapter 3

THE STUDY OF LANGUAGE FUNCTIONS

Thinking

Learner objectives: Chapter 3

Upon completion of this chapter, the reader should be able to:

1. Define the basic language functions.
2. Explain the importance of semantic relationships for learning to think.
3. Explain the preoperational and concrete levels of thinking.
4. Define expanded language functions.
5. Define extended language functions.
6. Define the relationship between thinking and speech acts.

To promise, to marry, to vow…
All of these language functions and many more…
Create more meaning than
words, sounds, and sentences.

Dora, the child in Chapter 1, learned to speak English structures because she lived in an environment where the speakers in Dora's world spoke English. The sounds, words, and sentence structures that Dora speaks are components of English that Dora learned from the speakers in her environment. These language structures are patterns. Chapter 2 explained how people learn patterns and how such patterns are, by themselves, a very low, imitative level of learning. For example, an Australian songbird, exposed to the trucks and sirens of rainforest loggers, began singing the siren sounds. Now the bird's song is the sound of a chainsaw. The bird is able to imitate acoustic patterns much like a parrot is able to imitate entire sentence structures such as "Polly wants a cracker." These patterns are structures, but acoustic patterns do not become concepts or thoughts. A parrot and this particular

Australian songbird are very good at imitating acoustic patterns, but their patterns do not become concepts or thoughts. However, in human beings other types of patterns overlap and develop thoughts or concepts. Language represents this thinking so that language is more than imitated structures; language includes the function of thinking.

Language functions solve problems, invent new tools, create living spaces in typically adverse locations such as Antarctica, create human artifacts such as clothes, tools, furniture, transportation forms, and so forth. Language functions allow a human to create a variety of cultural identities unique to the products of the human language learning system such as economic or political systems and rule-governed societies (e.g., Dance, 1985). *Language functions are the socio-cognitive processes of the human's Neuro-Semantic Language Learning System.* The socio (social) piece is the way that a person uses language to communicate with and to other people. And, the cognitive piece is the way a person thinks.

Activity: What does the socio-cognitive process of a language do?

Language functions are greater than the sum of their developmental patterns of language structures. For example, to "promise" to do a task is a very different function than to tell someone you will do the task, even though the language structures are similar. "I promise I will paint your house." "I tell you I will paint your house." Promise implies a guarantee that the person will paint the house. Even though the sentence structures are very similar, the *function* of "promise" is very different than the *function* of "tell."

The purpose of this chapter is to introduce the reader to the myriad of language *functions* of English that are so often overlooked in education and society. Language functions develop in complexity from those that are foundational or basic to those functions that are expanded in nature, that form speech acts and expand speech acts.

Activity: What is a language function? What aspect of the Neuro-Semantic Language Learning Theory is language function?

Language functions

As previously discussed, English speakers typically study language from a structural perspective. These structures include words, sounds, morphemes, phonemes, sentences, parts of speech, sentence order, sentence structures, and vocabulary. The primary assumption is that a speaker learns these structures in the process of acquiring language. Chapter 2 showed that the learner really acquires a hierarchy of semantic features from the sensory system to create patterns that form systems of concepts or language functions. The systems of concepts reflect what the learner is doing socially and cognitively. The learner acquires basic relationships that express the social and cognitive meaning.

Semantic relationships

Because all human beings develop the meaning of their environment as they acquire their language learning system, the basis of language, for all speakers, for all languages, consists of the meaning of those relationships about people, their actions, and their objects within a context or setting. For example, some of the first concepts that a child expresses reflect what the child knows about what he or she "can do." The child might say "my bottle" or "me do dat" or "no" to mean "I don't want that." These utterances are about the child; what the child can or cannot do or want. In other words, one of the *earliest functions* of language is to tell others about what the child understands about his or her own relationship to the environment (e.g., see Slobin, 2004).

Socially, children communicate about themselves in relationship to their environment. Cognitively, children think only about the way they act in relationship to the objects in their world. These meaningful relationships that a child possesses about his or her world are called ***semantic relationships***. These *semantic relationships function* to connect the child to his or her world and the child's world to the child's thinking. Early conceptual development expresses the meaning of the child's world to others and in turn the meaning of the world to the child. These semantic relationships function to assist the child's development socially and cognitively.

Activity: What is one of the earliest types of language function?

Because language represents a speaker's thinking, language also represents a learner's social and cognitive development. All conceptual learning is based in how language functions to represent both social and cognitive understanding. For basic, first developed, semantic relationships, the cognitive or thinking portion of the relationship represents what the child does to others or objects. The child is central to the action so the child is an *agent.* The concepts about how the child acts as an agent are social in nature because the acts are in relationship to others, and the child's actions are in relationship to the child. These social concepts about the child in relationship to others are concepts of *agency*. ***Agency*** is a basic function of early language acquisition.

Activity: What is agency?

Most of these early developing semantic relationships *function* to show the child's cognition or understanding of what the child does within the child's environment. As the child acts on this cognitive knowledge or "knowing" about one's actions, the caregivers assign meaning in return. For example, the child reaches for the juice cup and Mom says, "Do you want some more juice?" The child says, "Me juice." And Mom ***assigns meaning*** to the child's act: "Okay, here is some more cranberry juice." The infant develops enough meaning from the sensory and perceptual patterns to create some basic concepts about "him" and "the juice" and "Mom." When the child represented this socio-cognitive development as "Me juice," along with a non-verbal reach toward the cup, Mom assigns her meaning to the child's verbal and non-verbal acts by giving the child some more cranberry juice. As Mom responds non-verbally, she attaches the words that go with her acts. The child drinks the juice so Mom believes that her assigned meaning was the "correct" meaning. Until the child's language *functions* in a reciprocal way between Mom and the child, Mom's interpretation is a guess. The child could mean any of these possibilities: "I like cranberry juice." "I want some orange juice but I will drink the cranberry juice." "I don't want any orange juice so give me some cranberry juice." "I like my juice cup." "Where is my juice? The cup is empty." "Is this cup mine? I want to pour some juice into it." "Will you pour some juice into my cup?" "Who drank my juice?"

From looking at all of these possible structures and specific meanings, it is apparent that *the child's early language functions mean something more than just the words or sentence structures*. The child is expressing a relationship that connects the child, the cup, and the juice. The child is an ***agent*** who can act on the juice cup. The child, as an agent, performs an ***action*** in relationship to the ***object***, the juice cup. The child is learning the language about being an agent in relationship to performing actions on objects or with objects. The child is learning the basic semantic relationships of agent + action + object.

Activity: What is a basic semantic relationship (agent + action + object)?

The social component of these early semantic relationships is basic; it is about the child as an agent in relationship to his or her own environment. The cognitive component is how the child is learning to think about his or her world. Thinking about the world requires adding more semantic meaning with each experience. For example, when the baby is first born, the child is biologically ready to learn about his or her world (see Chapter 2) so the child is an ***extension*** of Mom's arms, the couch, the bed. Babies cannot separate themselves from the surfaces and must *learn* to sit up, crawl, walk, run, and so forth. As an extension of the environment, the child connects literally and physically to the world's surface. The child's body ***grounds*** physically to the surface of the object or person that is supporting the weight of the child's body. In essence the child "is grounded."

As the child cognitively acquires the perceptual patterns of the world's surfaces, the child also responds physically with gross motor movements so that the child's muscles develop strength, coordination, and muscle memory. With all of this growth and learning, the child begins to be able to separate physically his or her body from the surface of Mom's arms or the couch. The child can sit up and grounds physically to the surface that connects the child's body to the object or person on which the child is sitting. The child is learning as an agent to be separate from the objects and agents around the child. *The child's own thinking is developing from being an extension of others to being separate; from being a part of the ground to being able to sit independently.* These changes in physical development, such as sitting up separately from Mom, are not only the result of maturity, but also the result of the child's cognitive function. The child is learning to think.

Activity: What does extension mean?
What does grounded mean?

Each child's motor movement shows the observer what the child is learning. The child learns each motor act as part of the child's Neuro-Semantic Language Learning System. The newborn baby learns that he or she can move independently away (***social development***) from the ground or surface of a parent or object touching the child (***cognitive development***). The child learns the parent's patterns of language that represent their concepts. In this way, language development represents cognitive and social development. So, the child learns the English sound pattern for "juice cup" as long as the child is able to receive the sensory input and perceptually process the sensory patterns into *sound* patterns about things the child *sees*, then the child learns the basic semantic relationships about people or agents, their actions, and their objects.

Activity: When a child shows basic semantic relationships, what does the child know?

Problems with acquiring basic semantic relationships

A child who cannot receive the sensory input of spoken patterns (e.g., the child might have a hearing loss) or a child who is not able to turn the perceptual patterns into concepts (e.g., children with autism) may not develop the concepts easily and therefore will have difficulty acquiring language functions. In other words, a lack of language development affects the social and cognitive development of the child just like the lack of social and cognitive development affects language acquisition.

Activity: How does language acquisition relate to social and cognitive development?

It is important to remember that all languages utilize a basic understanding of one's environment. This basic understanding is referred to as semantic relationships among and between agents, their actions, and their objects. Once a child begins to acquire these basic semantic relationships (around 3–6 months) and can express them with sound patterns (9–12 months) then the child will begin to ***expand*** the ***language functions*** of the basic relationships. For example, a child may express a basic relationship, "mama cherries," which needs more refinement in order for the listener to understand that the child does not want more cherries; the child wants Mom to rake the cherries in the yard.

When the meaning of a basic semantic relationship expands, then the child develops higher thinking and therefore more acceptable social behavior. Note that for producing basic semantic relationships, the child can non-verbally point, reach, grab, shake; but for expanded semantic relationships, more language structures must be used. Language development structurally increases to show the development of the child's thinking. The meaning of the thinking extends beyond the basic single semantic relationship.

Activity: Does social and cognitive development affect language development?

Extended semantic relationships

Once a baby is able to express his or agency through non-verbal and basic verbal semantic relationships, then the baby begins to use these language *functions* in other ways. The baby grows into a child who is still acquiring a plethora of sensory patterns and is organizing these patterns into lots of meanings. Brain images show how these meanings are widely spread throughout the early childhood years (Bookheimer, 2004). These meanings do not function in just one way. For example, a child at 18 months says "me juice" but at 24 months the child more closely specifies his *intention* with the expression, "me want juice." This expression may still have many meanings but the child shows some *expanded* meaning by adding "want" to the utterance.

The purpose of the child adding an additional pattern is to expand the meaning of the utterance. These types of ***expansions*** allow the child to use language to "refer." The act of

referring is a *language function*. Being able to refer allows a speaker to be specific about the message the speaker wants to convey (e.g., Kasher, 1998). In the child's utterance, "Me want juice," the child refers to his relationship to juice. Because the child looks toward the adult's face as he speaks the phrase "Me want juice," and because he also reaches out an empty juice cup to Mom and then looks at the juice bottle next to Mom, the child is referring to an act that he ***intends*** Mom to complete. The child is expanding the utterance parallel to his ability to relate to the meaning of the world in relationship to him. The child is about 24 months old and is able to express a variety of intentions with these simple utterances paired with non-verbal acts. The child is learning how language functions to express his cognitive and social development which in turn results in others assigning meaning to what the child knows. The child's utterances are more than just structures; the child's words and acts represent the child's thinking and social development.

Activity: What is a basic language function called expansion? What is the act of referring?

The age at which many children are obviously learning to *extend* meaning is about age three. For example, a child is at the zoo. The child sees a four-legged animal with a tail and mane. The child says, "Mom, look at the horse!" Mom says, "That is not a horse. That is a zebra. See, it has black and white stripes." The child extends the early semantic features she has about "horse" to another situation where she sees the same semantic features of four legs, a tail, and a mane. Mom assigns meaning to the child's *language function* by correcting the semantic extension. This ***semantic correction*** by Mom increases the child's knowledge or meaning of the perceptual patterns that the child sees. In this way, the child develops a new concept, zebra. A zebra looks like a horse but has black and white stripes.

The interplay between what speakers and writers assign to the meaning of what a person says or writes provides a great socio-cognitive process of neuro-semantic development of *language function*. When meaning is given to what a person says or writes, then that meaning increases the concepts for higher cognitive development and the social use of language. Language represents the socio-cognitive development of the Neuro-Semantic Language Learning System. Semantic development allows a speaker to use language to perform a variety of pragmatic acts. These pragmatic acts often express ***social intentions***.

Activity: What is the age at which most children show the beginning of semantic extensions? What are semantic extensions?

SOCIAL INTENTIONS

As neuro-typically developing children express what they "know" from what they learn about their world, they begin to *refer* to a variety of ideas in a variety of ways. The various ways for *referring* relate to the way that children socially intend for their utterances to function (e.g., Bradford & National Research Council, 2000). Some of the social intentions for representing thinking through language functions include, but are not limited to, ***greeting***, ***rejecting***, ***denying***, ***existing***, ***negating***, and ***requesting***. The meaning of these language functions, like the acts of *referring* and *expanding*, are greater than the words or structures that the child uses. For example, when a three-year-old child, James, sees his grandma, he runs and hugs her and looks up at her face and says, "Grandma, come play." This utterance is not just a simple sentence; it is a *greeting* as well as a *request*. The child's non-verbal and verbal acts combine to create a *social intention. Social intentions* refer to the child's purpose for communicating with someone else, like Grandma. James relates his knowledge of Grandma to his play. In this example, Grandma interprets James's social intention as a *request* for Grandma to play. Other possible social intentions include: "No, Grandma, don't come in here. Don't look. I am playing." He *greets* her and then *rejects* her coming into his room where he is playing. He does not want her *existence* there and he *denies* her access and *negates* any overture she might make to play with him. These types of acts communicate more than the basic language structures provide. The child expresses an intention or semantic meaning of concepts that are social and therefore ***pragmatic*** in nature (Arwood, 1991a). The semantic and pragmatic development of language represents how the child thinks and acts.

Activity: What are some pragmatic ways that extend meaning from the basic semantic relationship for a child younger than seven years of age?

PREOPERATIONAL COGNITION

The child is learning more about how to relate to others (social development) as well as about how he or she thinks about play (cognitive development) than the child is learning sentence structures. Analyzing only the sentence structures does not explain how language functions for this child. To understand how a child thinks and how the child is able to socialize, the child's use of language for cognitive and social function is important to consider.

Activity: Why is language function important to consider in assessing language?

James is a neuro-typical, three-year-old boy who is learning language to represent his thinking and acting. In the previous example, his behavior and spoken utterances in relationship to his grandmother show that he has learned a lot of perceptual patterns that are becoming concepts about James, in relationship to other people, and what he and others in his world can do. He is able to extend the meaning of the basic semantic relationships of agents, actions, and objects from himself to Grandma.

Because James's thinking is beginning to become more complex, then his social intentions also increase in number and complexity of function. For example, James says, "Grandma, come play." Grandma says, "James, I came to talk with your mom about some adult concerns. When we are through talking, I will come and play with you. So, go play with your toys and I will come to play in a little while." Grandma uses a lot of good, rich, *functional language*. She explains what she can and cannot do in response to his request. James understands that Grandma is not going to play but he does not understand *why* she is not going to play because Grandma's language uses a lot of adult language. James does not know when she will play even though she says she will play. So, James tugs on Grandma's hand and tries to pull her in the direction of his toys. Grandma sets the limits of James's *language function*. She says, "No! I am not playing with you now. I am talking with Mom. Go play with your toys." James's social intention of greeting Grandma and getting Grandma to play have been less than completely successful. So, he hangs his lip and goes to play with his toys. Grandma talks with Mom for a few minutes and then goes over and sits down with James. She says, "Okay, I talked with Mom and now it is your turn. I want to play with you and your toys."

James is learning that when he initiates an intention, the other person may or may not accept the initiation at that moment. This development of language to explain social interaction is helping James learn the social rules of his community. He is beginning to learn that others have their separate needs, wants, and desires. Through *language function*, James is learning that there are other people who are agents performing actions in his environment. *Cognitively, he is beginning to see that even though he is central to his thinking, that his thinking affects other people. Socially, he is no longer an extension of his world, but he is separate from the world and others may act separately from him.*

James's response to sensory input (sensori-motor cognition) is expanding and his thinking is increasing in variety of social intentions. This is the beginning of the preoperational development of language functions for James.

Activity: When language function begins to expand, how does the thinking change?

In the aforementioned example, James, a neuro-typical three-year-old boy, shows the *social and cognitive function* of a child who is beginning the preoperational stage of *cognitive and social function*. The child's *language function* shows the child's social intention of learning in relationship to others in the child's environment. This three-year-old child will develop language that *functions* to show how James sees himself in relationship to others, their actions, and objects. This period of refining his thinking about himself in relationship to others and what they do will continue to develop during the next four years (between three and seven years).

Activity: What are the typical cognitive and social language functions of a three to seven-year-old neuro-typical learner?

Between the ages of three and seven years, James, who is neuro-typically learning the language system, thinks about ideas that he can see in the *here-and-now*. While he learns more and more about his environment, he uses his knowledge in a variety of ways. At three, he wants others to do what he does. At four, he wants to understand what others are doing so he asks many, many questions to try to understand what others do, and by age five he can tell you a story about what he knows others do. As a six-year-old, James begins to try to understand how others affect what he does. For example, "Sarah is my friend. She played with me on the swings today." Then the next day, James comes home and stomps his foot. "Sarah is not my friend." "Why is Sarah not your friend?" "She played with Sasha today. I had to play ball with Josh." The six-year-old James is trying to understand the social relationship of words like "friend" as it relates to his thinking about those who affect him. James is learning to think (cognitive language function) within what he can say and do. He intends to communicate socially from what he knows as an agent, acting within a context or setting that is present. He *operates* as if he is unaware of how his actions or those of others interrelate. James is using thinking that does not operate on the rules of society so he is said to show ***preoperational cognition***.

By seven years of age, James is able to use language to initiate play with a variety of people at various times and for various types of play. The seven-year-old child shows language that socially intends to create meaning between and among others and their actions. The child is developing the *social rules of how to fit into a group* which moves him from being the center of his mental pictures (preoperational thinking) to being part of a group who works and plays together.

Activity: What is characteristic of a child's social intentions of language function at three, four, five, six, and seven years of age?

Expanded language functions

The *expanded language functions* are probably the most important social and cognitive developments acquired by a child learning to think critically and problem solve. These *expanded language functions* move a child's communication from the here-and-now of juice cups to ideas that span time and place. Through these *expanded language functions*, a speaker can talk about ideas that cannot be seen, such as micro-organisms, or how to take a flight into space even though the person has never been there before, how to invent a new tool, create a one-of-a-kind masterpiece, or study ancient Babylon. These *expanded language functions* begin as soon as a child's cognitive development begins with the sensory input developing into patterns that form systems of concepts. But, it is only as the child develops semantic relations that the child's cognitive meaning extends past the here-and-now of physical objects or physical experiences (preoperational thinking) into expanded language functions.

Activity: What do expanded language functions do for a thinker?

All concepts expand in meaning through language function. For example, Mom tells her 18-month-old daughter to "put the cup on the table." While Mom speaks, she points to the cup and then to the table. The child looks at Mom and then at the place that Mom points to. The child then puts the only thing in her hand, the cup, on the table. There is distance between Mom's finger and the table. There is also distance between Mom's mouth that speaks the words and the table. This distance means that the child is learning that Mom's words or language functions to talk about things are at a distance from Mom or the child. Mom's language can refer to an idea across time and space. Mom's language *displaces* the objects she is talking about from her words. The child is learning that language functions as a form of ***displacement***.

Activity: What do expanded language functions provide for a speaker?

DISPLACEMENT

Children with neuro-typical language development acquire an adult grammar of language structures by seven or eight years of age. However, social intentions continue to expand and develop through a variety of language functions. Because language functions consist of a social and a cognitive component, this progression of development means that social and cognitive development continue to progress as well. From simple greetings in the here-and-now with Grandma, to greetings that occur across time through electronic or snail mail, the child continues to use language to create a variety of social and cognitive meanings. This change in referring to others and their actions in the here-and-now to referring to acts that are not seen or touched is another type of *language function* called *displacement*. Displacement is an important, expanded language function that begins early on and continues to expand throughout a person's thinking.

A child begins as an extension of his or her world which means the child is not displaced much from the parent's arms and then through learning begins to separate him- or herself from those people and objects supporting the child which provides more displacement. Then the child begins to act in relationship to others' acts realizing that there are others in the child's world and that they have needs and desires. Recognition of others' needs and desires increases the child's cognitive thinking about others who are more physically displaced from the child. This progression from physically being in contact with an adult to talking about people, their actions and objects that are no longer in the here-and-now helps develop the cognitive function of displacement.

Activity: What is displacement? Give an example.

Displacement is a language function that increases along with the increased development of conceptual meanings (***semanticity***), the use of semantic social intentions in a variety of ways (***flexibility***) to mean a variety of concepts (***productivity***) in a very efficient way (***redundancy***). These expanded language functions are important to the continued cognitive and social development of a child.

The child's concepts of "putting the cup on the table" continue to increase in meaning over time. As the child uses the cup in a variety of ways such as to shake juice, drink juice, and spill juice, the child's neurobiological language learning system continues to bring in information through more sensory input and more organized perceptual patterns. The input continues to ***overlap*** past experiences with present experiences. One use of "cup" adds to another use of "cup." The uses of the concept begin to ***layer***, one meaningful *function* on top of another meaningful *function. Overlapping* organized patterns *layer* the meanings of the concepts so the concepts become more complex. By the time the child is 30 months old, Mom can tell Shelly, who is in her bedroom, to go get the cup that is on the dining room table and Shelly complies. Shelly can also tell her mom, "Here is my cup." By five years of age, Shelly tells Grandpa, "Mom bought me a new cup. I wanted a Tinker Bell cup but Mom said the Tinker Bell cup scratches so I got a soft cup." Grandpa asks, "What do you mean the cup scratches?" Shelly says, "The cup bottom scratches a table, uh, Mom says…the Tinker Bell cup scratches, not my new cup." Shelly now can tell a story about a cup that the listener has never seen as it relates to Shelly and her ideas. By ten, Shelly can talk about even more *displaced* information. She can talk about various types of cups and how the cups for clothing differ in size, and so forth. By 15, Shelly can use cup in a formal meaning: "Mom, guess what? I won the President's Cup today! I finished first overall in cross country!" *Concepts increase in meaning allowing for more and more displaced language function. This increase in meaning results from the overlap and layering of semantic patterns through the Neuro-Semantic Language Learning System.*

Activity: What is overlapping and layering? How do these neuro-semantic processes increase the meaning of a concept?

As concepts increase in meaning, the *language function* increases the *displacement* of the meaning. The increase in conceptual meaning occurs as a result of overlapping and layering the concepts within the Neuro-Semantic Language Learning System. The increase in displacement occurs as a result of the speaker using language to relate ideas socially (cognition) that are no longer in the here-and-now. The speaker uses language to express these expanded relationships to others which in turn continues the increase of the meaning or semantic development of the concepts. In other words, when Shelly hears the coach talk about the President's Cup going to the most improved and best athletic performance, she is acquiring new meaning for "cup." Then, Shelly uses her language to assign meaning to the President's Cup. If she thinks in visual concepts, then she might think about what she would look like if her performance met the criteria for the cup. Mentally she would see herself running the race in a way that would show "the best athletic and most improved performance." This mental assignment of meaning might be in the form of a movie. Or, if Shelly processes the incoming patterns of the coach's voice into the sound of her own voice, then she might talk herself through what the most improved athletic performance would be like. The reader is reminded that not all people process sensory input into the same type of patterns and concepts. This ability to extend meaning through increasing the semantics of concepts helps displace ideas from the here-and-now to those that cannot be seen, touched, or felt.

Activity: Explain how the concept "cup" develops over time.

Semanticity

A child acquires the semantic features that become semantic relationships that represent concepts which overlap and layer to form more complex meanings. The representation of ideas is called ***lexical tags***. A ***lexicon*** refers to an individual's underlying meanings for what most adults call words. The child assigns meaning with a ***tag***, not really a word. This tag represents the child's own, unique meanings that result from the child's own unique experiences of learning patterns and concepts. Increasing complexity of meaning throughout life is a language function called *semanticity*. ***Semantic complexity*** *or semanticity increases over the life of a person so concepts increase in meaning and new meanings continue to develop as part of language function.*

Activity: What is the language function of semanticity?

Flexibility

Displacement and semanticity are two types of expanded language functions that take the basic semantic relationship of an agent, action, and object and move the meaning into complex ideas across time and space. These *language functions* allow the speaker to be more *flexible* with language. For example, a traveler is able to problem solve an unexpected situation through language. The traveler has been away from home on a business trip. She is sitting at the airport waiting for her plane, so she can fly home for an important meeting the next morning. As she waits to board her plane, she hears over the public announcement system, "I am sorry ladies and gentlemen but your flight is cancelled. Please see a travel assistant for rebooking your flight." The traveler goes to the gate counter and finds out from the travel assistant that the next flight to her home city is the next day at 1:00 p.m. But, this traveler has a very important meeting at 8:00 a.m. the next morning, so the traveler calls a nearby car rental company and books a car. Before she leaves the airport, she files paperwork for a reimbursement of the airplane ticket, and then she proceeds to the car rental where she rents a car and drives home, arriving at midnight so that she can make her 8:00 a.m. morning meeting. The traveler's ability to use language to think about her options and to problem solve provides this thinker with flexibility.

Flexibility is a language function. The traveler could have called and told her family and boss that her flight was cancelled and that she would miss the meeting. Although this is a solution to the problem, it leaves the responsibility for the meeting on others to cancel or rearrange. Furthermore, the content of the meeting was time sensitive so by not finding another way to get to the meeting as planned may have created a burden on somebody else. Only individuals who are able to think with maximum levels of language functions will have the displacement and semanticity needed to be maximally flexible.

Activity: What is flexibility?

Productivity

Flexibility, like displacement and semanticity, increases a person's ability to use language in a variety of ways for a variety of purposes. These expanded language functions help a person become more *productive*, because the person, who has maximum use of these *expanded language functions*, is able to use language to create a variety of linguistic forms for literacy. For example, to send a message to someone who is not in the here-and-now means that the message must be put in another form than just spoken language. Historically, scratches of meaning in the dirt or on rocks increased in complexity to form pictures, pictures with rules such as Hieroglyphs. Eventually, the language could be put into symbols that represent the spoken language either as an orthographic or written code of letters to sounds or as visual characters representative of expanded semantic relationships. These increased uses of language through writing are based on meaningful development of concepts. The language user has more than one way to use language production. This *productivity* develops as a *language function.* In fact, this is such an important *language function* that some students who cannot process sound into speech can learn concepts through the adult assigning meaning through writing rather than speaking. The adult pairs the written patterns with drawn concepts so that the child can develop language. More about these types of applications will be found in Part III of this book. The bottom line is that to be *productive* with language means that the user of language must also be able to *displace* the concept from the physical object, assigning meaning through the layering process of *semanticity* for greater *flexibility*.

> ***Activity:*** What is the language function of productivity?

Redundancy

There is one more very important expanded language function, *redundancy*. When a speaker continues to acquire meaning through the Neuro-Semantic Language Learning System, then the speaker may try to use more words to convey a particular meaning. For example, Daryl, a sixth grader, is trying to tell the teacher that the period of play, before school starts, is not called a recess. Daryl says, "Well, we went to the first recess, well it wasn't the first recess cuz if it had been the first recess then I would have been tremendously late. It wasn't a school recess. It was right before school. Then I did school. What was the next discussion on?"

Daryl's language is not easy to follow because he has to say one idea over and over. He lacks the maximum language functions of displacement and semanticity so his flexibility and productivity are reduced. In fact, he loses what he is talking about so he asks "What was the next discussion on?" which means, "What were we talking about?" Daryl's surface form of language becomes very *redundant*. Such *redundancy* occurs because Daryl's thinking (cognition) lacks sufficient meaning (semantics) to be able to use different words to mean different ideas. Socially, the listener has difficulty following Daryl's ideas.

This example is from a real student who lacks friends. His *external* language *redundancy* affects his thinking and therefore his social skills. If Daryl possessed more English, then he would have more meaning tied to his thinking. His language would sound like this: "Yesterday, I went to school early so I could play with my friends before the bell rang. Once the first bell rang, I went inside to do my work. Today, I came later to school so I didn't have time to play before school." An increase in Daryl's concepts increases his language function. The result is that his English functions with less external redundancy and is therefore more effective.

> ***Activity:*** What is the language function of redundancy? How can redundancy occur in the surface form of language as well as in the cognitive form of language?

Table 3.1 on the following page shows the expanded language functions.

Concrete cognition

The meaning of basic semantic relationships of people, their actions, and their objects increases through the neuro-semantic processes of overlapping and layering of patterns and concepts to form more complex concepts. These complex concepts increase the language functions of displacement, semanticity, flexibility, productivity, and redundancy from the child thinking in the here-and-now (preoperational thinking) to the child being able to think in the rules of societal expectations (concrete thinking). By 7–11 years of age, a child is able

Table 3.1 The expanded language functions

	Cognitive meaning	Social meaning	Language example
Displacement	Ideas are separate from the physical existence of a person, action, or object.	Communication with others can occur across space and time.	Jasmine, a nine-year-old third grader, is able to write about the 1800s and pioneers.
Semanticity	Concepts increase in complexity from the overlapping and layering of meaning.	More complex meanings can be shared about higher order thoughts.	Rialto is able to talk about freedom of speech as a US Constitutional basic right.
Flexibility	Concepts can be used in a variety of ways.	Communication with others takes on more variety.	Sharon is able to function actively at a meeting in an unknown venue that she has never seen.
Productivity	Concepts mean similar ideas whether they are in spoken or written form.	Concepts can be understood whether communicated through writing or speaking or drawing or numeracy.	Ashraf is able to read, write, talk, listen, view, think, and calculate in standard English.
Redundancy	Concepts increase in meaning to the point where they must become a new concept.	People can be very specific and efficient in conveying messages to others.	Clara's speaking is very effective because she is able to use English in a very efficient manner.

to relate other people (agents) and their actions to people that the child may or may not know through societal rules. "The sixth grade class is going to the theater on a field trip." These types of concrete relationships explain who is going, what they are doing, where they are going, and sometimes even a specific when, why, or how. "The sixth grade class is going by bus to the downtown theater to see *Pioneers* for a field trip because they are studying about the people who settled this area." This type of thinking expresses how others do their actions; the child no longer has to be central to the thinking.

Activity: How does concrete thinking differ from preoperational thinking?

As language functions express more meaning, the speaker's or the writer's cognitive and social development also increases. With an increase of conceptual meaning, the speaker or writer is able to use more advanced language structures and vocabulary. Structural complexity of natural language increases with an increase of underlying semantics or meaning. Similarly, *language structure drops complexity when the underlying meaning is not complex enough to support the structures.* For example, the following seven-year-old child uses very limited language structure: "My doggie'z big and bit him. She bad. She gots shots. She not like vet." From these utterances, it is difficult to know who the dog bit, if the dog is the "who" that is bad, when the dog went to the vet to get the shots, where the dog bit whom, and so forth. The basic semantic relationships are *not* well expanded to answer the basic who, what, where, when, why, or how questions.

A teacher works with this child and asks the child to draw out her ideas. To these drawings, the teacher helps the child answer the who, what, where, when, why, and how questions. The result is that the child writes:

> My dog's name is Milo. She chased a neighbor's cat and bit the cat. My neighbor had to take her cat to the vet for stitches. My neighbor was not happy about taking her cat to the vet. The doctor sewed up the cat's cut with 25 stitches. My mom says Milo was bad and that we have to pay our neighbor's vet bill.

The language is much easier to understand, and the child expresses more expanded meanings. The child's increase in language function comes from the educator who helped the child *extend* the meaning of her ideas through adding more meaning to speaking with drawing and writing. By ***extending*** the meanings through who, what, where, when, why, and how of basic semantic relationships, the child is better able to communicate her ideas socially. Cognitively, the child is showing an *extension* of language function through increased conceptualization. The concepts are moving away from the here-and-now to more *expanded language functions of concrete thinking.*

Activity: What is the language function of extension? How does extending meaning help develop ***concrete cognition***?

Expanded language functions allow for an increased meaning through extending meanings of basic concepts (e.g., Wittgenstein, 2001/1953). The result is more expanded language functions that also increase thinking for better problem solving, planning, decision making and so forth. At the concrete level of cognition, speakers are able to think clearly about others and what others are thinking about and therefore their language reflects the relationships. This concrete cognition results in expanded semantic language functions becoming more complex. One type of complex language function is the speech act (Brown, 1979; Dore, 1975; Lucas, 1978, 1980; Rowe & Levine, 2009; Searle, 1969).

Activity: What is an extension of meaning? How does extending meaning help develop the socio-cognitive process of language function?

Speech acts

Semantic development allows a speaker of English to use language to perform a variety of *functions* within a conversation. These conversational *language functions* or ***speech acts*** include the rules for the context, verbal and non-verbal characteristics of the speaker's utterance, and the effects on the listener. For example, an eight-year-old boy, Dexter, asks for help with his homework: "Dad, can you help me with my spelling?" Dad is busy working on his taxes. Dad says, "Not now." So, the context is that Dad is not ready to hear that Dexter wants help with his homework. Dad is not looking at Dexter. Dad is looking at his tax paperwork. In fact, Dad's back is to Dexter when Dexter asks for help.

For Dexter's utterance to work as a successful request for help with his spelling (Lucas, 1980), Dad would be looking toward Dexter and ready to hear what Dexter has to say. Dexter says his utterance with adequate grammatical structure, vocabulary, and appropriate intonation for Dad to hear him and to hear physically what Dexter says. But, because Dad is not ready to hear what Dexter says, Dad responds indicating he hears Dexter, but Dad is not accepting the request. Because Dad does not accept the utterance as a request, the speech act becomes a statement of information: Dexter wants help. For Dexter's utterance to perform a speech act of a request, Dad would have to respond that he accepted the request. Dad would say something like this: "Okay, let me finish this problem and I will then help you with your spelling."

For speech acts to be effective as intended by the speaker, they must affect the way the listener assigns meaning. This means that the speaker must understand that the listener (hearer) must be able to assign the meaning the speaker wants. Dexter is at a concrete level of understanding and realizes that Dad is not ready or able to help with the homework. Instead of Dexter performing a request, the speech act is completed as a statement of information: Dexter wants help and Dad is busy. They each know something that they did not know about each other prior to the exchange of words.

Activity: What semantic elements make up a speech act?

Expanded speech acts

As speakers engage in discourse, the language functions of the speech acts generate more and more meaning for the speakers and the listeners. The complexity of the *function* of language generates more than simple back and forth comments. In fact, probably the most complex type of *language function* occurs in a debate where two or more speakers are using a multitude of very sophisticated speech acts. The speakers present material that all speakers already know. These are simple *statements of information.* Each person of the debate wants to be sure that the other person knows that he or she knows the basic content of the topic to be debated. "We are here today to discuss the economic problems in the US." Then each speaker wants to let the others know that he or she has something to contribute that the other speakers do not know. This information occurs as a simple *assertion.* "Last year, I collected data on 20,000 households in my township." If this information is new to the other speakers, then the assertion is complete. The other speakers want to know more about the data, so someone asks a question about the data. "Was this self-reported data?" "Yes, the data was collected from tax statements." Another person asks, "Who collected the data?" Both speakers are *requesting information.* The statements of information, assertions, and requests of information are all types of speech acts.

In order for the speakers of the debate to use various speech acts to *argue* different opinions about the economic problems of the US, each speaker has to be able to *refer* (the act of referring was defined earlier in the chapter) to what another speaker said, and then create an *argument* about the topic. The argument is another assertion or statement of information or possibly a request. "Tax statements do not give a complete picture of a household's economic situation. There is data that may not be included such as how many children are in school athletics which affects how well a family is able to handle the economic times." The speaker's first utterance about a complete picture refers back to the data that the other speaker mentioned. Then the speaker adds a connecting speech act (statement of information) about school athletics which results in a conclusion about how the athletics may affect the family economics.

This type of connection between one argument that refers to a previous utterance and another argument is called a ***predication***. When two or more arguments are further predicated, the third idea is an ***auditory proposition*** (e.g., Arwood & Beggs, 1989; Grice, 1989; Lucas, 1978). For example: "Last month, I went to my farm out on the coast; but it was colder than usual, so I decided to stay at a cozy motel 30 miles on down the beach." The first argument is about the coast. The second argument is about the cold. The words "but" and "so" connect the first two arguments into explaining why the speaker stayed some place other than his own farm. These three arguments connect together into a proposition. English that is time-based, as expected, allows for these types of propositions to occur naturally in language function as a result of the use of temporal or time-based language. Propositions are important components of complex expanded speech acts.

Activity: What is a predication? What is an auditory proposition?

As a reader, you may be asking, why are all of these terms important? Well, the ability to problem solve at an adult level; the ability to understand words like freedom and respect; and the ability to understand spoken language so as to multi-task or follow through with an assignment are all products of a language user's ability to *predicate* cognitively. For example, a teacher says, "Your book reports are due in three weeks. Three weeks from today is December 5th. Put December 5th on your assignment due sheet." For a majority of students in this fifth grade class, the book reports are begun the night before they are due and most of the students have not read their books. About 30 percent of the class never turns in a book report. For another 30 percent, the teacher accepts late book reports. For about 30 percent of the class, they turn in a report that is either a summary of what they read on the computer or on the front or back cover, or in summary notes about the book. There are usually one or two students who not only read their books but also wrote the report on their own and in their own words and turned the reports in on time. These couple of students, who met the teacher's expectations, are able to use complex language functions in predicated propositions.

If schools want their students to be able to use their own words to debate, persuade, follow complex time-based activities, organize their work, complete multi-tasks on time; then they must give attention to these complex language functions. More about these types of functions for educational purposes will be reported in later chapters.

Activity: What is the educational purpose of knowing a complex speech act or predication to form an auditory proposition?

Summary

Chapter 1 provided the reader with an explanation for why most people emphasize the study of language structures over *language functions.* Culturally and linguistically, the "known" or "unmarked"[1] status quo relates language to the study and development of literacy based on language structures—sounds, words, morphemes, parts of speech, sentences, and so forth. These language structures are assumed to be the building blocks of language acquisition and language learning.

Language functions are greater in purpose and meaning than their representative structures. In order for educators to emphasize the meaning of language for cognitive and

1 Pairs or cognates are linguistically referred to as marked or unmarked. For example, one might say, "How hot is the water?" when waiting for a cup of tea. Hot is the unmarked member of "hot" and "cold" since one would not say, "How cold is the water?" when referring to a cup of brewed tea.

social development, they must learn about language functions (e.g., see Fry *et al.*, 1996). But *language functions* are not well known or studied or well described for educators to learn. Therefore, if educators do not understand language functions, they will not use language functions for the basis of literacy instruction in the schools. Since the emphasis on language structures over language functions is also a cultural phenomenon, parents must also emphasize language structures over language functions. Table 3.2 provides the reader with an example of a function as well as a structure for each of the areas of language study.

Table 3.2 Examples of the study of language structures compared to language functions

Area of study	**Examples of language structure**	**Examples of language function**	**Examples of expanded language functions**
Phonology	Sounds	*	*
Syntax	Word order; parts of speech	Semantic relationships; intentions	Speech acts
Semantics	Vocabulary	Lexical tags; referring; predicating, semantic relationships	Displacement, semanticity, flexibility, productivity, redundancy
Morphology	Endings, affixes, suffixes, infixes, etc.	Time, space, quantity, quality	Extension, expansion, modulation
Pragmatics	Turn taking narratives	Conversational roles—shared referents	Predication, auditory propositions

* Note that there is no language function listed under phonology: Remember that sound can be imitated without meaning or thinking and a language like American Sign Language can function without sound.

This chapter described several of the language functions that are important in the development of social and cognitive thinking.

Language functions expand and extend as well as change or modulate the basic semantic relationship to include more displacement, semanticity, flexibility, productivity, and redundancy so that the speaker can engage with a listener in complex speech acts that extend and predicate meaning for improved social and cognitive development. In order to improve social thinking for problem solving and academic learning for improved literacy, educators and parents must emphasize *language functions*.

Applications

- Listen to children and decide if they are using complex speech acts that connect their ideas together into time-based language.
- Check out some educational materials designed to teach literacy and determine how much of the curriculum expects students to use complex language functions.

PART II

ENGLISH LANGUAGE FUNCTIONS

How Do We Learn to Think?

Part I of this book provided the reader with three important elements to understanding the relationship between language structure and language function: First, language is traditionally studied from analyzing the structures; educators and parents can count structures and language structures include sounds, words, phrases, sentences, parts of speech, and so forth. Second, understanding how a child *acquires* language through the Neuro-Semantic Language Learning System offers insight to how children learn language as a set of functional processes, rather than as a set of additive structures. Third, language functions parallel the way a person uses language for thinking and learning; therefore, emphasis on language functions helps children become literate, to think more critically, and socially to maintain healthy relationships.

Part II of the book is set up for the reader to understand how the *thinking* (e.g., Gil, 2004) differences of language function help develop an assessment and intervention approach that is strength based. Chapter 4 describes the cultural properties of English function. Since most people think with a visual form of meta-cognition, but the dominant English speaking culture is a sound-based, auditory culture, Chapter 4 expands on the mismatch between how most students think and the way most teaching occurs. This mismatch suggests that a change in educational assessment, intervention, and curriculum may be necessary; see Chapter 5. The change is a cultural-linguistic paradigm shift that affects not only education but also the interpretation of research, assessment, and intervention. Chapter 6 provides an explanation of how the relationship between language function or thinking and literacy creates a basis to assessment and intervention for individuals (Part III) as well as for classroom education (Part IV).

While Part I of the book offered the reader knowledge about how learning to function with language is different than acquiring language structures, Part II provides the reader with the specific knowledge needed to understand that an emphasis on function, rather than structure of language, provides the basis to academic and social applications for more conceptual learning as discussed in Part III and Part IV.

Chapter 4

THE CULTURAL-LINGUISTIC PROPERTIES OF ENGLISH

Learner objectives: Chapter 4

Upon completion of this chapter, the reader should be able to:

1. Explain the properties of English as an auditory language.
2. Explain the properties of visual types of languages like ASL or Mandarin.
3. Explain the cultural-linguistic mismatch between English function and the majority of English speakers' thinking.
4. Explain restricted language function in terms of thinking.
5. Explain how culture influences the expectations of thinkers.

To think differently is to know a difference.
To speak with difference is to show one's thinking.
To think and to know
Is different than to study about language.

Because children learn language within their environment, they learn the meaning of what society *values*. For example, the speakers in Dora's environment assigned meaning with the English language (see Chapter 1). Therefore, Dora learned the value of speaking the English patterns of her culture. Dora learned to *imitate* the English language structures. As explained in Part I of the book, learning to imitate language structures does not provide conceptual learning. Neuro-typical children, like Dora, acquire concepts that represent the perceptions of what their society culturally values. Different environments provide different input and therefore differences in environments results in different values with different language patterns. People with different values produce different languages with different underlying properties that represent the people's differences in perceptions.

Different inputs from the different environments result in different perceptions for different people, which results in different cultures. These different cultures are the result of different perceptions of what is important. The perceptions overlap to create differences in thinking. Differences in thinking result in different linguistic needs and therefore differences in language structures as well as differences in language functions. This process is dynamically cyclic.

Linguistic differences are cultural in nature in that they represent the thinking of the population that uses the language. This chapter will describe the cultural properties of English, a time-based sound language that uses low context, followed by an explanation of the significance of a mismatch between English properties and most English speakers' thinking properties.

English: a time-based language

English is a time-based language (Traugott, 1975). The time or temporal component comes from the auditory processing (e.g., Moore & Shepherd, 2008; Overath, 2009; Sanda & Marsalek, 2009; Smith, 1978; Starr, Amlie, Martin, & Sanders, 1977) of the time component of the sound wave (Chapter 2).[1] Specifically, when a speaker talks, the sounds take time to produce. From the beginning of saying a word, such as "cat," to the last sound of the word, time elapses. In other words, it takes time to produce the sounds. English embeds these sounds into words. Not only do words take time to produce but also there are words created to conceptualize time, such as "today" and "tomorrow." English also represents time with changes in morphemes such as adding an "-ing" to a verb to mean "progressive action" or "ongoing." Furthermore, English uses small words of function or functors (Trask, 1992) such as conjunctions to join concepts such as "Mary" *and* "John." These types of functors are also time based. For example, the preposition "to" means that an action will occur as in "The boy walked *to* the store."

Basically, an English speaker uses two types of time: how events take time, and how the speaker moves through time (Arwood, 1991a). For example, a speaker might say, "The meeting will take about an hour" meaning that the meeting is an event that takes approximately an hour of time. From the beginning of the meeting to the end of the meeting will be about an hour. This is the kind of time that measures event time. But the English speaker can also show how time moves through the speaker by saying, "We planned for an hour of time but we have been in the meeting for an hour and I have more content to cover." In this case, time goes faster than the speaker wants. The speaker has more to do than the hour allows. The speaker might show his or her relationship to time by then saying, "I will fast forward the agenda and cover the essentials so we can go to lunch." Now the speaker is "moving" through time. By speeding up the agenda, the speaker is literally moving through the dimension of time. So, an English speaker can use English to represent thinking about how to complete an event within time or how to move through time: "The game takes two hours to play" or "I have to hurry and play so I can go home."

Activity: What are the two ways that time is used in English?

English that is time based on the surface reflects the speaker's underlying ability to organize time internally. For example, an English speaker might say, "Before I go home, I must run this transcript through the computer to see if this student needs to add a class before

1 The time element of the sound wave is processed by the auditory brain stem and by the way the cells function in the processes from receptor organ to the brain.

the deadline tomorrow." This utterance is "loaded" at the surface with time elements in relationship to one another. The time elements or temporal elements "*mark*" or assign meaning to the thinker's underlying cognition. The speaker's underlying thinking is quite complex and goes something like this:

> Because tomorrow is the deadline for registration changes that do not cost the students additional money, I need to stay at work and check to see if this last student needs to add a class to graduate. If the student needs one more class to graduate, based on what the student's transcript shows; then, I can add that class for the student tonight before I go home so that adding the class won't cost the student additional money. If I don't stay and check the student's record tonight and the student has to add the class tomorrow, it will cost the student more money to add the class tomorrow.

This complex thinking shows that the speaker understands her time and the student's time. In addition to understanding the time elements, this registration worker is able to use English to relate the different time needs of the constituents in a proactive way to solve a problem or prevent a problem. In this way, the speaker is considerate of the student's graduation needs, financial responsibilities, and is able to take the student's perspective, as if the registration worker were the student. This shows complex thinking and complex time-based linguistic social and cognitive function.

Activity: What is meant by time-based function of English?

Here is another scenario where the English speaker is *not* able to use the temporal properties of English. "It's five o'clock. Whew! I'm going out for a drink to celebrate the end of the semester! See ya' in two weeks. Happy Holidays!" Because the clock says it is five o'clock, the person goes home. Time is *externally* organized for this person, rather than internally part of this speaker's thinking. On this English speaker's desk is a special request submitted from a graduate student for a transcript to be sent after grades, but before the holidays, to another graduate school in order for the student's application to meet the application deadline to graduate school. The requesting student specified dates on the written initial request. Furthermore, the graduate student made the request in writing before grades were available, walked into the registrar's office after grades were posted to be sure that the request was going to be filled before office staff left for the holidays, and also called the registrar's office two days before the holiday break to remind them to be sure to send the transcript before they left for the holiday break. However, even with all of the reminders on the part of the student, the person responsible for sending out the transcript just went home because the clock said it was five o'clock. The worker never "got" to the request as she worked through all requests based on what she *saw* on her pile of requests.

Prioritizing requires a form of time-based language. This worker does not prioritize by time; instead, as requests came in they were added to her work pile. When the grades came out, the graduate student's request was on the bottom of the pile. So, earlier requests went to the bottom and later requests were sent out first. The student's graduate school never received the transcript before December 31, and so the student was not accepted into the program as her file was "incomplete."

The worker did not understand the urgency of sending the transcript before she left for the holidays because she did not literally see the request. It was on the bottom of the pile. This employee does not think in time but she thinks in the events of what she sees. As she cannot prioritize by time, she organizes her desk by what she *sees* needs to be done. As she does not have an internal time of urgency, everything has equal importance. So, when she arrives at work she starts to process what is on top of the pile. As new requests come in, she places them on top of the pile. A request placed early just never gets to the top of the pile.

Ironically, if the conscientious graduate student had waited until semester grades came out and then walked in *while* the staff person was processing transcripts, then the transcript would have been posted as the student stood there. The student expected the staff person to be able to think *in time* and therefore be able to use the *time* properties of English to *plan* and *prioritize* her work to meet the student's request. The student was trying to be considerate of the worker's time and not make a last minute request. The student was able to think about the worker but the worker was not able to think about the student.

Activity: How complex does the language function have to be to allow a person to think from another person's perspective?

The staff person thinks relationally and spatially, not temporally—this staff person thinks about what she needs to do in relationship to what the clock looks like, what the piles of paper look like, what the people look like that make requests—all in relationship to what she knows to do. The graduate student thinks in time, when something must happen in relationship to another activity in order to meet deadlines, others' requested timelines, and so forth. The graduate student is using a type of time-based thinking that matches with the time-based properties of English. The student assumed that if the worker spoke English that she would understand the time-based properties of the student's request. Because the worker has not learned about her visual way of processing events, she does not know that she is not prioritizing work by time.

Activity: How does time help a person understand how to prioritize activities? If a person does not use time for thinking about events, then what type of thinking does the person use to do activities within an event?

To be literate in a culture that values time as much as to have English represent time in so many ways, an English speaker should be able to think, listen, speak, read, write, view, and calculate using time concepts that allow for the person to go through time or to plan time around events. The following examples are *time-based properties of English literacy*:

- *Thinking* in time. A person is easily able to prioritize the urgency of events, move faster when in a hurry, organize multiple activities (multi-task), and put limits on what is not possible to do within a time frame. The registrar would have sent the student's request out in a timely fashion, before she left on holiday.
- *Listening* in time. English allows the content of wording to carry the sequence of time, not the syntax or word order. For example, "When the bell rings, be in your seat" means that the students sit down and then the bell rings. For students who do not have *literacy of time*, they might listen to the order of the clauses. Because

the first clause says, "When the bell rings," the student waits until the bell rings and then sits down. These students are tardy but do not know why they are tardy. Here is another example from a workplace. A furniture store is to deliver a couch between 2 o'clock and 4 o'clock on a specific Friday afternoon. The homeowner takes off time from work to be home during those hours. The deliverer does not show up. The homeowner calls the store and the store employee says that the couch is on its way. The homeowner explains that she is leaving home at 6 o'clock for a 7 o'clock meeting. The couch does not arrive by 6 o'clock. The homeowner has to leave. On Saturday morning, the homeowner calls the store and asks when the men will be delivering the couch. The men say they tried to deliver it on Friday but the homeowner was not home. The store employee is having trouble listening to time elements. After much discussion, the store employee said the couch would be delivered Saturday afternoon, but the couch showed up at 10:30 p.m. on *Sunday*. The store employee could see her job and she could mentally see the men delivering the couch, but she could not see the homeowner and therefore did not think from the homeowner's perspective of time. The store employee did not understand why the owner was not at home when the couch arrived in the evening on Friday or why the homeowner was upset with a couch being delivered so late at night on Sunday. Listening in elements of functional English means that the hearer is able to complete a task according to a timeline or an agreed upon time.

- *Speaking* is another process of literacy so being literate in time means that a speaker is able to use complex temporal markers such as those in the example about staying to check to see if a student needed a class before the deadline. If the speaker cannot think in time, then the surface of the language structures will be restricted and the time elements unclear. In later chapters, the author will show the reader how to use a spoken language sample to determine how literate a person is with the English time property.
- *Reading* and *writing* in time means that the English user is able to use the same spoken language in complex time relationships in reading and writing. For example, a written sample that does not contain time elements sounds like a list: "I like school. I like reading. I like my teacher." This type of writing is using restricted language function and therefore restricts the writer's thinking processes. Chapters 6, 11, and 15 provide the reader with more information on assessment and intervention based on spatial properties.
- *Viewing* in time literacy refers to the perspective that a person is able to take. In English speaking cultures, thinking about other people and their needs is considered a higher cognitive function than thinking of oneself. However, many children and adults who do not think with time properties of English do not view how their actions affect or influence others. For example, individuals diagnosed with autism spectrum disorders (ASD) do not view themselves in relationship to what others do or don't do, and are therefore considered to have social problems. One young adult diagnosed with ASD said that he was social because he stood out in the parking lot at school. However, on further exploration it was discovered that he never said hello to anybody who walked by. He did not realize that when the teacher said, "You need to hang out where the students come and go so that you can develop

some social skills interacting with others" that the teacher did not mean to stand in the parking lot. The teacher meant for the student to engage in conversation with students. This teen's viewpoint of his world did not include what others think or do, only what he thinks, based on what he sees and does. More about this will also be included in later chapters.

- *Calculating* in time has to do with distance versus space (Arwood, 1991a; Lucas, 1980; Wheeler, 1978). For example, when an English speaker who thinks in time merges into a fast moving traffic lane, the person thinks about her car in relationship to the speed of the other cars. So, the faster and closer the other cars are, the faster the driver accelerates to pull into the traffic. The driver is subconsciously calculating the time it takes for a car to travel at a given speed against the speed of her own car so that when she merges into traffic, the driver in the car behind her does not have to slam on his brakes.

English, as a time-based language, allows a person to think, speak, listen, read, write, view, and calculate using time as an internal property of cognition. This time-based property probably evolved as people developed English to represent their thinking about moving into other parts of the globe to preserve intangible values such as freedom, liberty, happiness, democracy, parliamentary decision making, and so forth. Time allows English to be very portable. A person can use English to represent ideas that are maximally *displaced*, not in the here-and-now (see Chapter 3) such as liberty, respect, freedom, and happiness.

Later in this chapter, the cultural mismatch between thinking with time and not thinking with time for about 85 percent of the English speaking population will be discussed. If 85 percent of the English speaking population do not understand time as an internal, sound-based function of the present, past, and future, then 85 percent of the population will need strategies or other ways to deal with the value of time or the culture will no longer value time.

Activity: What does time-based English mean in terms of being literate in time? What are some applications of time-based English to literacy activities?

English: an alphabetic, sound-based language

Another English property that makes English very portable is its alphabetic property (e.g., Holm & Dodd, 1996). An English speaker's words once were written as letters that represented the exact speaker's sounds. Oral English no longer mirrors the written or orthographic symbols of old English because oral language evolved more quickly than written language. Therefore, there is *not* an exact sound to letter match between spoken English and written English (Chapters 1 and 3). Even so, writers of English are able to take the letters that once represented a one-to-one correspondence to the spoken sounds of English and arrange them into infinitely new meanings. For example, "google" is made of the sounds and letters typically found in English arranged into a new word. This word, google, is a noun and a verb and is widely used. An English speaker combined English sounds together into a word and then wrote the letters that could correspond to the sounds of the pronounced word. Speakers, readers, and writers of English can use the new word. Eventually, with widespread use, google is put into a dictionary. People developed dictionaries to show the word's origin, pronunciation, and acceptable meanings.

The arrangement of English sounds and letters has no length requirement, only a consonant-vowel property so the word sounds like English. Sometimes the simpler the word is in sounds, the more meanings the word has in function. For example, the word "up" is a remarkable word. In most dictionaries, the word "up" fills more than a quarter-page of definitions because "up" has been used in so many ways—as a verb, a noun, an adjective, a preposition, and an adverb. The function of "up" continues to increase in meaning as well as use. "Up" consists of the simplest produced consonant (C) and vowel (V), in the simplest morpheme (CV) combination in the most varied uses. "Up" is easy to produce and therefore easy to use in a variety of ways. This is an example of a language function principle: *Simple structure allows for more complex function or meaning.*

Activity: Why does oral English not have a one-to-one correspondence between letters and sounds?

Using the alphabetic property of English assumes a sound processing element of the language. Each written word represents a spoken word. Each written set of letters has a pronunciation. Words like "up" are simple in oral production and therefore widespread in use. Such simplification leaves little left to change between its oral production and written representation. The word "up" is very different from most English words. Most English words consist of multiple strings of sound patterns that a speaker creates to mean a single idea such as "hamburger." Through time, the number of meanings increase which will simplify the production, but such simplification could take hundreds of years. In the meantime, speakers develop more words. Words are strings of sound.

Because words consist of strings of sound, educators and parents assume that English speakers are able to hear the sounds of the words. But, many English speakers hear sound and yet are not able to make the sound patterns they hear into conceptual meanings. For example, some children can orally read fluently by using phonic rules of sounds and letters, syllables, and words to say what they see on a page, and yet not understand what they read aloud. They are able to "word call" the names of the print without comprehension. Or, some children and adults are able to read a chapter silently with sub-vocal sound over and over, trying to make meaning out of the sounds but not really understand the sounds of the print they are reading. Or, some children can imitate a complete TV commercial verbatim and not know what the commercial means. Other English speakers hear the sound of people's speech but understand only the movement of the speakers' mouths. In other words, a speaker of English does not automatically have an innate sound-based system for understanding how letters connect with sounds to form the alphabet for literacy purposes.

Activity: What is the alphabetic property of English?

Individuals who cannot use the alphabetic property for acquiring conceptual meaning do not think in the sound of their own mental voice but in the mental picture or movies or graphics or shapes of what others say. This means that they do not have access to the alphabetic property of English for becoming literate. They struggle with literacy until they crack the visual code of what the words cognitively mean on the page; or, until they learn some coping mechanisms such as learning the meaning of printed words (reading) before they go to school so they do not need to learn how to turn sounds into mental pictures or other visual graphics. Parts III and IV will provide the reader with how to make English literacy visual so that children and adults who think in visual cognition can achieve the highest level of language function by matching the way they think to the way they learn to be literate.

To achieve a maximum conceptualization of an alphabetic language like English, visual thinkers must remove or ignore sound elements of English. The sound elements of English are removed and replaced by visual elements that are spatial and relational, rather than time-based and alphabetic. For example, a child can learn to write English words spatially as bubbles or shapes of ideas, rather than by putting sounds and letters together as a spelling task. Note: Most recent spelling bee contestants memorize the way thousands of words look. Today's spelling contestants are learning what the words or parts of words look like, not what they sound like. Most of today's spelling bee contestants are mentally seeing the word in their heads and are saying what they see. They are not sounding out the word and then attaching letters to the sounds, which is the way educators teach children to "spell."

Activity: What is meant by the English alphabetic property of spelling?

Changing the alphabetic properties of literacy programs into visual forms of thinking emphasizes language learning rather than sound-based production. The shift in education's emphasis, from teaching the sound-based parts of words to supporting students to learn to be literate in the way they think best, provides children the opportunities to think at their best. Because 85 percent of English speakers do not use sound to process what they understand, then 85 percent do not understand the use of the alphabetic properties that educators use to teach reading, writing, viewing, thinking, listening, and speaking. By using methods that match the visual thinker's learning system, then the learner acquires literacy in the way the learner thinks, which is the best of both thinking and learning.

Activity: How does the alphabetic property of English impact learning to be literate?

English: a low-context language

Since English is a sound-based, alphabetic language, speakers are able to speak words in isolation. For example, a young child starts to dart across a busy street and a parent yells, "Stop!" The child hears the concern in the louder than usual voice, and stops to turn and see what the parent wants. By then, the parent is alongside the child to keep the child from running across the street. The ability to use a single word to mean so much is beneficial to this child's welfare.

The dominant culture of English speakers retains the importance of "words." Educators and parents expect children to learn vocabulary as strings of words that make sentences. For example, early writing tasks might ask a child to write a word to fill in the blank, "I like____." The child writes: "I like orange." "I like me." "I like white." "I like tree." This string of sentences does not interconnect and really does not have a lot of shared meaning with someone who reads the sentences. But because the educational system values the use of sound-based words using an alphabetic property, this task of stringing words together is valid. Children and adults practice spelling words—putting sounds and letters together—not for the purpose of communicating but for the purpose of writing a correctly spelled word. Word walls are put up in classrooms so that children can see the words to practice. Schools provide grammar events daily where students practice how to rearrange random strings of words, and then punctuate the arrangement of the words based on the grammatical sentence that consists of words.

All of these types of word practices of English are sound based, using the alphabetic properties of words. Words are thought about as isolated meanings, meanings that the words carry *out of the context* of the environment. Because the dominant culture values the word and expects the meaning of the word to be carried within the sound of the word, then the culture uses words in isolation. For example, a teacher walks into the classroom and says, "Today we are studying Italy." This type of word use is like parachuting the concept of "Italy" into the classroom. The students are thinking of how they got to school, what their friends are doing, what they brought for lunch and suddenly "Italy" drops down in the middle of the classroom.

Activity: What are some uses of English words?

The ability to use words out of context makes English very portable. Business leaders who are able to think in the sound of words alone are able to sit down at a table and "do business" without knowing the other people or taking the time to create a shared event. Even with all of the emphasis on the value of English being an alphabetic, sound-based language that utilizes words to stand alone, the fact is that the majority of learners in school and the workplace do not think in the sound of words. So, when the teacher says, "Today we are studying Italy," the sound of the teacher's voice interrupts most of the students' mental pictures. They do not know what the teacher said or what they are to do, and so they begin to look around to see what others are doing, look for the written words on the board, and look for additional information from the teacher. The students are trying to create a *context.* A context includes the people, their actions, their objects, and their locations connected through language (e.g., Kramsch, 2004). Context provides for the meaning of the basic semantic relationships to connect the speaker to others.

Activity: Why do words not require context for meaning?

Because English speakers use words without creating the context, English is considered a *low-context* language. In the business world, doing business with words and little or no context may not be very effective in other cultures that value people relationships over words. These latter cultures are contextual in nature. Context includes an understanding of who, what, and where in relationship to the concepts. For example, with low context, a business person can say, "Let's start the meeting. First, we are going to vote on agenda item one." The context is inferred through the meaning of the words. However, the person who thinks in a high-context way would want to visit with the people in the meeting, finding out the names of people, something about families and where they are from, and so forth. In some cultures, business is not conducted until the context is satisfied; sometimes, this takes several meetings. Educational set-up and curricula based on English as a low-context language conducts minute by minute tasks of activities that are often not related throughout the school day. At 8:10 a.m. is daily oral language; 8:15 is math; 8:35 is silent reading, and so forth.

Since 85 percent of the English speaking population does not use words for their best communication, then 85 percent of the population prefers more contextual way of learning (see Chapter 16 regarding these numbers).

Activity: Why is English considered a low-context language?

English: a global language

Languages which are most portable, like English, expand in use and function from one group of people to another as the culture represented by English also spreads. In fact, English, at this time, is the only ***global language*** (e.g., see Rowe & Levine, 2009). The speakers of English no longer live in a small area of the globe, and the speakers of English no longer communicate in the past and present but into the future. As the cultures represented by English allow for expansion of ideas and experiences never seen, touched, or felt before, English spreads and the meaning of the ideas within the culture expand. The language increases its global function.

One of the reasons that English is a "global language" is that its properties represent cultural values that allow for easy ***portability***; that is, English properties allow for the language to be used in a variety of ways, for a variety of reasons, and by a variety of people for future, present, and past experiences. The basic properties of English (Chapters 1 and 3) that allow for its global function include the following: English functions as a *time-based, alphabetic*, *low-context*, and *sound-based or* ***auditory language***. The functional properties of the English language also represent the values of the dominant cultures that speak English. These properties help delineate the cultural values of societies that use English.

Activity: What is meant by English being a global language?

Other languages similar to English

English is not the only auditory language that represents the time-based, low-context, alphabetic sound properties of its speakers. Romance languages like Spanish, French, Latin, and Italian as well as the Germanic, Slavic languages, like Russian and German, use the sound-based, alphabetic properties that are also time-based and low in context. These cultures have a long history of alphabetic, time-based, auditory properties. Today's English evolved from the influence of these language families and became what we recognize as English just 400 years ago, a fairly recent development in the history of languages. In other words, English in its present form is a rather new language that evolved from other languages and the cross-fertilization of cultures that used an auditory, time-based, alphabetic approach to a low-context use of language.

These auditory properties represent a Western Psychological way of thinking. Because the people value the properties represented in these languages, they pass these values on to the next generation through language literacy. Adult members of the society assign meaning with language to children's experiences. Children acquire language through the Neuro-Semantic Language Learning System where their language represents their society's values. This means that all of the auditory cultures that utilize an auditory type of language like English value the auditory properties.

When children learn English and the other time-based, alphabetic and sound-based, low-context languages from the speakers in their environments, speakers expect the children to *hear* the sound of words and make meaning from these words. These meanings come from the overlap of sound with what the child sees when the adult talks. The overlap of sound and sight patterns from sensory inputs integrate in the auditory pathways to create auditory patterns that form auditory concepts that result in auditory properties of language such as the alphabetic property.

Auditory concepts develop from the overlap of sound and sight. Once an auditory thinker develops enough language concepts to use a grammatical form of the adult language (about seven to eight years of age), then the auditory thinker is able to create new concepts through his or her own mental sound of his or her own use of spoken words. This auditory thinker uses the sound of his or her own language, not the imitation of what someone else says. This auditory thinker also is able to create meaning from listening to someone speak the language without having to see their face or see what they are talking about or make mental or drawn pictures of what is said. A person who uses an auditory way of thinking and who speaks English or any other auditory language is expected to think in the way that his or her sound-based language functions—time based, alphabetic, and with low context.

Activity: What languages are auditory in nature? How does an auditory language function? What are some of the properties of an auditory language?

In today's English speaking cultures, about 10–15 percent of the speakers are able to use auditory thinking to match the auditory language they use for education and for the workplace. The other 85–90 percent of the population thinks in visual properties that are relational, high context based and spatial, rather than temporal in nature, even though their language is English, an auditory language.[2]

Activity: In what form do most speakers of English think?

2 This change from time-based thinking consistent with the properties of English to a more visual-based thinking that does not match the written properties of English could be attributed to several changes in the environment including: first, a need for better use of environmental space rather than the need to explore in future time; second, children used to die from middle ear infections but with the advent of antibiotics used to cure infections allows children to live but the fluid in the middle ear takes 8–12 weeks to reabsorb so infants with middle ear infections hear spoken patterns as if they are listening to sounds in water; third, society uses more visual-motor language inputs and less oral language for assigning meaning and the brain research shows that input affects the way the brain organizes data; and fourth, a person who has a visual system is more likely to pass that thinking onto his or her children so a phenotype becomes a genotype.

Thinking: a relational process of visual language

This section compares the cultural-linguistic values of English to the *thinking* properties of most English speakers. English is alphabetic and so people expect speakers of English to use sounds as words without context. But, if a thinker does not use the sound of words to think, the thinker has to create concepts in some other way. One way is to think about what a person sees as it *relates* to mental pictures or graphics. For example, the listener sees the speaker's mouth move. Mouth movements form a shape that the speaker recognizes as a meaningful idea. This shape is a visual mental picture. In this way, the person who uses visual patterns for creating visual concepts thinks in the meaning of the visual pictures that represent the meaning of the language. In order to make a visual picture very specific, the visual pictures must be in *relationship* to past and present pictures. For example, in a travel brochure with a picture of a tropical destination like Hawaii on it, a person might think about lots of options: Hawaii is beautiful and I should visit or I wonder if that is Hawaii or I wonder on which Hawaiian island that picture was taken? For every single picture, there are lots of interpretations (Arwood, Kaulitz, & Brown, 2009).

In order to understand the specific meaning of the picture on the brochure without words, there would need to be several pictures that showed not only the location in Hawaii but who was going to that location in Hawaii and when they were going and how they were going, like a mini-movie. In other words, *relational* language (e.g., Caffarel, Martin, & Matthiessen, 2004) uses visuals in context to explain an idea or event (Arwood & Kaulitz, 2007).

Another way to understand the concept of *relational* language is to recall the old-fashioned sketched pictures in little books. Each picture by itself had limited meaning but when a person quickly flipped the pictures, the characters began to move and the movement of pictures created a movie clip. One picture *relates* to the next picture which *relates* to the next picture and so forth. ***Relational languages*** connect all people into a circle of life that represents how people live together as a community.

Activity: What is relational language like?

Instead of words or pictures standing alone, relational languages or cultures connect multiple visual events to form the whole meaning. Storytelling is very important in *relational* cultures because the stories over time create a picture of the values of the people of the culture (e.g., Simmons, 2002; Verschueren, 1999). People are therefore more important than words, because people and their actions represent the *relationships* among stories. Because relational languages connect events through stories (e.g., Simmons, 2002) and through people and their lives, then context is imperative. Remember from Chapters 2 and 3, *semantic relationships* are the bases to all languages. Context consists of basic semantic relationships (e.g., see Kernan, 1970; Lust & Foley, 2004). In an auditory language, these *relationships* are explained through the use of time-based words like "of," "so," "will," "might," "to," "for," "yesterday," "while," "during," and even "so forth." In a *relational* language, these types of time-based function words are typically not used. Instead, people's roles, purposes, and relationships are central to the story of an event.

Activity: What is a relational property of language?

Thinking: a high-context process of visual language

Whereas English is considered a low-context language, Mandarin Chinese and other visually rich and relational languages like American Sign Language, Hopi, or Chamorro utilize context for maximum language function. In English, speakers use words, often alone or in phrases or single sentences, for meaning. In relational languages, the speakers tell stories about people, what people do, where people do what they do, how and why they do what they do as important components to everyday life and doing business. For example, in English a person can perform a greeting with a single word spoken out of context, "Hi!" In a culture that values context and therefore relationships, the speaker who said, "Hi!" and walked on would be considered rude. A proper greeting would create a context, such as asking about a person's family members, what each person was doing, about the day, about what they did that day, etc.

Only by creating context can a person, who uses a relational property of language, feel comfortable with the communication. In other words, to make individual visual concepts mentally move into meaningful mental pictures or stories, there has to be a sufficient number of related pictures to make the individual frames form a movie. The *relationships* among people, their actions, and their objects expand from simple, basic semantic *relationships* to complex stories. Instead of using sound words to stand alone, most people think in how ideas relate together to form stories about people and what people do.

Activity: What is context? Why is English a low-context language? What is relational context like?

Thinking: a spatial process of visual language

English is a time-based language but relational languages represent cultures that create a whole picture, independent of the time frame. Until the task is complete, there is no task. If a person in a ***high-context*** culture has items to sell, then when the sun comes up, the person goes to the marketplace and stays there until all the items are sold or the sun goes down. The task is selling the items. The time it takes to sell the items does not figure into the selling. Likewise, the hours a person must spend to complete a task also is not as important as doing the task until it is completed. This type of event-based culture uses visual processing for determining when to do what (e.g., Emmorey, 1993).

Auditory cultures use languages that are time based, like English, and therefore their people expect to sell as many items as possible, in as little time as possible. The people in these cultures have a significant value placed on a person's time. Likewise, this value on time appears in their language which is auditory, time based, and alphabetic.

Activity: What is the difference between an event-based culture and a time-based culture? Which one uses an auditory form of processing to conceptualize or think? Which culture uses a visual form of processing to conceptualize or think?

Because some cultures are not time based and their languages are therefore not time based, the use of the *context* of events determines what the person does according to the *space* that the person is in. These non-auditory languages are ***spatial*** in nature. They use people, their actions, objects, and events to create ***referents*** for language function. For example, "I know it is Tuesday; I am at school." The event of going to school tells me where "I" am. Chapter 5 will expand on the differences between visual and auditory languages and what it is like to live in an auditory world but think with a visual system.

Spatial thinking derives from the spatial planes of existence. So, a person who thinks in these spatial planes typically lives in a culture that puts people into roles in relationship to other people. Spatial thinking represents the way ideas relate to others and their roles within the community. For example, a person is a part of a family and the family is a whole. Any action that affects the person, affects the family. Another example of thinking with the visual use of space (not time) may be found in education. Most school-aged children think with a visual, spatial language function; so, even with intensive instruction about how to write letters from the top to the bottom, most children will write their letters from the space they are in; they write in relationship to their bodies. The adult sees this writing as writing the letters from the bottom of the paper to the top. Children with spatial thinking use the space of their bodies in relationship to their papers. Therefore, where the paper is in relationship to the child's body is more important for a visual thinker than the direction of making a letter. More about using the knowledge of thinking with spatial properties will be provided in the intervention chapters of Parts III and IV.

Activity: What is a spatial property like?

Cultural properties of English

As explained in Chapter 2, children acquire language by members of a culture assigning meaning to what they say and do, which is then processed as part of their neuro-semantic learning system. So, children in an English speaking culture learn the meaning of not just the words but also the thinking behind the words (e.g., García & Otheguy, 1989). Because English is a time-based, alphabetic, low-context, and sound-based language, the dominant culture expects adults and children to learn new concepts by thinking in the *sound* of words that are time based, non-contextual, and alphabetic (word based). For example, children are expected to learn the *sounds* of words, to talk with words, and to think in the *sound* of their own voice. English speaking children are expected to learn to speak through assembling *sounds* followed by using those *sounds* with letters that correspond to the sounds for learning to read and write. Children are taught the *alphabetic* properties of sounds to letters to write by spelling; that is using the same spoken *sounds* aligned with letters to form written words. Furthermore, educators teach children in a dominant English speaking culture to memorize *sound*-based language structures such as spelling words, multiplication tables, vocabulary, and parts of speech, to name a few units. Furthermore, educators expect English speaking children to learn how to plan their work by using the *sound* of words in *time* for organization, following directions, and executing tasks. Likewise, employers expect employees to produce work in a *timely* way, where assignments and pay for work are *spoken* without historical or relational context, and where most business is completed with *spoken* and written words. *The dominant culture values a time-based, alphabetic, sound-based culture even though the majority of people think in a spatial, relational, high-context, visual form.*

This means that educators and employers who speak English assume that the majority of their learners and workers think in the time-based, alphabetic, low-context, sound properties of English. However, at least 85 percent (Arwood, 1991a, 1991b; Arwood & Brown, 1999, 2001. 2002; Arwood, Brown, & Robb, 2005; Arwood & Kaakinen, 2004, 2008, 2009; Arwood, Kaakinen, & Wynne, 2002; also see Chapter 16) of English speakers *do not use the sound-based, alphabetic, low-context, time properties of English when thinking.* The majority of people "think" in contextual, spatial, relational, and visual thoughts.

Activity: What are the assumed properties of English thinkers? Do most English speakers think in the English properties?

Implications of the mismatch between English properties and cultural expectations

Because the functional properties of English represent dominant cultural values, educational teaching programs, employers, and families assume these properties as important values in teaching and learning. For example, most English literacy programs use an alphabetic, sound-based approach. And, most businesses use a time-based work value when reimbursing employees. However, because learners of these cultures do not think in these assumed properties, there exists a mismatch between the way children and adults think when they learn new concepts and the way they are taught in the schools, in the workplace, and at home.

Because the dominant culture values time, sound, low context, and the word (alphabetic property), then the dominant culture *pushes* the teaching of patterns (see Chapter 2) or products that represent the time-based, low-context, alphabetic, sound-based properties of English. These taught patterns or products include words, sounds, letters, vocabulary, definitions, reading aloud, memorizing words for multiple-choice tests, and regurgitating the content of spoken or printed words. As English speakers produce more of these memorized patterns, through imitation, copying, and regurgitation, the less the learners conceptualize or actually learn for later use. The mismatch between thinking and learning results in lower abilities to use English for critical thinking, problem solving, literacy, work ethics, and creating a solution-directed culture. Emphasizing the cultural values of an alphabetic, sound-based, low-context approach to education and the workplace when the majority of learners think in a visually spatial, contextual, and relational process *restricts* the function of the English language. More about how to reconcile this mismatch is offered throughout later chapters.

Activity: Why does the dominant culture emphasize the teaching of words, sounds, letters, vocabulary, definitions, reading aloud, and memorizing content for copying?

RESTRICTED LANGUAGE FUNCTION

As previously described, language functions represent the way a person thinks. So, a person's thinking determines how well the *person's language functions* (e.g., Angus, 1977). To determine how well a person's language functions, a test of the "strength of the grammar" will help. Testing for only the language structures is a ***weak test of grammar***. For example, chimpanzees are capable of producing language structures such as symbols arranged in new situations for simple problem solving of the past or immediate present. The trainer provides the symbols and then later observes that the chimpanzee uses these symbols in a structure such as "want cookie" to get a treat. The chimpanzee's request is limited to what the listener is able to infer from the situation. For example, does the chimpanzee mean that he wants the trainer to give him a cookie or that he doesn't want any more cookies or that there aren't any cookies around or does he want to know where are the cookies? The chimpanzee's use of symbols in a structure is *restricted* to interpretation. *When listeners must do more than half of the interpretation of meaning for conversation, then the language is restricted in language function.* Therefore, according to the weak test of grammar, a chimpanzee is capable of learning a grammar but the structures are restricted in linguistic function. The chimpanzee uses symbols that are limited in their linguistic function.

Activity: What is a weak test of grammar?

On the other hand, displaced language that shares in the communication of ideas that can't be seen and touched, such as concepts about government, liberty, outer space, ancient Egypt, or respect, provides complex meaning (semanticity) across cultures, places, and times (flexibility and productivity)[3] and suggests a "strong" language function of grammar. In other words, a ***strong test of grammar*** means that the function of the language is greater than the surface forms of patterns of words, phrases, and sentences. Language function that meets a strong test of grammar allows for a conversational ability between the speaker and listener. Within a strong grammar, each speaker is capable of initiating, maintaining conversation, and adding to the meanings of others' language function. In essence, a strong grammar is one that allows a speaker and listener to share in the most *displaced, productive, flexible, and complex semantic functions.*

Activity: What is a weak grammar? What is a strong grammar?

There are a number of examples of restricted language function in today's society. For example, technology has brought in rapid message forms such as texting, which is often very *restricted* to the present time and to those who are interpreting the text according to a shared code. If the code is not shared, then "LOL" could be laughing out loud, lots of love, or luck out Louie. These types of restrictions lack the complexity of thinking that represents the formal cognition of ideas such as respect or liberty, and are not designed for such abstract thinking. Since there are so many people who think visually, the use of visuals without language is also increasing. For example, speakers use fewer words and more bullets, lists, and more pictures to tell others about products and ideas. Instructional manuals sometimes are all pictures and no words, even though no two people have the same pictures for an idea. When the use of English words is limited or restricted to explain a process (remember the word is the sound-based unit), then language function is also limited. For example, a brochure might say "Visit soon." The person looking at the brochure recognizes the background picture of Hawaii and puts the picture with the words. But, do the limited words and picture mean to book a trip with your local travel agency to Hawaii? Which part of Hawaii? And is the picture on the brochure of a specific place to visit in Hawaii, or any place in Hawaii, or a destination like Hawaii? Or maybe the brochure is

3 Chapter 3 provided the reader with an explanation of the linguistic functions of displacement, semanticity, flexibility, productivity, and redundancy.

not really about Hawaii but taking time out for yourself by sitting in a lounge chair in your office and thinking about a place you love to visit. *Restricted use of language limits the specific meanings of the language.* The listener must think for the speaker. The speaker must assume the listener's context. In the case of the Hawaiian brochure, the person looking at the brochure is the listener; the listener must try to think about what the speaker or writer means by "visit soon." With speakers limiting their use of English, then English becomes less flexible and productive, and less global in function.

Activity: What is an example of restricted language function?

Structural changes in the use of English such as the use of fewer words while adding more pictures represent changes in the underlying thinking of the speakers of the culture. As more people think with visual parameters of language, more people restrict the use of language. Without the full use of the language grammar for maximum linguistic function, thinking becomes restricted. Restricted function affects speakers' abilities to think critically and to problem solve in their culture. Restricted language function affects the way that employees think in the workplace. For example, a worker is sent out to complete what should take the time and resources of a single service visit. When the service worker, with restricted language function, arrives at the customer's house and *sees* the job, he then leaves the house to go get the tools and materials he needs. From his perspective, that is how he is able to complete the job. From the customer's perspective, the worker was told on the phone (sound-based) what job was to be completed and it was assumed that the service worker would know what materials would be needed. Therefore, during the contractual phone call, when the service worker said it would be a half morning job, the customer expected the job to be completed the first time (the first half day) the service worker came to perform the job. But, when the worker arrives and has to leave to get the tools and the materials for the job, the job has to be rescheduled and the customer is still waiting for the job's completion. This actual job may take several visits because the worker literally has to *see* what needs to be done each time before he can do the next step of the job. The service worker does not have enough *language function* to be able to use his language to *think* about what he needs to do before he comes to do the job or the next step of the job. The worker's ability to problem solve is restricted by his mismatch between thinking differently than what the culture expects.

Activity: Give an example of a mismatch between culture and thinking.

For the service worker, the sounds of words by phone do not make mental pictures. By phone, the worker can't see the job so he doesn't have any pictures in his head to ask questions on the phone about what he needs. On the phone, he cannot see the job. Because the worker does not think about the job before he sees the job, the worker is not using a time-based form of thinking. He sees no reason to think ahead (in the future), to plan, or to organize from the customer's perspective. There exists a cultural mismatch between the way the worker thinks about the job and the way the customer expects the work to be completed. This mismatch obviously results in a loss of income or profits by the service worker's employer. Multiply this loss by thousands of businesses and their employees and the inefficiency of the workplace begins to be noticed by the national, global economies.

Another cultural mismatch exists between teachers who expect their students to be able to use a sound-based and time-based language for thinking about homework, and the actual way students are able to use language to complete and turn-in homework. The number one complaint of teachers and parents about school-age children to this author is that the children do homework and do not turn the homework in to the teacher. The second most common teacher complaint is that the children know how to do the work but don't have the time management or organizational skills needed to complete the work. Students who think in visual cognition do not think in time properties. Therefore, they do not know how much time a task takes or when to do the task. And, if they don't know how to remember seeing themselves do the homework, then they don't even remember to do it. Furthermore, they may have a picture of what their social studies work is but when the parent or educator asks if they have "homework" to do, they will say "no" because "homework" is a different mental picture than "social studies."

Activity: What are some ways that the cultural-linguistic mismatch, between assumed expectations of thinking and actual ways to think, affects education and/or society?

Visual thinking but English is auditory

The reader may be wondering what the surface language of a speaker who uses a restricted form of language function looks like. Below is a language sample from two 19-year-old males, matched by age, gender, college level, social economic status (SES), IQ, position in family, and family structure. The question posed to each of the speakers was, "What do you do on a typical day?" This is an auditory, time-based question that requires a spoken response. This exact question is part of the *Temporal Analysis of Propositions* (*TEMPRO*: Arwood & Beggs, 1989) assessment. The speaker's language was audio recorded and then exactly transcribed. Boxes 4.1 and 4.2 give the two language transcriptions.

Box 4.1 Speaker One's typical day

What do you do on a typical day?

I get, I would get up and usually not take a shower because I was too lazy. I put a cap on so my hair wouldn't look too nappy and go to class. And, uh, after I got out of class, I would go back to my room and sometimes watch TV for a while, sometimes study and I, and I would just do that for most of the afternoon, read or something, and I would go down (cafeteria in dorm) and eat and then I would go to work and I would usually be there anywhere from two to three or four hours. I'd usually get back around ten, eleven, twelve, depending on which night it was and then I would study some more and listen to records for a while, sometimes write most of the night.

Analysis of Speaker One: He is able to use English words to take the reader back and forth in time, from the dorm, to school, to the dorm, to work. He connects his ideas in time and he makes a parallel in time between how long he works and what day it is. He is able to refer to the question of what "typical day" actually means and therefore he actually answers the question. The listener "gets" the idea of what his typical day is like: He goes to class, he studies, he works, he studies, and so forth. This speaker's function meets the "strong test" of a grammar because the listener does not have to interpret or guess what the speaker means. The first speaker is able to use English as a time-based, sound-produced language of words that refer to events in time and with time for maximum displacement, semanticity, flexibility, productivity, and limited surface redundancy. He casually, but succinctly, answers the question.

Box 4.2 Speaker Two's typical day

What do you do on a typical day?

Usually I'll sleep in and, and, and uh, if I get the chance, if the television's on I'll go right for it but otherwise I'll read and I like to read. If I have a good book, I'll read 'til midnight, from morning 'til midnight but other than that I'll read science magazines or I might go and something, if I'm real curious about something I might go to the library and look it up there. And study it some. Sometimes I get into little patterns where I can't get out of and I find something interesting and it leads to other things and that I could spend my whole day doing that or it can go that I don't feel like doing anything and I'll watch TV. I kinda' hate that thing...

(The speaker continued on and on about "things" until the person collecting the sample said, "I get the idea. I think I have plenty of language to transcribe.")

Analysis of Speaker Two: He does not understand the time-based concept of "typical day" so he refers to "typical day" as "usually" he "sleeps in." Culturally, "sleeps in" means it is not a typical day. He does not use his words to take the reader through a "typical day." The reader has to interpret the non-specific meanings of "things" or "stuff." Speaker Two does not provide specific information about "who," "what," "where," "when," "why," or "how." This speaker talked about things he does but he does not refer to his job (which he has), his school work, or his activities before or after school, which would describe "his typical day." And, this speaker did not know when he had answered the question; so, he was not succinct or efficient in his use of words. It should be noted that there was another "paragraph" of the same type of utterances which were not transcribed as they did not add to the meaning of what this speaker said. In fact, the person collecting the sample finally had to tell this speaker to stop talking by politely saying, "I think you have answered the question. Thank you!" Speaker Two's language function is restricted because even though he has a lot of grammatical types of structures, his language does not maintain a shared conversational referent where the listener understands the words without having to take on the speaker's responsibility for thinking.

Activity: What are the differences in language function between Speaker One and Speaker Two?

Summary

A speaker of a global language like English should not show restricted function like Speaker Two. Languages like English allow for maximum displacement, semanticity, productivity, and flexibility through limited redundancy as a result of the alphabetic, time-based use of non-contextual words.[4] If a speaker of English cannot access the sound-based, alphabetic properties to think in a time-based function of English, then the speaker's language becomes restricted which limits thinking and problem solving as well as decision making and planning. With as many as 85 percent of the population lacking a strong grammatical use of English, then the thinking properties change as the culture changes. There are two options for dealing with the mismatch between language expectations and thinking differences: First, either develop compensatory strategies that match the thinker's way of learning so as to assist in translating the ***visual thinking*** into English that retains the auditory properties of the language; or, second, the language and culture continue to evolve over a long time so that there is less of a mismatch between thinking and being able to learn the valued concepts of the culture. The latter option does not support the culture or the presently accepted values. Currently, the dominant culture of English speaking groups still values the alphabetic, sound-based, time-based, and low-contextual language functions, even though the majority of English speakers' cognition is visual and relational (spatial, not temporal) in nature. More about the implication of restricted language function will be provided in later chapters. Chapters 7–10 will provide assessment and intervention suggestions while Chapters 13–15 will provide a variety of classroom applications. These strategies are aimed at teaching English speakers to use their learning system to acquire new concepts in the way they think, not the assumed way they think. In this way, ***visual language*** methods are used to help English speakers translate their thinking into English for reading, writing, thinking, viewing, speaking, listening, and calculating while retaining the maximum function.

Applications

- Look at three different marketing advertisements used by the dominant culture and decide if the language meets a strong test or weak test of language function.
- Think about a business service experience that was not satisfactory. Was there any communication breakdown as a result of differences between expectations and the worker's (workers') thinking?

4 It should be noted that some languages have restricted properties because the language is limited to a geographic area and/or specific cultural uses. Most of these languages are not written and become secondary or extinct when another culture that possesses a time-based, alphabetic language moves into the same area where speakers are using the restricted language.

Chapter 5

LIVING WITH A VISUAL BRAIN IN AN AUDITORY WORLD

A Paradigm Shift

Learner objectives: Chapter 5

Upon completion of this chapter, the reader should be able to:

1. Define the paradigm shift from teaching to learning with emphasis on thinking.
2. Explain why there is sometimes a mismatch between the majority of thinkers and the cultural thinking expectations.
3. Explain how thinking and learning concepts relate.
4. Explain the relationship between emphasis on sound production for literacy and the way most people think to form concepts.
5. Explain why sound does not need to be the basis for English literacy.

I see what I know.
I know what I see.
But I do not know what I don't see
Because what I see and hear do not connect.

Language studies were prolific in the 1960s and 1970s. Researchers (e.g., Bloom & Lahey, 1978; Brown, 1973; Gleason, Berko, & Weintraub, 1976; Klima & Bellugi, 1979) defined child language and attempted to determine where language originated. Without access to the brain, researchers could not go beyond speculation and philosophy or beliefs about the acquisition of language (e.g., Arwood, 1983; Bruner, 1983). When non-invasive brain research methods began to surface in the 1990s, new models of language study (e.g., Bookheimer, 2004; Damasio, 1994) began to address the relationship between the brain and the mind.

Researchers wanted to know where in the brain does reading and writing originate? Where do language structures like word order develop in the brain? Where does emotion stem from? When a child struggles to learn to read or write, where is the breakdown in the brain? Most of the studies that address these questions focus on examining language structures or the products of the learning language system rather than focusing on the processes of language function. One possible way to discover more of the way language cognitively functions is to explore the neuro-semantic processes of sensory input, perceptual integration, and conceptual feedback as language functions between thinking and learning.

Chapters 1–3 provided the reader with knowledge about how the neuro-semantic learning of language occurs. Dora, who was introduced in Chapter 1, *learns* to speak. She also learns to read, write, think, view, calculate, and listen. Without a typical Neuro-Semantic Language Learning System, Dora would struggle acquiring the products of these processes. As pointed out in Chapter 4, the meaning of language represents the cultural values of society. Dora learns the values of her society through language. Each language represents society's values. Furthermore, English is an auditory, sound-based language that is temporal and word-based or low in context. Subsequently, the dominant culture of society not only expects that Dora, but also assumes that Dora and the majority of people, value these sound-based characteristics because they think in these qualities. But, the majority of people do not think in the sound-based properties of the English language. Therefore, a cultural-linguistic mismatch exists between thinking and learning for those people who think in visual meta-cognition while living in an auditory culture. This mismatch affects research interpretation, educational programming, curriculum, assessment practices, and intervention for learning language or literacy. This chapter addresses the effects of this cultural-linguistic mismatch between thinking in visual concepts while living in an auditory culture.

Cultural and linguistic paradigm bias in research

As human beings use their own language systems as cognitive tools for setting up research, asking research questions, and for interpreting research findings, the values of language are used as a lens when engaging in research, setting up education curriculum, and so forth. For example, because English is a low-context language where the word is able to stand alone, parts of language such as sounds, letters, and words are valued. Therefore, most educators and researchers of language acquisition view language as an additive set of observable parts or structures (Chapter 1): The child produces sounds; sounds form words; the child uses the sounds; the sounds form words; words and sounds of words develop literacy tasks such as listening, reading, and writing. Yet, in Chapter 2, the reader learned that the child actually learns the features of sound and light waves, not words.

This cultural bias results in assumptions about the parts of language making up the whole. Similarly, brain studies follow the same cultural assumptions: Scientists look for specific parts of the brain that are responsible for specific skills such as saying words or reading letters. The cultural assumption is that by adding together the parts, the scientists could understand the function of the whole brain. As more brain research is collected, it is surprising to many scientists (e.g., Schmidt, 2008) that the brain is much more synergistic or holistic in its functioning (e.g., Malafouris, 2010).

For any given task, several areas of the brain can be stimulated, not just one area of the brain and not in the exact same location in different people. In other words, the research does not support the particular research bias that specific parts of the brain are *explicitly* responsible for *specific* words or parts of words as many assume about language structure development. Complex language functions represent the dynamic processes of thinking that involve the whole brain.

Activity: English is described as an auditory, sound-based, alphabetic language. How would these properties of English affect the way a scientist might interpret research?

The cultural assumptions about language and the brain also result in assessment and intervention that is driven by the belief that testing and teaching the parts is the *only* way to learn to be literate efficiently. For example, as neuroscientists mapped (e.g., Merzenich *et al.*, 1998, 1999) and discovered problems between the use of sounds and letters (Shaywitz, Pugh, Fulbright, Constable, Mencl, Shankweiler, *et al.*, 1998), it was also *assumed* that the deficit in the parts should be "fixed." The essential key to an assumed auditory type of literacy is to train or teach more of the sound-based parts. For example, if a person has a problem speaking, programs for developing speaking such as practice on producing sounds or words are put in place. In this way, these programs provide opportunities for children and adults to work on producing the parts that are assumed to develop the whole. These programmed parts parallel the assumed values of an auditory culture; sounds in sequence of time without context. Programs drill the practice of such sound patterns as a way to add the sounds to form words, to speak, read, and/or write. Underlying this approach to education is the auditory assumption that most learners think in an auditory meta-cognition. Hence, there are numerous programs and research studies designed to *prove* the very essence of the assumptions: Teaching auditory parts is the only way and the most efficient way to make children literate. Even though many of the studies are critiqued, the main assumption that literacy consists of learning English properties or parts remains dominant (McGuinness, 2005).

Activity: How does cultural bias about linguistic function result in bias in deciding how to teach literacy?

The brain and its complex systems of neurology are physical in nature, and so a lot of brain-based language research aims at trying to find how to "fix" those parts of the brain responsible for learning differences or problems. This certainly makes sense when the research approach attempts to find a physical cause for multiple sclerosis or a brain tumor and therefore find a cure. Physical diseases with a single organic, physical cause may be approached from a straight physical research bias: Find the cause and develop a cure. However, many scientists are finding that diseases are often more complex and involve multiple interactions such as the need to map genomes for individual cancers. Similarly, higher order thinking and learning utilizes many physical sites of origin as a result of the interaction of *unique* stimulation from *unique* outside input coupled with the genetic factors of the learner's system. So, while the brain is physical, the mind is an outcome of neuro-physical learning in the brain mediated by the *function* of language. Therefore, research about learning and literacy needs to consider the way the system functions synergistically, not just from a developmental, additive approach of parts to whole. Thinking about literacy as a developmental set of products that result from an acquisition of learning language and later from language that assigns meaning to develop higher order concepts requires more of a dynamic or synergistic paradigm.

Activity: Why does higher order thinking necessitate a more dynamic approach to learning?

Because the brain does not produce a one-to-one correspondence between parts and products, then the synergy of the brain results in the function of the brain being greater than its parts (Arwood, 1983; Peirce, 2000). For example, a child may learn the words "I want more cheese" but not be able to ask why goat cheese is seasonal. An English speaking teen may learn all of the vocabulary and grammar of the French language but not be able to order a meal in French. An eight-year-old child may be able to say all the words in an oral reading task of a college book but not be able to ask to go to the bathroom. A college student may be able to get an A in chemistry but not be able to make meaning out of the chemistry textbook. A secondary education student may be able to read the history book, but the student may not know what she read when she has finished the reading.[1] *Producing the pieces does not add up to the whole function of language for literacy processes of speaking, reading, writing, listening, thinking, viewing, and calculating. The function of the brain is synergistic and so is language function. Remember: How a person thinks represents the way language functions.*

Activity: Give examples to show how literacy functions are greater than the additive parts.

The synergy of the brain allows for more function than just the structures or parts are able to create; the synergy of the brain allows for the systems of cellular meaning to interact to form cerebral cortical networks of what people know as images or concepts. And, language patterns or structures represent those concepts (see Chapters 1–3 for an explanation of this type of learning system). The underlying concepts are basic to language function. The cultural-linguistic bias in research that suggests that the brain functions as parts to form a whole and therefore the educational programs also teach a set of additive parts must be questioned. A paradigm shift away from teaching additive parts to emphasizing the processes of learning (Chapter 4) must be considered, if thinking and problem solving are valued parts of what it means to be literate. This shift necessitates an understanding of the relationship between how a person becomes literate and how the learner's literacy functions is important.

Activity: Why should research assumptions that are based on auditory language properties be challenged?

Language and literacy in auditory-based research

Some view literacy as an outcome of an input system. When a child lacks the development of the products, the child's physical input system is checked. If the eyes and ears are okay, it is assumed that the child's input is okay and that the problem is in the output. So, the child is

1 These examples are from actual people who have shown this mismatch between learning products and their ability to think or conceptualize.

taught those products as additive units. The child is taught to "speak, "read," and/or "write" the parts. The child is given drills to practice the development of patterns or structures of language such as saying sounds, word calling printed patterns, writing sentence patterns, and so forth. Input the sound patterns and practice producing the sounds.

Research looks at whether or not a child is then able to produce the taught patterns. As the brain functions only with patterns, educators who provide programs for teaching patterns can show effective outcomes of patterns. What is put into the learning system as a pattern can be measured as a pattern. However, it is apparent, from what really happens in classrooms, at home, and in the workplace, increasing patterns does not always result in the learning of concepts for higher order thinking, problem solving, or literacy function. For example, children can often recite rules when in trouble, fluently read, and show that they can do their papers, but they may not understand the conceptual meaning of the rules, comprehend what they read, or know how to organize their homework so that they do the homework and they turn the homework into the teacher.

Activity: What are some problems in learning patterns without comprehension?

In this type of input-output model, teaching what comes out as a direct input process works. However, there is always the possibility that a person can learn to imitate, copy, or regurgitate the patterns of words in speech, reading, or writing but not be able to understand the meaning of the concepts talked about, read about, or written about. Higher order language functions require conceptual meaning that is greater than the sum of the taught parts or patterns. Conceptual meaning or language functions are higher synergistic organizations of neural networks that are greater than the two-tier Western Psychological Model of sensory input to form patterns of output.

Figure 5.1 shows the basic two-tier model used in much of the Western European-American Psychological Model.

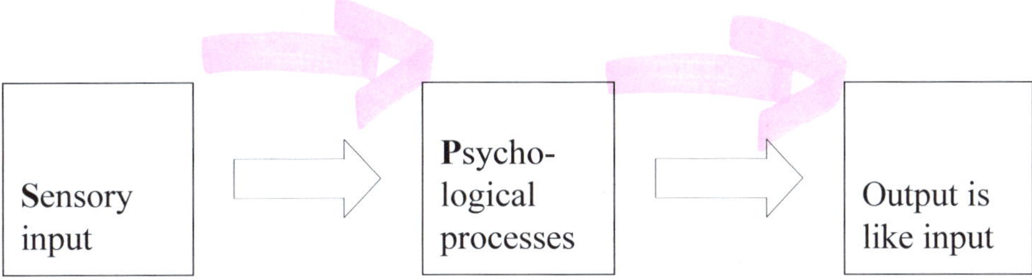

Figure 5.1 Two-tier Western Psychological Model

In this two-tier model, there are the inputs sometimes described by the neuroscientists as sensory input or described by other professionals as the stimulus or the probe. At the second level, there is everything that results from this input—memory, attention, focus, motivation, impulsivity, comprehension, imitation, production, language, reading and writing processes, and so forth. This model allows for teaching to the test which includes learning to imitate patterns for oral fluency testing; recognizing patterns for naming letters; spelling words;

regurgitating definitions; scribing vocabulary definitions; most multiple-choice testing; pattern matching; filling-in the blank; most true-false tests; completing homework that necessitates reading the question at the end of the chapter and matching the patterns of the question to patterns in the chapter; imitating others' writings; copying ideas; and so forth.

Activity: What is the two-tier model like?

With this type of model, there is the input to the learner and the psychological processes as the result or product of the input. These two steps result in output such as behavior, writing, reading, and speaking. If the learner has difficulty producing the outcomes, the logical conclusion is that the learner needs the input to be given in a different way or practiced until the input results in the desired output. The learner is trained or taught to produce the expected outcome. For example, in the case of auditory language, language is broken into its sound parts and the parts are taught (input) in additive steps to form larger units such as words and sentences. Tests and assessment measures are developed to ascertain the functioning of psychological processes involved such as memory or imitation. These measures provide a score that tells how well one child or student produced the outcomes in relationship to other children on which the test was standardized. In this two-tier model, literacy is the output of how well the various psychological processes function.

This two-tier model does not account for how neurobiological learning within the brain forms systems of concepts that are greater than their meaningful parts; nor does this two-tier model account for the power of *language function.* Remember in Chapter 2, the human *function* of thinking is different than the thinking in other animals. When a person has a problem to solve, he or she uses a type of thinking that is different than a chimpanzee, for example. The human builds upon the past experiences creating something that previously did not exist. The human takes a stick and turns it into a tool that is carried in a newly developed pouch whereas the chimpanzee discards the stick and must find a new one when presented with the same problem of reaching the bananas at a later time. This *displaced* type of human thinking allows for *flexibility* and *productivity* beyond the here-and-now in meaningful ways that allows for new inventions and explorations in the future. Linguistic functions like displacement allow for maximized problem solving which is greater than the additive parts of structures. These functions represent thinking! Each person thinks in the development of concepts. And, language (complex function of neural networks) represents the underlying development of the networks (concepts).

Activity: How do humans differ in their thinking from a chimpanzee?

These neurobiological systems of concepts continue to add meaning throughout a human being's lifelong plasticity of the brain. This leads to the second way that language may be treated: Because the concepts have to be learned, the focus on language in academia for literacy should be on conceptual development, not the teaching of language patterns or surface structures.

Teaching the language patterns or surface structures will not develop the underlying concepts. On the other hand, learning concepts will develop more surface structures. Earlier in this chapter, a paradigm shift from fixing the parts to emphasizing the whole was suggested. Within this paradigm shift, there is the need to understand that a person learns the concepts underlying language which results in something greater than just producing the structures or patterns. The Neuro-Semantic Language Learning System consists of more than just an input that produces patterns or statements of belief; the learning systems of the brain meaningfully produce concepts which *language functions* to use for thinking, problem solving, planning, organizing, and so forth. There are four tiers. Figure 5.2 shows the model.

Sensory input → Perceptual patterns → Concepts ↔ Language

Figure 5.2 Four-tier Neuro-Semantic Language Learning Theory Model

There is a two-way arrow between concepts and language because language represents conceptual meaning and when a child has developed the adult-like language structures around age seven or eight years, the child can begin to use language as a way to increase the meaning of previous concepts. In other words, language mediates learning for the older child, so the child can use language for learning concepts that cannot be seen, touched, or felt like the concepts of government, freedom, parliament, royalty, liberty, and respect. *In this way, language mediates the mind while also representing cognition or the concepts.*

Activity: How is the two-tier model different from the four-tier model?

Literacy, in this four-tier model, is a function of reading, writing, thinking, viewing, speaking, calculating, and listening to the concepts of language. Increases in language functions increase literacy. Note that the standard definition of literacy includes "viewing" and the majority of English speakers "view" the world from a visual linguistic perspective, even though the culture is still auditory in nature. If becoming literate is the goal of an educated society, then learning to think in the way one views the world is paramount. Learning to be literate would parallel a person's thinking. It would be counterintuitive to teach a person the products of literacy in a way that is different than the way a person thinks. In other words, a person thinking in a visual way needs to learn to read in a way that matches a visual way of thinking. So, educational emphasis needs to consider the synergy of the human brain as well as the way a person forms concepts with which to think.

Activity: Explain the four-tier model of learning language.

Philosophy behind a paradigm shift in research assumptions

The philosophical notion that the whole is greater than the parts is not new. In the 1800s, Charles S. Peirce called this concept *pragmaticism*. He showed through numerous writings and mathematical calculations that thinking produced more than the sum of the developmental parts. An application of pragmaticism to education (Arwood, 1983) suggests that a child has a learning system that functions to produce social and cognitive development that is greater than what results from the additive teaching of social and cognitive skills. For example, Bonnie Robb, a first grade teacher,[2] emphasizes language acquisition in her classroom. Language represents underlying conceptualization or cognitive development. If the principle of pragmaticism pertains to education, Robb's emphasis on language function rather than practicing the splinter skills, such as drilling on sounds and letters for reading and writing, should result in greater outcomes. Her results show that this principle of pragmaticism is pertinent to the classroom. The students in her classroom do pass the skill-based district tests in math, writing, and reading at over a 90 percent rate, often at a 100 percent passing rate even when she does not teach the skills on the test. The students often jump two or more levels of language function in less than an academic year, and, socially, the students change from believing they can't do well academically to students who function with high academic self-esteem and positive self-concept. Obviously, the philosophical assumption that students must be taught the splinter skills to achieve academically (Western Psychological Two-Tier Model) should be challenged. Utilizing a more holistic learning approach to children's development of literacy, as suggested by a pragmaticism philosophy, shifts the educational assumptions from teaching of products and skills (Chapter 4) to the learning of language (Chapters 1–3) representative of concepts related to reading, writing, speaking, listening, viewing, thinking, and calculating. Table 5.1 shows the paradigm shift.

Table 5.1 Educational paradigm shift

Current educational paradigm	Future educational paradigm
Teaching	Learning
Language structures: additive parts	Language functions: whole is greater than parts
Low context (auditory methods)	High context (visual methods)
Western Psychological (two-tier)	Neuro-Semantic Language Learning (four-tier)

Activity: What are the differences between the current educational paradigm and a proposed educational paradigm shift?

Research on the brain and on learning typically follows the cultural-linguistic and philosophical assumptions of the two-tier model: Give the subject an auditory task and see where in the brain that task occurs, or *if* the brain is designed to do the task. For example, some research suggests that the human brain is not set up to multi-task. That is probably true in a two-tier model where input goes to output. The subject is given a multi-task set and then images of how the brain functions in response (input-output) are collected. The conclusion of this type of experimentation is that the subjects have brains that are not set up to multi-task (see Chapter 16 regarding this research).

Now consider the results from a more holistic perspective. The majority of English speakers do not think in a time-based system; they think in a relational system of context of events (not events in time). So, if research studies on multi-tasking do not consider how

2 She teaches at a Title I school with 78 percent free and reduced lunch; 30 different languages with 7–8 different languages per classroom; with over 50 percent mobility rate.

subjects conceptually use language to think, the interpretation of the results of their study could be biased. The subjects do not use time-based auditory language for multi-tasking and the brain research on these subjects supports the way the subjects function. But what if these subjects learned to use English as a tool for multi-tasking; would their brains also show the ability to multi-task? In other words, research studies that conclude that human brains are not designed to multi-task are probably looking at subjects whose thinking is visual or spatial, not temporal, without consideration for the impact of language on learning in the brain. Furthermore, the dominant culture has not provided these visual thinkers with tools that match their learning system so that they are able to use their visual way of thinking to maximize their functioning in an auditory culture. Brain studies on learning need to consider whether or not they are assuming a Two-Tier Western Psychological Model in setting up their research questions. Again, remember that brain research shows that the function of the brain is synergistic and greater than its parts. Researchers need to consider the subjects' abilities to use auditory language and their cognitive way to develop concepts in setting up studies because language function may influence interpretation of brain research.

Activity: How does the assumption that the learning system is an input-output system affect brain studies of learning and cognition?

Educational curriculum changes to match paradigm shift

Because the dominant culture utilizes a sound-based, time-based, low-context language, English, for teaching children to be literate, educational curricula in this culture tends to focus on teaching the sound products of English within a low-context design. This focus is logical because adults in the dominant culture are unaware of the fact that children do not learn English as a set of language structures, as adults tend to assume that there exists a two-tier model of input the sounds and output the sounds for reading and writing and speaking. But this assumption that children learn language as an additive process of structures is not valid for the acquisition of *language functions* (Chapters 2 and 3). Language functions have to do with how a person thinks and makes choices based on thinking. Language functions have to do with the socio-cognitive linguistic properties of displacement, semanticity, flexibility, productivity, and efficiency (less external redundancy). Language functions reflect the way society assigns meaning to the social and cultural way of being socially competent.

Training the brain to produce the products does not account for how well a person thinks with those products, nor does programming the products account for how a person thinks or is able to use those products to initiate and maintain healthy relationships. *Language structures and language functions are not the same!*

Activity: What is the assumed basis to literacy in an auditory culture?

It is also important to realize that as the majority of children and adults do not think in the sound properties of the English language, they also do not use the sound properties of English for language function. *In other words, language structures do not develop language functions.*

Curriculum programs designed to encourage children to practice products, such as the teaching of sounds for speaking, reading, or writing, assumes that such programming will help develop language function. However, teaching the sound-based products to a child who thinks in visual cognition approaches education from a *deficit approach*; that is, the more practice on what a child cannot do is aimed at training the child's thinking to be something that the child's learning system is not wired to do. If a child does not show these types of alphabetic sound-based properties for literacy, programming those properties through intervention provides the child with the *opportunity to learn what the child cannot do.* It is true that the child may learn to imitate and produce the perceptual patterns of the sensory input. For example, a child may learn to say "ma" with extensive imitative practice or brain training or programming. But, this child may still not be able to think with maximum displacement about "monuments." Note: The word "monuments" begins with the same first syllable of sound but the meaning is different than "ma." The typical goal of these sound-based programs is to eliminate the deficits by adding missing parts. The assumed thinking process for the child is auditory. So, the assumption is that teaching the auditory properties of language structures will help children better function with English!

Activity: What is the deficit approach to teaching literacy?

Teaching a sound-based approach to English will help develop the products of the English language, but not necessarily produce a better way for the child to think or problem solve with English. *Thinking and problem solving develops through language that functions for better literacy, not through the training or teaching of additive properties of language structures.* This author believes that language function for higher order thinking and learning would be better served if the deficit-based programs designed to develop an auditory structural foundation to English literacy were replaced by a strength-based approach. This strength model would involve utilizing the cognitive properties of the child's learning systems. Furthermore, since the majority of the English speaking population does not think in the sound properties of English, instead of working on sounds and words, working on making meaning visual through drawings and shapes enhances the way the learner develops concepts the best. Working on the way the majority of learners create concepts rather than on the sound deficits also compensates for learners' weaknesses. Educational curricula should be based on the learner's needs. Therefore, the curriculum structure should shift to match the way most learners think and acquire concepts.

Activity: Why are today's literacy programs aimed at improving sound-based structures? What would a strength-based approach to literacy focus on?

A cultural-linguistic shift in curriculum to match most thinkers' learning systems

Since the late 1960s, this author has been working with children and adults who learn with a visual system of thinking. In the 1980s, this author found that 60–90 percent of the school population did not think in sound. In the early 1990s, when she wrote this statistic (Arwood, 1991a), many people were amazed at that high a percentage, as most educational practices assumed auditory thinking. Since then, the author and her colleagues have collected data from a number of groups, including young adults and professionals. The numbers are really much higher (see Chapter 16): closer to 85 percent of the general child and adult population thinks with a visual system (Arwood & Kaakinen, 2008). And, when the author tells teachers and parents that around 85 percent or more of today's regular school population as well as young adults think in a visual way, very few people question this notion. The fact that so many people think in visual properties seems logical because the people listening to the author are mostly visual thinkers themselves. Most people think in the form of visual graphics like pictures, mental movies, slides, prints, and so forth.

For some populations the number of individuals who do not think with sound is even higher than 85 percent. For example, Bonnie Robb (Arwood & Robb, 2008), a first grade teacher in a Title I school where 78 percent of the students receive free and reduced lunch, where the mobility rate is 50 percent or greater, where more than 30 languages are spoken by ***English language learners (ELLs)***, and where literacy is always a struggle, 124 out of 125 children in her classroom across five years thought with visual properties. In other words, over 99 percent of her students thought with visual properties of a language (Chapter 4), even though the school adopted alphabetic sound-based programs for teaching the population to be literate. It is apparent that the learning system for how people think is changing. *Learning to be literate can no longer be assumed to be sound based, auditory in nature. An auditory, alphabetic, part-to-whole curriculum does not meet the majority of students' thinking or learning needs.*

Activity: Why can educators and parents no longer assume that learning to be literate is an auditory, sound-based process?

There is a mismatch culturally between how children think to learn to be literate (visual) and how schools assume that children learn (auditory). There are several options for how to ameliorate this mismatch. Three of the most frequent or logical approaches include the following:

- Program the deficit sounds so that the brain changes to accommodate sound, as English is a sound-based language.
- Use more visual ways of seeing the sounds so that children learn the sounds visually.
- Use the visual properties of thinking to teach concepts, as conceptual thinking is greater than the sum of the parts.

Each of these approaches will be discussed in the following section of this chapter.

Teaching deficit sounds through programs

The brain is synergistic in that it adapts to whatever input it processes (Begley, 2007; Merzenich *et al.*, 1998). Because the brain only recognizes patterns, programming the sounds of English into computer patterns is an effective way of providing children with the sounds (Miller, Linn, Tallal, Merzenich, & Jenkins, 1999). Without the sophistication of a computer, numerous curriculum programs attempt to teach elements of literacy through teaching a sequence of sound and letters into words that are decoded (read) or encoded (spelled and written) in sentence structures. These sound-based auditory methods are effective at teaching sound patterns to the majority of students. With the emphasis on sound, children may show immediate progress at learning the sounds for reading. In fact, children will often show an immediate two years of sound growth when tested to determine if they have learned the sounds in a variety of literacy tasks from reading orally to showing pattern recognition of words. For example, the child is asked to point to a picture of the spoken word: "Harvey, point to the picture of the closet." The child recognizes the patterns of the spoken word, "closet," and is able to point to the right picture of a closet. Or the child orally reads a grade level passage to show oral fluency of saying the sounds of words on the page.

These types of tasks require the learner to use sound-based patterns. Patterns or skills do not automatically form the concepts for thinking. Pattern learning is quite extensive in the schools and even the workplace today. Pattern learning is a form of recognition by imitation or copying (see Chapter 2). These programs teach the learner to copy and practice the patterns. After a period of practice, children are tested on whether they can use the patterns. If the children can recognize or produce the taught patterns, the program did what the educators expected. For example, the children learned how to identify the acoustic patterns that make up words for reading, writing, or even speaking.

Activity: Why do many literacy programs emphasize the pieces of language such as sounds?

Another assumption underlies the use of these approaches to literacy: Students will use their new-found sound-based skills for problem solving, critical thinking, and living in the auditory world. But students may not be able to make the learned patterns into usable concepts for better language function. Curricula that are based on teaching patterns are not teaching children to think or use language for thinking. In fact, the author's research indicates that the learning of language structures such as sounds, words, and sentences does not improve a visual thinking child's or adult's ability to problem solve in an auditory world. Critical thinking and problem solving require the acquisition of socio-cognitive *concepts* (not patterns) related to the problem or issue at hand. Once again, thinking or language function is greater than the sum of its parts.

Activity: What do sound-based literacy programs assume?

All learners acquire the meaning of concepts in the way their neuro-semantic learning system turns patterns into concepts. So, if a student thinks visually, then programming sounds for literacy helps the student do the language structural tasks of sound patterns but does not necessarily change the way the student is able to develop concepts from the patterns. Furthermore, a two-year gain in sounds only takes the student to the point of being able to decode and encode sounds for speaking, reading, and writing but does not progress the child to the point of being able to comprehend for analyzing or understanding what the student reads, for problem solving a real-life crisis, for pro-socially developing relationships, and so forth. In other words, learning to use auditory patterns does not mean that the student will use these sounds as the basis to learning or thinking in concepts. Because language represents concepts or thinking, higher order conceptual thinking, problem solving, organizing, planning, creating, or designing must occur in the way a person is able to create concepts.

Activity: Does programming sounds necessarily change the way a person thinks?

Programming sounds and words provides many children with a change in how well they are able to use sounds for the same types of tasks. But learners' ability to use sound for thinking or learning new concepts rests with how well learners can connect their visual way of thinking to the sounds of spoken or read language. For example, some people who think in visual graphics like pictures are able to connect what they hear in the sound of their voice or other voices to their pictures. They think in pictures and then translate their pictures to sounds. Or, if they have to read aloud, they scan the print with their eyes to make mental pictures before they begin orally reading. In this way, they preserve their thinking while still performing the sound-based auditory task of reading aloud for the educator or parent.

The author has found that in most Kindergarten through college age classrooms, 30 percent or greater of the students *are not able* to connect their visual thoughts to the sounds of what people say or the sounds of what they read in texts. For Bonnie Robb's classroom, the number of students who cannot think in the sounds of others' spoken words ranges from 40 to 70 percent. Without some other options for learning to be literate than the typical sound-based curriculum, these students' abilities to think will be restricted along with their conceptual learning for problem solving. As these visual thinkers in auditory literacy programs become older, their abilities do not change. By middle school, where they are expected to use language for learning content, their abilities drop because they are not afforded educational alternatives to the auditory patterns. In other words, they do not learn how to use their language for thinking and problem solving. As young adults in college classes, they do not comprehend what they read in texts, so they don't read texts. They do not understand the sound words of the course syllabus, so they ask for examples of assignments so they can imitate or copy what they see. They do not know that what they copied from the book is exactly what the author meant so they appear to be plagiarizing.

If a visual thinker is taught with sound-based auditory assumptions, then learning to use visual thinking may not happen. *Thinking is the basis to language functions. Language functions provide the best critical thinking and problem solving. Therefore, for most people who think visually, an effective approach to literacy is also an effective thinking approach to learning.* Teaching a person who thinks visually to learn visually provides the person with a strength, rather than deficit, approach to thinking and learning, while maintaining the cultural values of an auditory culture (Chapter 4).

Activity: Why does working on sounds become a deficit approach to literacy? Why does working on the visual strengths of visual thinking affect learning to think?

Seeing the sounds

Many educators, parents, and researchers have noticed that a straight sound and word approach to literacy does not work with the majority of students (approximately 85%), so educators and parents have developed visual ways for students to *see* sounds. For example, a letter "A" might be connected with a body position of a child or a hand position or a mouth position or in a rhyme. The letter "A" is translated into what a child can see or into the shape of what the child can physically feel. Another example comes from deaf education where a program, Signing Exact English (SEE), translates auditory English into seeing the sounds on the hands, rather than teaching American Sign Language, a visual language. Thinking with letters to form sounds to form words uses the auditory properties of being alphabetic (Chapter 4). Putting the sounds of words onto the hands uses the auditory properties of an alphabetic, sound-based language. This is a part to a whole, sound-based approach.

The assumption of making sounds visual is that if the sounds are taught "visually," then the child changes his or her way of thinking. The child who thinks in visual concepts may have the tools to perform the educator's tasks such as sounding out practiced words but may still, and probably will, think with visual concepts, not the sounds of words. Furthermore, learning the parts such as the sounds as visuals or letters as movements is an auditory, curricular approach: teaching the input is tested as output.

Remember that in the Neuro-Semantic Language Learning System, there are four levels of learning: sensory, perceptual patterns, concepts, and language. Making a letter visual does not mean that the person is able to use concepts and language that are sound based. Making sounds visual is still auditory in language function. Using words or parts of words is always out of context and is therefore auditory in nature. Furthermore, this approach to trying to make the parts visual or felt is sensory at best; it does not reach the higher order thinking and language functioning that represents the concepts.

Activity: Why does seeing sounds not make the activity visual in thinking?

Seeing ideas rather than making sounds visual

Visuals come in different forms (Arwood *et al.*, 2009). Because the dominant culture thinks of visuals as what a person sees or can copy, then the concepts and language that are visual do not gain much notice. Table 5.2 shows the various ways that the dominant culture uses the word "visual."

From looking at Table 5.2, it is no wonder that people are confused about what the term "visual" means. The bottom line is that *thinking is the way a person will function; and, the way a person learns concepts is the way that a person thinks*. Educational curricula for people who think visually should follow what the visual thinking properties are for a non-auditory type of language like Mandarin Chinese or American Sign Language. In this way, visual thinkers are able to conceptualize or think at their highest level and will also then be able to use the auditory language, English, in a way that matches their thinking.

Table 5.2 Different uses of visuals

Visual term	Meaning	Educational purpose	Educational implication
Visual style	Educated preference or belief of how one learns	Personal preference for teaching materials	Visual style or visual learner may not match thinking or learning system
Visual modality	Input-output method	Used for teaching	Visual modality is external, not internal
Visual materials	Something that can be seen to be used for education or learning	If a material can be seen, it is considered visual	Seeing is not necessarily "knowing"
Visual learning system	How a human neurobiologically learns concepts that language represents	Visual perceptual or motor perceptual patterns overlap to form concepts for thinking	Internal "knowing" is language based
Visual discrimination	Acuity	Measure of what eyes physically do	Seeing isn't knowing
Visual perception	Recognition of internal sensory input	Meaning is limited to recognition of patterns	Can replicate, imitate, regurgitate, fill-in-the-blank, model, practice pattern, develop skills; but perception is not "knowing"
Visual concepts	Mentally thinking in graphic forms such as pictures, movies, organizers of words such as a rolodex[3] print	Learning of concepts represent the way a person thinks…visual concepts occur through the overlap of visual and motor patterns	Input for learning matches the way the person forms concepts for maximum thinking and learning
Visual language	Technology uses this term but so does education; visual languages are contextual and relational in aspect	Understand that the characteristics of a visual language match the concept formation of a visual thinker (Chinese is a visual language; English is an auditory language)	Thinking occurs in the way that visual languages function
Viconic Language Methods™ *	Impose visual language functions onto auditory English language characteristics	Translate auditory culture into visual thinking	Provides a student with a visual way of thinking that matches with strategies for learning in an auditory world

Source: The use of visuals is adapted from Arwood *et al.* (2009) *Visual thinking strategies for individuals with autism spectrum disorders: The language of pictures.*

* This term is coined by Ellyn Arwood and should be referenced when used. Trademark has been applied for.

1 A rolodex is a generic term for paper or computer formats that organize contact information. A paper organizer like this can physically be "spun" or "rolled" to the chosen entry.

Activity: Why do programs that emphasize making sounds visual utilize auditory properties of language? Why would a visual approach to visual thinking help a person learn to think and use language better?

Using visuals in a way that a person thinks is a strength-based model whereas a reductionist, deficit approach to teaching auditory parts results in restricting language function. This restricted function further restricts adults' expectations. For example, when students are not able to show an acquisition of sound-based English products, educators often reduce expectations or subtract some of the skills. If a child cannot spell, for example, the teacher might give the child 10 spelling words to practice while the rest of the class receives 20 spelling words. In this way, the expectations for the child are cut in half. Furthermore, spending the primary grades on sound-based, word assumptions for teaching literacy, results in a limited number of students who are able to develop enough sound-based tools by fifth grade to assign meaning with language when they read or write. As a result, the number of students who are able to function with sound-based tested literacy by eighth grade in the US is quite dismal. According to the Rand Corporation, less than 33 percent of the students are able to read and write and do math at grade level (McCombs, Kirby, Barney, Darilek, & Magee, 2005). This is because the US continues to teach in a deficit manner, making sound or sound-based products the ultimate purpose of literacy education. But the majority cannot think in sound, so this approach *restricts* how a child is able to think as a productive member of society. *Individuals who need to learn in the way they see what they think benefit from language learning that is based on how they visually conceptualize.*

Activity: Why does rehearsing or practicing sound elements for a person who visually thinks not result in seeing or thinking in ideas or concepts?

Seeing ideas rather than imitating products

Beacuse a deficit approach to literacy is limited in its effectiveness to make the English language function in an auditory culture, using a strength approach that allows children *to see what they think* allows individuals to learn not only the products of literacy but also how to think or conceptualize. As mentioned in Chapter 4, the reason for teaching an auditory language like English, in a way that a visual thinker is able to conceptualize, allows the learner not only to "learn to think" but also to "think to learn." Providing visual thinking as a way to learn to be literate in English allows the learner to acquire English literacy at his or her potential. English then becomes a tool for higher order thinking. English is a flexible, highly displaced, productive, and rich semantic language (see functions in Chapter 3). Allowing each person to develop his or her best language function of English helps develop not only literacy but also language functions necessary for independence within societal expectations. This proactive approach to English literacy suggests that learning English, as a complex language with maximum language function, allows a learner also to develop the best thinking. In this way, language for becoming literate need not be "dumbed down," but students should be provided English literacy through the way they learn concepts for thinking.

In order to make auditory English language learning match a visual thinker's way of developing new concepts, knowledge about visual properties of languages can be utilized. Arwood and Brown (2002) developed multiple literacy methods that utilize visual properties of language that match most English speakers' visual ways of thinking. The author calls these methods Viconic Language Methods™ (VLM)—visual language processes of thinking to facilitate the learning of an auditory language, English. For example, a visual thinker may find learning to write English easier when he or she draws out his or her visual concepts first, then translates those drawings into the written words. More about VLM will be found in Parts III and IV of this book.

Activity: What are some ways to help children learn to think with the sound-based properties of an auditory language like English?

The relationship between thinking and language

Thinking and *language* are intertwined. *Language* affects the way a person *thinks* and thinking develops differences in language (Arwood, 1983; Gil, 2004; Vygotsky, 1962/1934). Language is learned within the context of a specific environment. And the language function is the result of how a person thinks. This interdependence between language and thinking provides the basis for effectively teaching children to *learn* to use *language* to *think* within the values of society.

Activity: What is the relationship between thinking and language?

Different peoples have different needs, environmentally and culturally. These differences in how the people think and function in their environments result in differences in thinking values (see Whorfian Hypothesis: Carroll, 1956). For example, a culture may not have a word for war because they do not value war. Or, a culture may have 20 different words for rain because they live in a rainforest. As shown in Chapter 2, language represents the way people think (Arwood, 1983, 1991a, 1991b). Therefore, educators and parents really need to know how language development represents learning and how to adjust programs for language literacy to meet the way that learners think. To approach all language users as having the same thought processes is naive. Just because a child comes from an English speaking home does not mean the child thinks with the properties that define English. Or, just because a child does not come from an English speaking home does not mean the child does not think in sound. Furthermore, changes in the way a child is able to process the sensory input of the world influences the way a child thinks. For example, a child who is born deaf cannot receive the sound of a speaker's voice, so the child will not develop English without intervention. Furthermore, this child's thinking will not be based on the use of sound, even if the child learns to make the sounds of English. This person's learning system is visual in the way the child is able to process the meaning of the child's environment.

Activity: How does the environment affect the meaning of language concepts?

Thinking to learn

In Chapter 2, the reader learned about the Neuro-Semantic Language Learning Theory, where sensory input becomes organized into patterns. There are a limited number of ways that input from the distance senses of the eyes and ears can organize the patterns to form concepts. The reader learned that *the overlap of acoustic input with acoustic input results in imitation, not conceptual learning.* So, English is more than organized acoustic patterns. English is a complete language that represents conceptual learning. Visual patterns of input to the eye could overlap neurologically with past visual patterns such as seeing the shape of the mouth or hands or print. *These overlapping, integrated visual patterns will form visual thinking concepts.*

Language represents concepts so a language that uses visual patterns would use visual concepts for thinking. For example, American Sign Language (ASL) uses the overlap of what a person sees with assigned meaning from seeing hand movements in relationship to past and present visual patterns to create visual concepts. ASL is a visual language. By integrating overlapping patterns, a person learns to think in the language used to connect the environment to thinking.

Activity: What is the difference in learning between overlapping acoustic patterns and overlapping visual patterns?

English uses sound (acoustic information) to convey meaning. For example, add the sound /s/ to the end of "dog" and there is a new meaning, "dogs" or more than one dog. English also uses visual meaning. For example, for a child to understand the difference between a cat and a dog, the adult might point out that the cat has a different coat, is a different size, and so forth. So, meaning also comes from what the child sees. If the child's Neuro-Semantic Language Learning System is able to connect what the child hears *simultaneously* with what the child sees, the child is thinking in the sound of his or her own language which means the child is thinking in an auditory set of properties (about 1–15% of today's population). If a child's Neuro-Semantic Language Learning System thinks in the way that the child sees what people say or do, then the child has a visual way of thinking (about 85–100% of the population).

Because the dominant culture uses English, an auditory language, then it is important that all members of that culture are able to use English with all of its functions. The only way for a person who thinks visually to be able to use English with maximum function (Chapter 4) is for that visual thinker to form visual concepts from organized patterns of visual sensory input. Figure 5.3 shows two different thinkers in a classroom.

If a learner's environment does not provide the sensory input in the way the learner forms patterns to create concepts, the learner will not develop the concepts that other children in the same environment might develop. If the child cannot develop the concepts, the child's thinking is restricted. In other words, a child who thinks in the visual movement of the mouth or hand, but who never receives reading or writing instruction in the way the child *visually* learns concepts, may not learn to read and write. Instruction in learning to read and write with sounds may provide this child the opportunity to word call fluently; and yet, the child may not be able to make meaning of the sound patterns. For example, an eight-year-old child diagnosed with Down syndrome had a lot of really good instruction with sound: Sounds for speech, sounds for reading, and sounds for writing. When she was first evaluated by the author, the child could orally read (word call) a college level text *fluently*, but she did

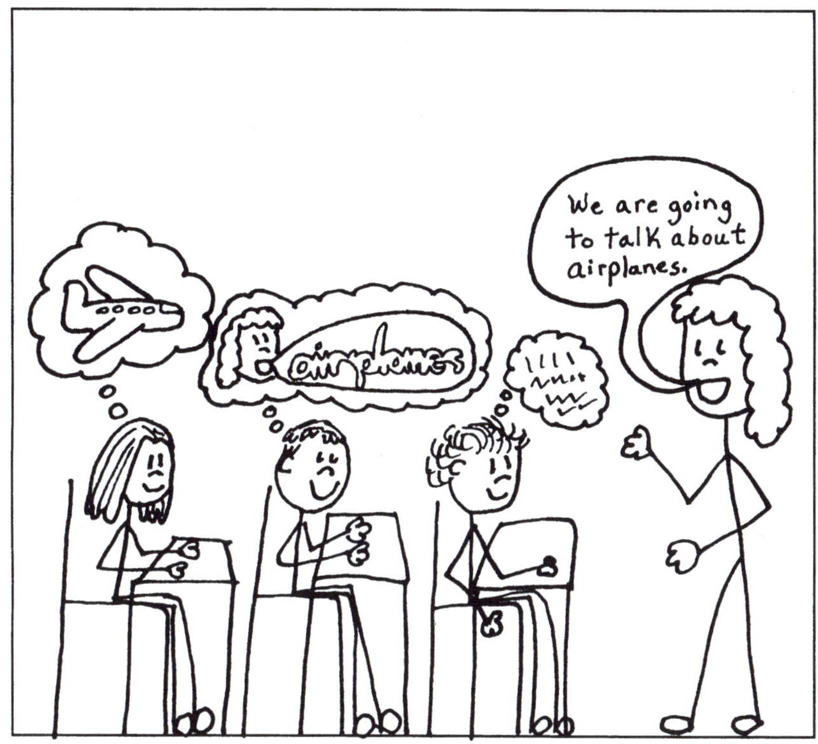

Figure 5.3 A visual thinker and an auditory thinker

not have enough language to ask to go to the bathroom. She often recited rhymes and finger plays in response to a simple question such as, "What did you do today at school?" or "How is your cat?" or "What does your cat do?" She had learned to imitate, copy, and regurgitate sound patterns, but she had not developed the visual concepts that went with the sound patterns. Her auditory world did not provide much meaning, as her thinking system was visual. Without intervention matching her visual learning system for concept acquisition, this young lady functioned at a very low level.

Activity: Why does conceptual instruction have to be in the way a person thinks?

There are many other examples from those with diagnosed or non-diagnosed disabilities. For example, many individuals who are diagnosed on the autism spectrum are often given instruction in how to produce sounds for speech and read fluently with sounds, but these individuals do not think in sound (Arwood & Kaulitz, 2007). This mismatch of instruction in their environment does not help them develop speech or learn to think at a developmentally appropriate level for cognitive or social concepts. The result is that many of the individuals who are diagnosed with autism do not receive the appropriate type of visual input to learn concepts. As these individuals grow bigger and get older, they show less and less of the expected conceptual development resulting in a secondary diagnosis of intellectual disability or cognitive impairment (some report as high as 80%).

On the other hand, some individuals who begin school with little language but who receive appropriate language learning in the way they conceptualize develop visual concepts that they can then use as the basis for their English literacy. One child who was diagnosed in first grade with an IQ of 65 showed an IQ of 90 by the end of the year and an above average IQ of 120 by the time she was in middle school. This student had a parent who advocated for the school to provide instruction for literacy (reading, writing, speaking, listening, thinking, viewing, and calculating) in the properties of the way this child thought. The child thought in the visual shapes of movements of people's hands for writing and of people's mouths for speech so the child learned to create concepts mentally from these visual shapes. She progressed through regular education because her parents and teachers provided her visual strength, not training on the sound-based deficit.

Learning language in the way a person forms neuro-semantic concepts is critical for students to become literate. Using the auditory assumptions of adult English in an additive, deficit model does not help develop the thinking language functions of a visual thinker. However, providing students with literacy instruction in the way they learn concepts helps them think at a higher developmental level. Therefore, students who think with visual concepts need visual language education to develop auditory English with expanded language functions for higher order thinking and problem solving.

Activity: Why does teaching a visual thinker with a visual approach to literacy help the visual thinker become literate?

Learning to think with visual concepts in an auditory culture[3]

To think with visual concepts means to embrace all of the literacy processes with a visual mind. In other words, a person who thinks in visual concepts will also speak, read, listen, write, view, and calculate with a visual mind. Because different environments provide different amounts of various inputs, learners will acquire unique ways to think visually. For example, some adults who think visually refer to thoughts as taking different forms. Some think in pictures like a slide show most of the time, unless it is a familiar topic and then the pictures create a mental movie. Some adults say that the better they know a topic, the greater the depth of conceptual development so they may have multiple mental movie screens. The greater the number of pictures or mental movies that a person possesses, the greater the person can use the mental, visual concepts for language functions (Chapter 3). Some individuals say they think in a mental rolodex: The rolodex spins and up "comes" the pictured word.[4] Some people who think with visual concepts talk about the markee (mental billboards) in their heads where the print of words goes across their forehead or where they dream in a tickertape of words or think in the scroll of subtitles. Some people talk about the

3 This heading is similar in meaning to a title of a book *Learning with a visual brain in an auditory world: Language strategies for individuals with autism spectrum disorders* (Arwood & Kaulitz, 2007) but is not just limited to those who are diagnosed with autism spectrum disorders.

4 This reference to a rolodex means that the thinker was mentally able to see the words flip as if they were on pieces of paper that spun from one word to the next.

flowchart of words or boxes that they can see mentally and move the ideas or words around into diagrams. Others talk about the exact rewinding of past seen ideas or events in a copied or photographic form.

There are some commonalities among the development of visual concepts: First, people who think in visual concepts are able to *mentally see* their thoughts. Individuals with auditory mental concepts hear the sound of their own voices but see only visual images, not clear visual concepts. People who learn concepts visually are able to make clearly distinguishable visual concepts from shapes or sights. The mind is visual for those who create new concepts from mental visual constructs.

Second, there is a developmental hierarchy to the development and organization of visual concepts,[5] similar to the hierarchy of auditory development:

- Individual pictures or shapes come first.
- Multiple, randomly ordered, pictures then develop as meaning increases for a concept; or, the visual thinker learns the position of ideas like a jigsaw puzzle or a mental drafting board.
- Multiple pictures about an idea must become organized into a cartoon, movie, mental file drawer, flowchart, and/or replaced by the usually written words. Many adults say that they see the written word for those topics for which they have the most information or the most mental pictures. Some visual thinkers use the *movement of their mouths* or the movements of other body parts such as the hand for writing as a way to organize the shapes of ideas into concepts so they constantly talk to be able to organize their thinking.
- Organized pictures such as files, rolodexes, movies, and graphics allow for the most language function. Many talk about putting multiple ideas into space such as separate chapters of content onto separate fingers where they look at the right index finger, for example, and can mentally pull up an entire lecture or chapter.

Third, visual concepts need the same spiral or scaffold (e.g., Coltman, Petyaeva, & Anghileri, 2002) of learning development to refine conceptual meaning. This scaffolding and refining comes from environmental feedback similar to the feedback that speakers provide auditory thinkers.

Finally, visual concepts have characteristics of visual properties. For example, time as a visual concept is clock or external time, not internal time. Therefore, the spoken language of a visual thinker will demonstrate external time, not internal time. Spoken language represents how the person thinks; so, the spoken language that represents a visual thinker's concepts is different in language function (e.g., displacement) than auditory spoken language. For example, a visual thinker sees the sun (external time) come up so it is time to go to market. Whereas an auditory thinker "knows" it is about dinner time so it is time to eat dinner. Chapters 7–9 discuss how to assess these differences.

Activity: What are some of the developmental stages of visual concepts?

5 Note that the developmental hierarchy for the acquisition of language structures provided to the reader in Chapter 2 assumed an auditory system of thinking. Most developmental milestone charts for language make the same assumption where the sounds and words are the unit of development, not the features of the sensory system and the meaning of the patterns forming concepts.

Living with a visual brain in an auditory world

Because language represents concepts, a visual thinker uses an auditory language like English often in a visual way. For example, since English is an auditory language, the dominant culture values the use of time. The entire US economy has been based on a time factor. People are paid for their time to perform a task or are paid to do a task within a time frame. A wage worker is paid by the hour. A salary worker is paid by the job. And, some people, such as National Football League (NFL) players, are paid for a job others cannot do. Because there are few people who can do what an NFL player can do, these people are paid money based on what the market can afford. As long as the NFL is popular, large amounts of money are available to the players. The US economy has been an auditory, time-based economy, based on the auditory assumptions of the properties of English. *The culture is auditory in the properties of linguistic functions even though most people think in the visual properties of a language.*

A person who learns concepts in a visual way, but who lives in an auditory culture, may struggle in society. For example, the reader is probably able to recall at least one situation where the delivery of a service or good took more time and therefore cost more money than expected. In the US, this is a common current practice. The following is a typical example. A homeowner calls a number of roofers who advertise that they inspect, repair, and replace roofs. The homeowner asks others in the neighborhood, checks references, and even checks some of the Internet sites available for a roofing company that will do the job they say they will do for a fair price at the time they say they will do the job. After much time on the part of the homeowner, she calls three companies and asks for bids from the three companies for a job to remove moss from the cedar shingles, inspect the roof, replace broken shingles, and apply a moss prevention agent. The homeowner is a professional so time away from her job costs the professional owner money. So, contracting with a roofing company that will do what they say they will do, when they say they will do, is an issue of not only time but also cost.

The homeowner accepts the middle bid because that company sent a person out within days of the call and the inspector who came out climbed up and "looked at the roof" and gave a reasonable bid. He was efficient and thorough. The bid was several thousand less than the top bidder, who came two weeks later and did not come on time. But the bid was a middle bid as the lowest bid was several thousand less, which was offered by a worker who came late one evening and eyeballed the roof without climbing up on the roof.

The company who was contracted to do the roofing job sent individuals who did not have the right equipment to do the job. The bidder knew what the roof looked like but he did not think about what the workers knew about the job. The workers made two more trips on two more days to do the job. This meant two more days for the professional to take time from work. However, even after the company did the work, the job was not effective. After two years of ineffective treatments, multiple phone calls by the homeowner as well as written correspondence, and spending more money than originally contracted for the bidder to bring in a different crew of workers and their equipment, the homeowner hired another company which was paid a similar amount as the original bid: This meant the homeowner paid twice for the same job. This second company came when they said they would and did the job right the first time. They obviously could *mentally see* what they said they could do. In other words, their mental pictures matched their words. They could think and use language to represent their words about being able to do the job. Interestingly, the first bidder said he would "remove the moss" but the workers said the job was to "treat the moss." They did treat the moss but the moss was not removed. However, the effective company said they would "remove the moss by hand" and then "treat it so that it would not grow back." Notice that the meaning of the language used by the second company is quite different. Their actions matched their words.

This type of mismatch between mental thoughts and words is quite prevalent in English speaking countries, which results in a time-based culture becoming less efficient and more costly. The author cannot help but wonder what some of the big company executives were mentally thinking when they borrowed money they did not possess in order to pay themselves incredibly well for jobs that did not take into consideration the well-being of their constituents. This mismatch between the executives' well-being and the well-being of their constituents may easily be explained by a cultural mismatch between values and abilities to think about others. To think about others means that an employer or executive is able to see the needs of others. When the executives of banks and mortgage companies sold mortgages to people who could not make the increased payments when interest rates increased, were they thinking of these people or only of themselves? Were they able to understand or see others' needs? Did they see how their actions affected others? Do they see other people as mentally part of their pictures? Or, were these executives the only people in their pictures?

To this author, there appears to be a number of people who can see themselves and their actions in their mental pictures and have learned the material values of the US culture, but who do not see others in their pictures. Seeing others in one's mental pictures, and seeing how one's acts affect others, means that the thinker must be able to equate his or her job to what others are spending or are able to spend for the job. The job is worth only what others can afford to pay. And the culture pays based on time spent and valued for jobs completed. When a roofing company, for example, continues to send their employees out to do a job, there is lost time for both the homeowner and the company; lost revenue means someone has to work harder. Working harder results in more time spent and less value for a job. Eventually, the company cannot stop the leak in its revenue and goes out of business. Since the late 1990s, the number of bankrupt companies in the US has hit a record high. People cannot afford to function in a time-based culture where the majority of the culture cannot think in economic time of an auditory culture because the majority of the culture has not learned to "see" what the auditory culture values.

Activity: What is the relationship between living in an auditory culture where most people think visually?

The reader might be thinking what do these adult examples have to do with education? Well, the children learn to think with language at home and in the first few years of school. After the age of seven or eight years, they learn to use language for problem solving. If educational programming and curriculum designs do not integrate thinking and language, those who think visually, but live in an auditory culture, will have restricted problem solving and social development as an adult. Meanwhile, the education systems continue to treat learners as having an auditory way of thinking, not providing the cultural tools for the learners who are visual thinkers.

Activity: How does living in an auditory culture affect education?

Auditory culture and visual thinking

Internal, auditory time is the basis to the economic values of the US. Goods and services are valued based on the time and cost to make and sell. What is the role of education in an auditory, English speaking, culture who possesses primarily auditory thinkers? If the role of education is based on strengths, not deficits, then the role of the US education should be to provide the opportunity for all children to use the dominant culture's values for living in society. As the society is auditory in values, educators should be spending time on teaching children how to use their visual thinking for living in the time-based auditory culture. In this way, students grow up understanding how their actions affect others and how their use of time affects others. For example, as previously mentioned, the number one complaint of teachers and parents is that children do homework that they do not turn in. This means that there are many children who are not learning to *see* that their teachers do not know how they did on the homework unless the teacher *sees* the homework. There are also a number of students who don't do homework. They are not learning that doing their homework is a contribution that they make to the classroom.

A child's cultural job in school is to think in a way to become language literate. Children must learn to see others in their mental pictures with them. They need to learn that whether or not they do their jobs affects how others think of them and how others are able to work with them. Later, as adults in society, they must develop higher order concepts while also having language strategies to use their visual concepts to meet their expectations of the auditory culture, if the values of the auditory culture are to be retained.

The dominant culture of English speaking cultures is auditory in nature. This means that English speakers talk about the future because they can think about the future. Setting goals, planning events, anticipating outcomes, exploring the unknown, prioritizing, and even doing homework are all future types of tasks. It is no wonder that today's children have difficulty doing these types of activities, that adults pay millions of dollars each year for organizational help, and new businesses aimed at helping people clean out their "junk" continue to emerge. Even some neuro-scientists argue that language-based thinking accounts for the present and past but not the future. This interpretation suggests that there is physical evidence for "time-based" thinking no longer to be present in the majority of the population. If this is true, the culture or the language will change to match the thinking unless there is an explicit attempt to protect the auditory cultural values. For example, auditory language function takes a person into future learning of Ancient Greece. Ancient Greece occurred in the past but the thinking about Ancient Greece occurs in the future. Or, auditory thinking takes the person into planning and organizing based on what could be, not what has already happened.

Auditory cultures also allow for temporal portability or multi-tasking. As previously reported, neuro-scientists indicate that today's brain is not wired to multi-task. Multi-tasking requires time—the time to think about what one is doing while planning to do something else. So, maybe what a person is able to do with his or her brain affects the way the brain is able to function (Begley, 2007). If this is the case, providing children with language literacy in the way that children think is a necessary part of education, if the dominant culture expects its members to be able to multi-task. For example, being able to hold a job, raise a family, volunteer in the community, and plan for future needs such as retirement are examples of everyday multi-tasking. The parent who comes home from work and begins to cook the evening meal will find interruptions from children needing assistance, from the phone ringing, from the other parent coming home, and possibly from neighbors as well as from co-workers. Multi-tasking is valued as an economic, time-based ability. This type of multi-tasking is easier for a person who has advanced language functions that allow the person to displace (Chapters 3 and 4) from the event, prioritize activities based on urgency and need, which results in the ability to organize activities in multiple ways. English, an auditory language, uses time-based elements that represent this type of thinking. But the majority of English speakers think with the visual properties of space, what they see, not time. Therefore, educators need to rethink the way to make auditory values visual so that all visual thinkers have equal access to thrive successfully in an auditory culture.

> ***Activity:*** What are some examples of the use of time in an auditory culture?

Summary

Language function represents the way people think...differences in language function represent differences in cognitive thinking. Approximately 85 percent or more of English speaking people do not think in the English thinking properties of time, sound, low context, and the alphabet for being literate. *The majority of English speakers think with visual concepts that develop from contextual, space, sight, and graphic types of learning. Therefore there exists a mismatch between educational expectations of the auditory culture and the way that most learners think.* This mismatch results in difficulty for those who expect time-based sound use of the language for economic, educational, and organizational purposes.

A paradigm shift suggests that education emphasize helping individuals think visually while retaining the auditory function of English. This type of shift in focus suggests that the dominant culture values auditory properties while thinking with visual properties. Table 5.3 shows this shift.

Table 5.3 Proposed shift in educational paradigm

Current educational paradigm	Future educational paradigm
Teaching	Learning
Language structures: additive parts	Language functions: whole is greater than parts
Low context (auditory methods)	High context (visual methods)
Western Psychological (two-tier)	Neuro-Semantic Language Learning (four-tier)

Higher order thinking and problem solving requires the best function of language for thinking. As educators and parents begin to recognize that a strength model for teaching children to be literate provides for maximum language and thinking, their cultural auditory bias will shift to allow children other ways to learn and therefore be successful. Chapter 6 will expand on the relationship between thinking and literacy.

Part III of this book will provide methods to show how to shift the educational parameters to allow for both a functional use of English as well as higher order thinking and problem solving for all learners through visually based assessment and intervention.

Applications

- Discuss some examples of the mismatch between auditory cultural values and a thinker's abilities to use auditory properties like time.
- Discuss some ways to take a classroom lesson plan and make it more visual in thinking.

Chapter 6

LANGUAGE, LITERACY, AND THINKING

Learner objectives: Chapter 6

Upon completion of this chapter, the reader should be able to:

1. Explain how language and literacy interrelate.
2. Explain how reading and writing are not just sounds on a page.
3. Explain how viewing and listening are not just hearing.
4. Explain how speaking and writing are not self-talk.
5. Explain how calculating is a language function.
6. Explain how literacy and thinking interconnect.

Knowing to read and write,
Learning to speak and listen,
Viewing ideas of spoken thought,
Develop the language of literacy.

Researchers and scholars continue to discuss whether or not cognitive ability is static or dynamic. Does a person's cognitive ability change over time? Or, is cognitive ability inherited and therefore static? In other words, can a person's cognitive ability change over time? A logical approach to these questions provides an answer that reflects both the person's genetic as well as environmental opportunity to learn to think and function.

Cognitive ability is conceptual development. Because a child learns concepts through the Neuro-Semantic Language Learning System (Chapters 1–3), a baby brings to the learning setting the biological predisposition to acquire concepts through his or her environment. Consequently, children learn as well as their neurobiological system allows, and children acquire the meaning of concepts from their environment. As stated in Chapters 2–5, the child learns to think with language functions. Through ongoing learning, children learn to use language that represents increasingly more complex, higher order thinking or conceptual development. *As language increases, so does a person's ability to use language as a tool for acquiring more layers of conceptual development. In this way, an increase in conceptual development increases cognitive ability. An increase in language increases higher order thinking.*

The purpose of this chapter is to show how language function or cognition relates to becoming literate. Case studies will provide examples.

Language concepts of literacy

As the reader may recall, in Chapter 2, the Neuro-Semantic Language Learning System presented a model of how a child learns concepts. Chapter 3 showed how the first concepts are basic, relational concepts that increase in meaning over time. Chapters 4 and 5 showed that most people think in visual concepts that necessitate a layering of visual (not sound-based) input. This chapter provides the basis to how concepts increase in functional complexity over time. For example, a two-year-old "knows" table as a place for a toy or bottle. But, a six-year-old "knows" table as a four-legged object that is used for coloring, eating, and other tasks. A 10-year-old "knows" table as a piece of furniture that comes in a variety of sizes and types for a variety of functions (e.g., dining room table, teacher's work table, card table). And a 15-year-old knows that the concept table does not need to be literal, but can also be figurative: "Let's table the motion until next meeting." *In this way, concepts layer meaning and so language function increases in depth or complexity.*

Structural language complexity plateaus at about seven or eight years of age. By this age, a child with solid language development has the structural language complexity of an adult. The child can use complex sentences in a variety of ways. But, language functions continue to increase throughout life. In fact, language function is a major tool in the continued development of conceptual meaning. With adult structural language tools, a seven to eight-year-old child will begin to use language to assign more meaning to the concepts so that the concepts increase in complexity. Parallel to the beginning of this ability to use language for increased concept learning, children at about eight years of age show a higher level of cognitive development than their younger, three to seven-year-old counterparts. Between 7 and about 11 years of age, a child's brain (e.g., Bookheimer, 2004) is actively using language to acquire lots of meanings that are added to the child's basic early childhood meanings. This preadolescence (7–11) period allows a child also to learn how to use language as a tool for literacy. Literacy consists of the psychological processes for constructing meaning to be able to read, write, think, view, listen, speak, and calculate (Cooper, 2006). *This means that language is a tool of literacy.* Therefore, a child should have the complex language structures of an adult (7–8 years) to access the functions of language such as those in literacy. The following sections of this chapter show the relationship between specific areas of literacy and language functions.

Activity: Does language function increase beyond the years of structural language development? Explain.

Reading

Reading is more than decoding and encoding of sounds into words and sentence structures. As Heilman (2005/1964) and others have pointed out, a child learns to read what a child "knows." In other words, a reader brings his or her language to the reading task. For example, consider reading an article about something you know "little" about. You can say the names of most of the words with good sound decoding but the sounds of the "said" words mean little. You read, and reread, and reread. You still do not know what the article means. So, having the language of the concepts on the page is essential to the literacy of "reading." In fact, ***reading*** is a process by which a reader uses his or her language as a tool to interpret the meaning of the ideas on a page. In other words, the reader thinks in the ideas of what the reader knows about what is "said" on the page.

Activity: What is the language definition of reading?

As scholars and practitioners have developed tools for "naming" the sounds of words for oral fluency, the basic assumption has been that sound is the unit of interpretation of meaning. Chapters 4 and 5 provided the reader with knowledge about how readers of English do not think in sound but in visual concepts. Therefore, it is logical that tools for assisting a child to learn how to "see" the meaning on a page would help a child learn how to use what he or she knows to "read." But, for a child to "see" the meaning of the words on a page, a child must "know" the meaning of the concepts on the page. The more language a child possesses, the better the concept development of the child. In other words, *a "good reader" is not a child who can say the names of the words, but a child who "knows" the meaning of the concepts underlying the words that the child sees on the page.* This definition of reading supports the paradigm shift from teaching to learning, from products to processes, from skills or patterns to concepts that increase in meaning through the lifespan.

Activity: What is a good reader?

By understanding how the Neuro-Semantic Language Learning System works, it allows educators and parents to understand that a child learns the language system, parallel to the development of concepts. A child acquires meaning of recognizable patterns that become concepts. And, language represents those concepts. The natural acquisition of language structures represents the child's underlying thinking. The more concepts a child is allowed to learn in the way a child thinks, the better the child functions in thinking.

The process of reading to understand works this way: First, the majority of children, about 85 percent, see the print on a page because they can recognize the patterns of the print. Then they convert the print to mental pictures which are the concepts. Last, they share with others what they "know" about what they read. Sharing could be accomplished by talking, drawing, and/or writing. Many visual thinkers actually can draw more of what they see on the page than they are able to talk about what they "see" or read. From the drawings comes the writing, a visual way to represent concepts in print.

Activity: What is the process of reading like for most children?

The assumption of most scholars who develop "learning to read" or "reading" programs is that the patterns are made of sounds. So, it is not surprising that the majority of initial reading programs emphasize a phonic, phonetic, sound type of emphasis, not a thinking-language approach. The purpose of these programs is to develop a "recognizable" sound to letter patterns in the child. In this way, the child looks at the print on the page. The child is able to see the print as recognized sound-letter combinations. The child says those sound-based patterns, and it is assumed by the auditory culture that the child will know the patterns as sound-based concepts already stored in memory as part of the cognitive language system.

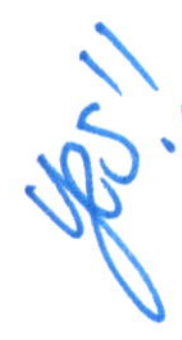

As described in Chapters 4 and 5, most children (about 85% or more) do not form concepts from sound. So, the result of these types of sound-based reading programs is that the majority of children learn to say the sounds but not necessarily understand what they say. Through years of sound practice, about 55 percent of the students who make visual concepts learn to connect the sound of spoken words to their visual mental concepts for which they have already developed language. But as they become older and what they read is more abstract, they less they understand (see Chapter 5 for explanation of statistics). For another 30 percent of children who think in visual concepts, sound actually "gets in the way" of mentally seeing their ideas. In other words, the sound of the teacher's voice reading or the sound of the student's own reading voice makes their mental pictures disappear. These students continue to struggle with comprehension of reading. Is it possible to read with some other form of patterns other than the sounds of letters?

As mentioned in previous chapters, the neuro-typical learning language system has a limited number of ways to create a concept. One way would be to integrate sound and sight together like with phonics, but only 15 percent or less integrate the sounds and sights for thinking. Another option for pattern recognition would be to integrate visual patterns with other visual patterns such as the pictures of stories with the print. For example, Dick and Jane types of books were able to do this when the teacher provided the language of the picture and made sure students had the concepts for thinking about the pictures. With this method, a picture of a typical task, such as a boy riding a bicycle, would be connected to the print that said what the picture was about. The assumption was that the students reading the book had the language and experience to understand the meaning of the pictures, and therefore also the meaning of the print. The print would "say" what the picture said. "See Dick. See Jane. See Dick ride his bicycle. See Jane ride her bicycle." Note that the book has a relational visual property of language in that the book is contextually based on a story about people doing actions that children would typically recognize.[1]

Before the children were exposed to the print, a gifted teacher would start with a story about what she did with her bicycle, using very rich language. For example, the teacher's story might go like this:

> Yesterday, I took my green and white bicycle out of the garage because I wanted to ride it to the park. I got on my bicycle and rode to the park to watch my brother play baseball. When I arrived at the park, I got off my bicycle and put my bicycle by the tree so I could walk over to the baseball field where my brother was playing ball. When I first walked into the park, I looked out in the field and saw my brother playing short stop.

Then the teacher would ask the children about their bicycle experiences. After two or three students told about their bicycle experiences, the teacher would read the picture in her Dick and Jane book while she pointed to the parts of the pictures that matched her oral words. The children, who usually worked in small groups, would each tell their stories for the teacher's pictures. The teacher would then have each child open his or her book. The teacher would

1 Visual language properties are relational, spatial, and contextual.

give each child a half sheet of paper to cover the words and look at the picture. Each child would talk about the picture before they read the print. In this way, the children had the language for the pictures. Then the teacher would have the children move the paper to see the first words, "See Dick." The teacher would say something like this: "Let's see what the author of this book says about Dick. The author says, 'See Dick.' What does the person who wrote this book say?" The students would answer together and then the teacher would ask each student in the group the same question to be sure each child saw the pattern that went with the picture.

The teacher worked between the children's language knowledge and the meaning of the concepts in the pictures. To the visual concepts of the pictures, the teacher showed the print or visual patterns of the words. Because the children had the language for the pictures, the children could "read" or recognize the printed patterns of the picture concepts. This approach worked well for teaching many, many children to read. Children learned that the print on the page meant something. What the print meant had to do with what the children knew. Later the print would bring new ideas that children did not know.

However, there are a number of factors that can make this type of reading difficult for some students. If the teacher does not make a language connection between the child's own experience and the pictures, the child who does not have Dick and Jane experiences will not have the concepts or language for being able to understand the meaning or the relevance. For example, children from other than Dick and Jane cultural backgrounds would need the teacher's ability to make language connections as well as different stories. Or, children who do not have adequate development of language would have difficulty, if the teacher were not skilled in providing the language. For example, some of these story books are used as "basal readers." Teachers "say the sounds" or read the print and expect the students to do the same. The children may not even know that the print goes with the pictures. Today, many primary books have pictures and words that do not match which would not work well as a material for this type of connection between visual patterns of print and visual concepts of language. Using visual print to go with visual concepts of pictures provides the purpose of reading. But, many educators struggle with the notion of what does a child do when a child sees a word that the child does not know? Or, what happens when there are no pictures? So, many educators developed methods to "sound out" the word. The assumption was that if the child could "hear" the sounds, the child would know the word and therefore the meaning. This works only as long as the child has enough language to support the words orally produced. For example, a child might "sound out" the word "defy," but unless the child has the meaning for this word, it is just a sound pattern.

Activity: How do language and reading go together to create the meaning of print? What are some strategies for connecting meaning to the print?

The grade at which many students begin to lose the language to support the sounding out of words is about third grade. By fifth grade, reading is designed to provide new information about content material. The majority of students past fifth grade, educated in the US, struggle with reading comprehension; they do not have the language to support the way they have been "taught to read." They do not make concepts from the sound of their auditory culture and auditory classroom, and they have not developed strategies to align their thinking with the auditory way to read. The result is that their reading scores decline in the fifth to eighth grades. Most students will not read for information because they do not have the mental pictures to understand what the words mean and they do not have the strategies to translate the auditory sounds of words to pictures. More about how to provide visual strategies for translating auditory skills into visual concepts will be provided in later chapters. Many of these same students do read novels for entertainment, as they already have the language for the words and can create mental movies when they read this type of material.

Activity: What does reading comprehension require?

How does a student who thinks visually become a great reader in an auditory culture? There is a simple answer and a complex answer to this question. The simple answer is that the visual thinker learns to recognize the print as mental visual concepts. So, the visual thinker looks at the page of print and sees the mental visual ideas that match the print patterns. Most college students who are good readers and who think visually tell this author that they could "read" before they went to school. This means that they learned what print meant based on their well-developed language before they were introduced to letters and sounds in the schools. Most of them also say they can recite the phonic rules but have no idea what they really mean because they don't read with sound; they read with visual mental language! They look at the print and make a mental picture, graphic, and/or movie.

Activity: What is the simple answer to how people with visual thinking read?

The complex answer includes more of a theoretical explanation of how language functions for literacy, specifically for reading, as well as an understanding of what the reading task is about. Language represents thinking. A visual thinker uses visual language types of properties (Chapters 4 and 5) in their conceptualization or thinking. For example, a person who thinks visually depends on the context for interpretation of meaning. So, the visual thinker uses more context than a person who thinks in the sound of what they see, an auditory thinker. This means that a person who thinks visually prefers to look at large segments of print, such as whole pages, in order to "see" the context. Reading silently allows for such visual scanning of seeing the whole. Just as in speech reading or reading the hand movements of American Sign Language, as in a ***gloss*** of the context, the whole context matters. ***Decoding*** the meaning for a visual thinker comes not from being able to say a word mentally or orally. For the visual thinker, decoding comes from putting the print into the context of who is speaking, what the person or author is talking about, where this story is taking place, and when is this "story" or information relevant or important. Visual strategies, based on this type of contextual decoding, are a lot more effective for visual thinkers than sound-based decoding. Of course, this is assuming that the purpose of reading is for accessing meaning.

Activity: What are some of the ways that a visual thinker decodes written material for meaning?

For most visual thinkers, reading with sound takes away mental pictures, interferes with the development of meaning, and slows down the language process of acquiring more complex meaning. On the other hand, reading the print of the visual idea in *context* allows the child quickly to access the meaning on the page in the way the child learns concepts the best. Chapters 10–15 will provide a more in-depth explanation of how to teach reading as a visual task that results in auditory, well developed English for all literacy processes.

Remember that language represents thinking and that a baby learns the meaning of his or her community through the assigned meaning of those around the child. Language represents the acquisition of the meaning of those in the child's environment up to age seven or eight. Then, the child can begin to use his or her own language to acquire meaning from other sources such as books, the Internet, the teacher, newspapers, articles, and so forth. With sufficient language structures that function to represent the access of more advanced conceptualization, the child can use his or her language to assign meaning to what he or she is able to read. In this way, the function of language for reading is about learning to access meaning from the print so as to learn academically.

Activity: Why do visual thinkers do better reading contextually than by sequencing words into sound?

It is logical to see how reading programs that emphasize sounds first developed. Reading was viewed as a translation of the oral language of auditory English into graphemes that are alphabetic in sounds. So, reading is orally saying what the graphemes show. Unfortunately, there are too many children who are not able to translate those sounds on the page into their language system for one of the following reasons: they are not able to use the sounds to create concepts; they do not have sufficient language structure to support the assignment of meaning through print; and/or they do not understand how the oral reading becomes a visual thinking task.

Activity: Why are auditory-based reading programs popular in an English speaking culture? What are some of the reasons that sound-based reading programs are not successful for reading comprehension?

Case 6.1: Cheryl

There are many students who cannot use sound for learning new concepts. *Some* of these individuals are diagnosed with special needs labels such as attention deficit hyperactivity disorders (ADHD), autism spectrum disorders (ASD), mildly cognitive impaired (MCI), learning language disabilities (LLD) including specific disabilities such as dyslexia, dysgraphia, dyscalculia, and dysnomia, central auditory processing (CAP) difficulties, and so forth. On the other hand, some people, who cannot use sound for learning new concepts, are quite successful professionally and have never been diagnosed as having a *problem*.

Cheryl was a college student in education. She learned to read before she went to school by watching her mother's and father's mouths move as they read picture books to her. Cheryl figured out that specific mouth movements meant that the speaker was referring to specific concepts in the pictures. Her parents would also point to the words so Cheryl realized that mouth movements "talked" about the environment and that print on the page told the story. By the time she went to school, she had learned a lot of language. In fact, some of her language learning came from "seeing" how print made ideas about concepts that she could see, like the people in her world. And her language learning helped her mentally "see" concepts that cannot be physically seen, such as the concept of love or friendship. Cheryl had phonics instruction and did not do well with it but the schools "overlooked" her poor performance because she was reading two or three years above grade level. After all, the higher grade level books have more content which means better language and better context. For Cheryl, these higher level books were actually more enjoyable because they were easier for her to see the ideas as a story than the rhyming, non-relational reading practice books. Books that did not create context and therefore few pictures sounded like this: "The cat is big. The cat is not small. The small cat is not big. I like the big cat." Or, "I like ice cream. I like pickles. I like snow." These simple sentence types of books made no sense to Cheryl, who often struggled to read orally any of these out of context, low-content books. But Cheryl could read about a family's adventures to the city or about how trees are graded in the woods for logging because these were written with good language function and with the purpose of advancing conceptual meaning.

Activity: Where did Cheryl learn to read? Why were the more advanced books easier for her to understand?

Cheryl went through school with good grades, no tutoring or special education, and no diagnostic labels. She was socially active and went on to college. In college, she discovered, in her college education classes, that others could connect sound to their visual concepts or could use sound for *thinking, speaking, reading, writing, viewing, listening, and calculating.* Cheryl cannot use sound or connect sound to any of the language functions of literacy. For ***thinking***, she thinks in complex pictures, movies, and printed words. For ***speaking***, she does not hear her own words. She knows she is producing sound but the sound is not connected to her mouth movements. She watches others' faces to see if what she is saying is resonating with others. When she teaches, she writes out her complete lesson ahead of class so that she can *see* what she will *say.* As a child she often talked a lot and had no idea why others were "bothered" by her mouth moving. She literally did not know she was making sound that they could hear. In middle school, her friends told her that she was loud. But she had no idea that she was making that much sound. Cheryl was using her mouth movements as ways to process what she was thinking. When she was excited she used bigger mouth movements or louder sound. Please note there is nothing physically "wrong" with her ears. She hears sound but she does not process sound for language function. And, Cheryl is a bright, capable person without any diagnostic label.

For ***reading***, Cheryl makes pictures in her head. She prefers novels that create mental movies over textbooks. But Cheryl has learned to use visual methods of scanning and creating visual pictures before reading a textbook so that she has the language as mental pictures to help her understand what she sees on the page. When Cheryl first entered college, she had many sound-based strategies for ***writing***, which meant she could not spell well and she could not edit well. She learned to make a mental picture of each word so that she could write the idea the way the shape of the idea looks, not the way words sound. Cheryl learned to edit her writing through drawing. Because writing is a visual-motor task, not a sound based task, writing became a strength for Cheryl (these strategies will be explained in Parts III and IV of this book).

For ***viewing*** or seeing the world from others' perspectives, Cheryl is mentally able to put herself in others' situations and attach the written (visual) words to the event. Being "respectful" creates multiple mental pictures of different ways that Cheryl shows "respect." Fortunately, she was raised in a home with lots of language to explain appropriate behavior models and high expectations for behavior, and expected social skills. Cheryl's ability to see others from mentally stepping in their shoes comes in handy for other spatial rotation tasks. For example, if she is playing a trivia game and the question asks for geography, she can mentally see herself anywhere on the globe.

Listening is the most difficult language function of literacy for Cheryl. In class, Cheryl always sits at the back of a room so that she can see the sides of other students' faces and the face of the teacher because she listens by seeing the mouths move. If she cannot see the mouth, she cannot listen more than about 10 minutes without her processing becoming overwhelmed and her thinking beginning to shut down. If lights are turned off for a slide demonstration, she can copy down the print on the slides but hears nothing that the speaker says, because she cannot see the mouth of the speaker. If there is an overhead, she can copy the print of the overhead but will not also be able to watch the speaker's face or hand move on the overhead. She is an excellent teacher of middle school math and she has learned to tell the students that she needs to see their faces when they ask a question. And, like all higher functioning literate people, more language is always better than less language. When the student asks a question using a lot of language, Cheryl has more context from which to understand the student's request.

Calculating has always been easy because Cheryl could mentally see and manipulate the visual patterns. However, when she entered college, she had difficulty understanding the concepts of numbers because she had never learned the meaning of the mathematical patterns. Cheryl learned to draw out the meaning of numerical concepts and put that meaning to the visual patterns of numbers.

Cheryl was able to use her well-developed language to "figure" out the code of the auditory world so that she could read and perform other literacy tasks well, even though she did not learn the way the schools taught her. Other children are not always as fortunate as Cheryl because they either do not have enough language when they come to school or they do not come from an environment that supports them in helping to figure out the visual code of sound.

Activity: How does Cheryl think for reading, writing, thinking, speaking, listening, calculating, and viewing? Why was Cheryl unable to use sound but able to function in a literate community?

Cheryl's case study highlights several factors related to how well language functions for literacy. The following section expands on the relationship between thinking and language for becoming literate.

Language thinking for literacy

One of the most serious issues in today's auditory culture is that fewer people are using language to assign meaning to children's behavior, academics, and social development. Language is learned from those who are in a child's environment. If the speakers in a child's environment use little language in any of the behavioral, academic, or social areas, then a child will not acquire the language concepts related to behavioral, academic, and/or social development. For example, a parent who never explains why a child cannot behave a certain way will have many more discipline problems that a parent who explains why a child cannot stand on a chair or why a child cannot run into the street, and so forth. A teacher who does not explain why students are doing a particular task will also have more discipline and probably academic problems than a teacher who makes tasks relevant for the students. A parent who does not explain the social tools of a community will have children who must socialize from others. If the child socializes with those who are ***pro-social***, then the child is more skilled socially than those who have parents who engage in anti-social behavior or who must learn how to socialize from ***anti-social*** peers.

As a result of too little language being used, there are some populations where many of the children do not possess sufficient language development to support literacy. Later, in Chapters 13–15, the reader will be introduced to teachers who are effective in creating language-based classrooms that first develop language and then literacy for their students. For many schools, this order of teaching is imperative. *The students must have adequate language functions to mediate the development of literacy. In this way, language development is more important than the teaching of specific products of literacy.*

Activity: Why do children need sufficient language to engage in literacy activities in schools such as reading, writing, and math?

The reader may be asking, "Why are the children coming to school without sufficient language function for literacy?" Because most people are visual, but live in an auditory culture, they are not taught visual strategies for higher language function in their homes. This mismatch between culture and language function results in a number of language-literacy issues that affect all aspects of conceptual learning, not just reading:

- People who think in visuals do not realize that others do not have the same mental pictures so they see no reason to use oral language to explain their actions, their behavior, their choices, and so forth. Parents and educators just don't do a lot of talking that explains choices, reasons, etc.
- Because most people are visual, their literacy function is best when it is visual. So, writing should be a strength but because writing is taught as an auditory task, then many people do not find writing an easy task. People can learn concepts through writing very functional language but they must have the visual-motor strategies for making writing a visual way of thinking, not an auditory way of spelling words on a piece of paper. For example, letters written today are more like lists or text messages, not the travel logs or long monologues of past decades produced as an art of letter writing.

- Because language function, not language structure, helps develop cognition, then a person who thinks visually needs visual strategies for obtaining the highest levels of literacy; but, people are taught auditory strategies which do not develop concepts and therefore limit language development. Without educators and parents using visual strategies to help children acquire concepts, language function remains limited. Furthermore, when language *is* taught or emphasized it is taught as a series of additive structures, not cognitive functions.
- Because people with visual ways to conceptualize are not given literacy strategies that match their learning systems, they do not achieve good language function of literacy and therefore do not recognize good language. For example, one professor could not tell when a student was making coherent arguments in an essay format or was just writing grammatical sentences, because the professor could not recognize good language function. She had learned only language structures. So, she looked for the words that matched her visual mental patterns. If even the best educated people in the culture are not trained to understand how language functions to help a person become literate, then it is no wonder that the average educated person does not see the purpose in increasing the use of language for higher order thinking and learning. For example, some companies use pictures only for advertising or pictures only for assembling an object. Remember that pictures are conceptual but are not language tools. And, pictures are never conventional; no two people have the same mental concept for the same spoken or written idea.

Activity: Why do some children come to school with or without adequate language?

Reading is not oral language on the page

Some children cannot convert the oral reading into concepts. Therefore, they do not figure out that oral reading represents thinking. For example, an 11-year-old attended summer session with the author. He said he could not read. When the class members chose books to look through to gain ideas about the classroom content, China, this student picked a book on kites. The author went over to him and asked him about one of the pictures in the book. He said he did not know anything about the picture because he could not read. The author told him that the picture had no words and that whatever he saw in the picture was the meaning of the picture. He said he saw a kite. The author pointed out how the kite had many tails on it and wondered aloud about who made the kite. The student said that he did not know. So, the author pointed out to the student that the words on the page told them about who made the kite, why they made the kite, how they made the kite, and so forth. She added, "Whenever you see this pattern written like this, kite, it means 'kite'." Then she asked him if he could find that idea, kite, or pattern on the page. He said he couldn't. So the author quickly took a pencil and circled the word, kite, and said, "This idea says, 'kite.' Here is the same pattern, kite. Every time you see this pattern, it is always the same idea." She had him copy the pattern by writing it. She bubbled the word (see Figure 6.1) so he could see the shape. She took the letters out of the word and he said he finally saw "kite."

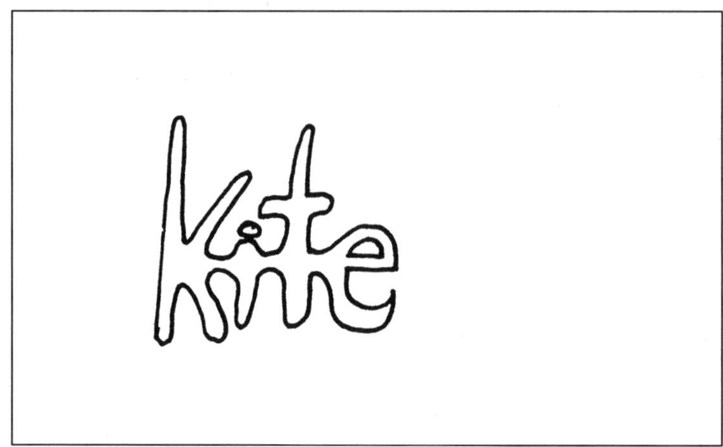

Figure 6.1 The shape of the word, kite

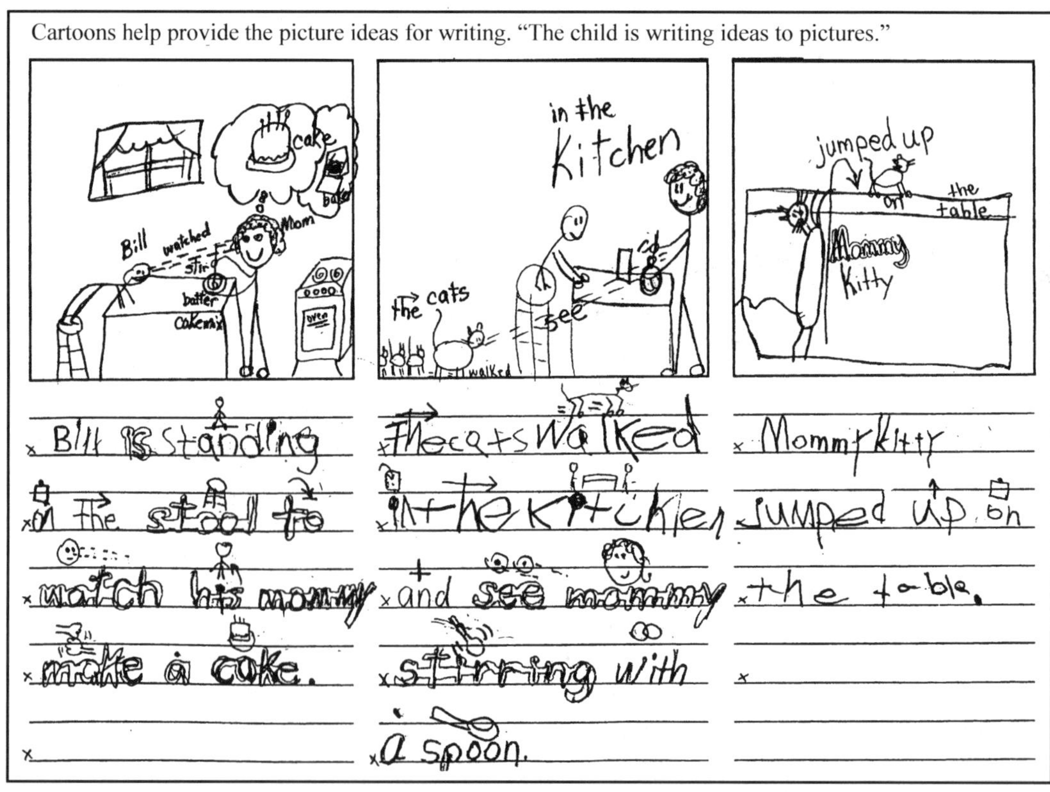

Figure 6.2 Draw before write

This 11-year-old had spent so much time working on letters and sounds that he did not realize that he could see the meaning of a word as a shape or as a concept, a picture. Unless educators teach students to use language functions that match the way students' learning system creates concepts, students do not necessarily learn the function of the reading task, to find and learn about what others write.

Activity: Why do some students not understand why reading is a literacy (constructing meaning) task?

Writing is not sounds on a page

As previously discussed, writing can be a visual-motor task: The writer uses movements of the hand to create the mental shapes of visual concepts. Writing does not have to be an act of spelling words in a sound-letter sequence. Like reading, writing can be putting on paper the shapes of ideas that represent visual thoughts.

To be a visual thinker, who writes with English language function, the visual writer must convert his or her mental thoughts to written word shapes. The easiest way to convert mental visual pictures or movies or images to printed form is to draw the concepts first, then write the patterns (printed words) that match those concepts. Figure 6.2 shows an example. First, the student draws his ideas, then he writes the print that goes with the drawn concepts.

Because the eye is able to see light reflect off the surface of an object, the eye also is capable of seeing the edge of the surface of an object (see Chapter 2). The edge of the object creates a shape. A shape is one entire concept. So, individuals who have difficulty with sound do better seeing the shape of an idea. Figure 6.3 shows a study guide for a student learning science vocabulary as well as spelling.

This student sees the shape and attaches a picture to the shape to create meaning of the visual shape. Because the student assigned his own understanding or meaning to the shapes of concepts, he can mentally recall the way the concept looks as well as the concept's meaning. He is visually recording the way the concepts look, rather than trying to spell, which is an auditory task that he cannot do and does not need to do. This particular student received the highest grade in his ninth grade science class out of 125 students. Prior to learning how to write with the shape of ideas, he was diagnosed with a writing disability.

Activity: Why do shapes provide meaning for a visual thinker to use for writing?

Spelling is often a process of ***encoding*** the decoded sounds and letters as a way to write. As the reader may already know, national spelling bee contestants prepare by "memorizing" thousands of words. Most of the spelling bee contestants are not learning the spelling of the words which requires sounds and letters, but they are memorizing the way a word or parts of words look according to their meaning. When the student is given a word, the sentence provides context for the student to recall the word as a visual pattern that is connected to the meaning. Other meaningful cues come from derivations, suffixes, prefixes, and infixes that the best "spellers" use for remembering the way the word "looks." Seeing a written pattern as a shape allows the shape to be part of the relational, contextual language—a visual way of thinking. More examples will be provided in subsequent chapters.

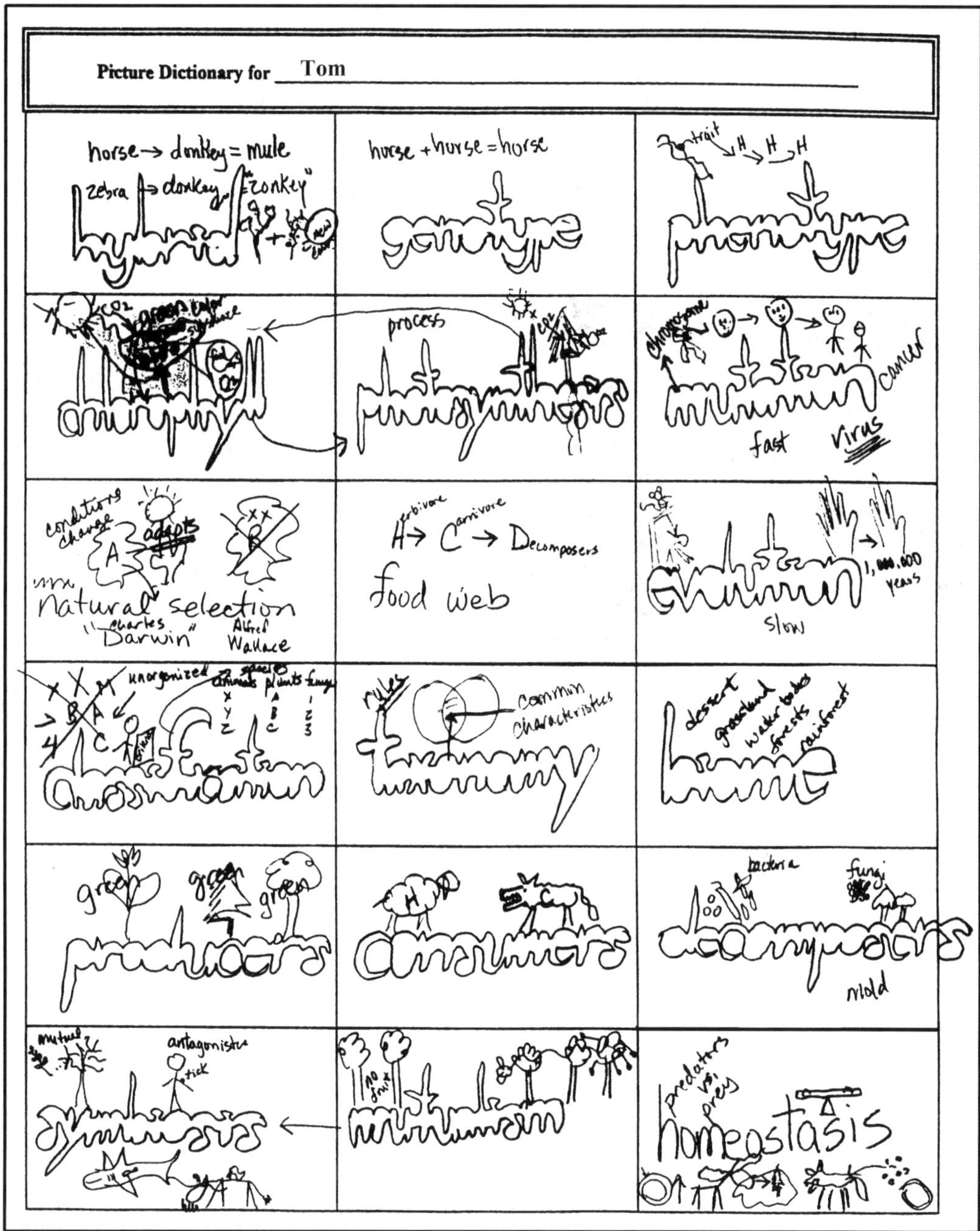

Figure 6.3 Seeing the ideas as shapes of meaning

Activity: How can spelling be a visual thinking task?

Writing by "sounding out" the spelling of words limits the task to only 10–15 percent of the population. Strategies for writing by shapes and by context of meaning will be provided in Parts III and IV. Also, some students who do not have good oral language learn from print through the process of writing. These students' cognitive development increases over time. Examples of these students will be found later in the book.

Writing should be a way for students who learn visual concepts to use English, an auditory language for thinking and for increasing the development of thinking. Writing allows many students to conceptualize at a higher level of thinking. In this way, the *writing* of English is what both auditory and visual thinkers have in common. For example, when students take an essay test, they often say that if they were to retake the test, they know they would do better. That common statement is the result of the student actually learning from writing the essay. As the student writes the essay, writing requires the student to use language to assign meaning to what the student knows. The more the student writes, the more the student knows. This is also why the end of an essay is often much better conceptualized than the beginning of an essay. By the end of the essay, the student has learned a lot from the writing language function.

Activity: How does writing as a language function increase language and thinking or cognition?

Thinking is not self-talk

In addition to reading and writing, thinking is also a language function of literacy. A person thinks in the way that he or she learns new concepts. So, when a person learns a new concept by overlapping visual patterns or shape patterns, then the person thinks in visual concepts (Chapter 2). This thinking is not about how the input comes into the learner and out again (modality), but is about how the person thinks. Concepts develop from the "meaning" of the world that the learner can recognize. So, the person who thinks with visual concepts uses a lot of context or events to understand, plan, and organize his or her activities. Whereas, a person who thinks with the sound of one's own voice assigns meaning to others' words with his or her own self-talk.

Remember the dominant culture expects the time-based way of thinking, but in reality, the majority of people think by the visual components of an event. How do these differences in thinking affect literacy? If the number one complaint of teachers and parents is that students do not turn in homework or do not do homework, it is because families and school continue to use "sound" or speech to tell students how to plan and organize. If students don't develop tools for planning and organizing, they become adults who work jobs in an economic market based on time but who do not have strategies for understanding time as a complex language function. They do not see how to hurry up, be efficient, and do the job the correct way the first time, how what they do affects the time of others, or how what they do affects the economy of the community. They are *thinking* in a culture that is not the way they are supposed to be working.

The more language a person obtains about how to translate thinking into actions, the more tools a person has for making choices. For example, the visual thinker language that an educator uses with a student might sound like this:

> During art, sometimes scraps of paper fall onto the floor. If we do not pick up the papers before we leave the room then the students who come in to our room after we leave will have to pick up the papers. But, when the next class of students

> comes into the room, they want to be able to start their art work as soon as they read the assignment on the board; so that they are finished with their art work when the bell rings at the end of class. But, if they have to pick up the papers that fell on the floor when we were doing art, then they cannot start to do their work. If they do not start to do their work when they come into the room because they have to pick up the paper scraps that we left on the floor, then they will not have their work completed when the bell rings so that they can go home. So, John, when you pick up the papers off the floor after art and put them into the recycling box you are being kind to the students who use the room after we leave. You are also being respectful of the space you work in and you are being considerate of others' needs.

This language function is *redundant* (Chapter 3). On the surface of the language, the structures overlap. But this overlap of surface words helps the visual thinker to make mental pictures. In this way, the student has the language necessary to work in an auditory world but visually think in the way that the student best learns concepts. The use of lots of language by the teacher helps John learn the higher social concepts such as kind and respectful which also increases cognitive language function.

Activity: How is thinking a language function?

Viewing is not hearing

Being able to "see" the world is both a language function and a form of literacy. As a person develops more language and uses more language, concepts increase in complexity and so does literacy. One of these functions of literacy, viewing, develops in the social as well as cognitive domains. Viewing has to do with being able to see the world from different perspectives. And, a person's ability to take different perspectives is a function of social and cognitive development. Language function increases a person's ability to be a perspective taker.

Nathan is an eight-year-old boy who is in the second grade. He often appears "angry" as he uses a loud voice and unkind words to tell other people what to do. "Jason, you go play with Ralph." When he does something that others don't like such as hitting, he blames others. "You made me hit you." When an activity is his responsibility but he does not do the task, he has an excuse. "You didn't tell me to do the spelling." When his mother wants him to perform an action such as ordering his own drink at a local coffee shop, he refuses to do the task. "I am not ordering a drink." But, when his mother tells him that the drink is not for him but for her and that he needs to order his own drink, he yells and pouts. "I told you that you can order my drink. I am not talking."

Nathan is not capable of taking others' perspectives. He does not realize how his actions and words affect others. He does not have enough language about his choices, his thoughts, and his behaviors to know that others are affected. Nathan's behavior can be rewarded or punished and his desired behavior be reinforced but that will still not give him the language he needs to function socially in a proactive way. Figure 6.4 gives an example of how oral language is changed to picture concepts that have writing attached to help Nathan learn the language he needs to view the world from others' perspectives. Developmentally, language provides the social tool for moving from not seeing one's body separate from the rest of the world, to seeing one's body central to an event in a single picture, to seeing how one interacts and works with others, to seeing how to walk in others' shoes.

0–2
I am an extension of others.
3–7
I am the center of my universe.
7–11
I think about what others think about my actions.
11+
I can figuratively walk in another person's shoes.

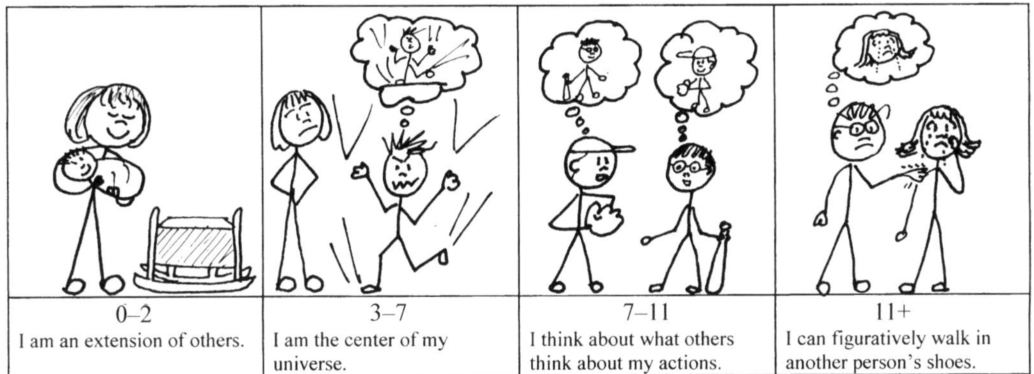

Figure 6.4 Viewing the world

Activity: What is the literacy language function of viewing?

Listening is not just sound

Listening as a language function of literacy has already been addressed to some extent. Remember Cheryl? She was not able to use sound to listen to another's spoken message. Instead, she watched the speaker's mouth movements and because her family helped her learn to use print for reading, she learned to see what the print meant and how that meaning could be seen on a speaker's face. Listening may be watching! Listening can also be hearing the sound of the speaker's voice as an acoustic signal.

Hearing what another person says is acoustic in nature. Like a parrot imitating the speech sounds of a person's voice, acoustic input can be copied. For example, Charles is a 12-year-old male in middle school. The principal saw him climb through a window and into a computer lab on a weekend. She unlocked the building, called the sheriff's department, and walked to the lab to find Charles smashing computers. She said, "Charles, what are you doing?" He replied, "Nothing." The principal said, "Are you alone?" He said, "Well, no. I live with my mom." She said, "Why are you destroying the computers?" He said, "Jake said we needed to get rid of the computers. They take away people's jobs." Over the next few months, the sheriff's department employees, the detention center employees, the principal, and community members could not understand how Charles could take Jake's (adult friend of Charles's mom) words so literally. Charles held onto the belief that he did not do anything wrong because the window had been left unlocked and he was doing something to help Jake who lost his job.

Charles was capable of hearing sound, but he did not have the language function of listening to be able to hear the intended meaning of what Jake said. Listening requires more than the ability to hear sound; it also requires the ability to have enough language to understand the message content at an appropriate developmental level. By 12, Charles should have been able to understand Jake's words from a formal or figurative perspective. If Charles's language functioned at a ***concrete operations*** to ***formal operations*** level,[2] then he would not have heard the literal interpretation of Jake's words. Listening is a language function of literacy that is dependent on the cognitive and social level of the hearer's language.

Activity: How does listening work as a language function of literacy?

Speaking is not saying sounds

The act of speaking is purely an acoustic-motor set of patterns. The person speaking has to be able to hear the acoustic pattern and then have the apparatus to produce the patterns motorically. This is why birds, like parrots, who have a biological apparatus for speech, can imitate the speaking patterns of human adults. However, for speaking to be a language function of literacy, the spoken utterances must have concepts underlying their production. So, the importance of speaking is that the person who produces the speech understands what he or she says, and the speaker has an intended purpose for producing speech.

There is a developmental hierarchy to acquiring the speech patterns of English, as well as other languages. This hierarchy is based on how well the speaker can hear what others say, match those sounds, and then produce those sounds. When children do not acquire speech as developmentally expected, many parents, educators, and specialists attempt to work on the sounds and the sound patterns. From a language function perspective, working on sounds without language does not make sense. Speech is oral language. Oral language represents underlying concepts. Children are able to show their understanding of concepts through non-verbal gestures ***gestural signs*** and actions before they will typically be able to speak about their underlying concepts. Working on sounds in children who do not show or cannot show their basic understanding of the world around them suggests that the child may learn to imitate sounds but still not talk because the child does not have any language to use.

Activity: What is the literacy function of speech?

On the other hand, children with lots of language who occasionally misarticulate sounds will also benefit by emphasis on the meaning of language rather than on the production of sound. In fact, learning to write and read helps many students learn to see what the sounds look like. Overall, working on sound patterns will not connect the speaking to the language function and therefore will not necessarily become part of the cognitive development. Those children who cannot physically hear or who have physical, organic problems affecting production do need help in how to produce sounds, but for the purpose of a language function.

Activity: How is speaking a language function?

2 Piaget (1952) identified four cognitive stages: sensori-motor, preoperational, concrete, and formal. These stages provide a framework for evaluating the meaning of ideas or behaviors (Arwood, 1991a; Lucas, 1980).

Calculating is not just patterns

Calculating as a language function is more than "doing mathematics." Mathematic operations can be imitated or copied patterns whereas calculating implies understanding a problem that requires a solution. Most of the everyday mathematical problems have solutions in language. For example, an 18–24-month-old child with good language development knows how to obtain "more juice," or how to obtain "one more" cookie, or how to obtain "another" toy from the box, or how to stack "more than one" block. These are all additive problems of early numeracy. These young children are developing the language concepts related to the meaning of quantitative concepts. More about quantification will be found in later chapters.

Likewise, a young child also knows how to take away something. Early language concepts in this semantic area include stopping an action (***cessation***), not wanting something (***rejection***), and recognizing the absence or presence of something (***existence*** or ***non-existence***). These types of concepts are part of the development of numeracy. Like all concepts, these numeracy concepts continue to layer and add more meaning. At some point, an adult shows the child what the "numbers" look like that pair up with the language. In this way, the numbers also have language function.

Early language development supports the conceptual understanding of numbers. For example, a five-year-old can divide a sandwich in half, creating two halves from a whole. Or, a five-year-old can sort buttons and other objects into sets; those buttons that have one small hole from those with two small holes, or by different colors, and so forth. Even five-year-olds can find the unknown. For example, Grandma gives a child a candy bar. Mom tells the child to share the candy bar with his two siblings. A five-year-old with good language will keep "dividing" the bar until all three children have an "equal" amount. His language will include words like more, bigger, smaller, another piece, a little more, and so forth.

Too often, the adults in a child's environment try to teach mathematical operations or algorithms as language structures of mathematics without capitalizing on the language functions of what children already know. Helping children see the shapes, measures, and amounts all around their environments allow children to develop the language function or thinking necessary to understand the concepts for calculating. Operations are patterns that when supported by language functions represent the child's cognition.

Activity: What makes calculating a language function of literacy?

Summary

Learning language as a series of neuro-semantic layers of meaning provides the acquisition of language for learning. In other words, children spend the first seven to eight years acquiring language structures that represent underlying basic relational concepts in the way they think or are able to form concepts. In order for children to gain higher order thinking, they must learn to gain meaning from other sources than what caregivers assign during the first years of dependence. A learner's own language functions as a tool for assigning meaning to increase the complexity of conceptual meaning.

Sources of access to meaningful ways to increase conceptual development include the various forms of literacy: reading, writing, thinking, speaking, listening, viewing, and calculating. In this way, a learner with grammatical language structures that function to share meaning can use his or her own language for reading, writing, thinking, speaking, listening, viewing, and calculating. Whenever a learner uses his or her own language for these literacy functions, then his or her own cognition increases. These cognitive increases occur because language function represents the underlying concepts. So, a child who can read, write, and talk about a topic will also show increases in thinking, viewing, and listening about the same topic. Cognition parallels the use of language for learning to be literate. Chapters 7–9 discuss how to assess language function followed by a section on how to intervene to help develop visual ways of becoming literate in an auditory world.

Applications

- Talk to an adult about how he or she thinks for the various processes of literacy (thinking, viewing, listening, reading, writing, speaking, and calculating).
- Talk to different age children about how they mentally think.

PART III

LANGUAGE

How Do We Assess and Intervene?

Language structures are easy to identify, count, and teach. For example, a parent may want to know how many different words her child uses in comparison to other children of the same age. To answer this question, an educator collects an oral language sample from the child, transcribes the child's oral language, counts the number of different words for the sample, and then compares the child's average number of different words in the sample to normative data collected on a group of children the same age who perform the same task. From this data, the educator has an idea of how many different words the child uses. Words, parts of speech, the alphabet, spelling, counting, multiplication tables, grammatical rules, oral fluency, and vocabulary are all examples of language structures, products that come from a child's learning system. Educators may easily identify, count, and compare products. Furthermore, educators can easily teach the language structures through imitation and repetition or practice. *Language structures are patterns and products of a child's learning system. Educators often test and teach these structures as evidence of literacy.*

Language functions represent a child's thinking processes. Because language functions are internal, educators have trouble "seeing" the language functions. And most professionals and parents do not know what language functions are. Therefore, most educators and support specialists like language pathologists do not examine a child's language function for how well the child is able to ***displace*** an idea, ***flexibly*** converse, ***productively*** use a variety of ways to be literate, use concepts for ***referring*** and ***predicating (semanticity***) to plan and organize one's life, and/or how well a child is able to ***perform speech acts*** to promise, vow, or pretend, for example, or to understand others' perspectives (***redundancy***). Most professionals know about language structures and therefore consider only the language structures.

Most educators and support specialists emphasize assessing and teaching of language structures such as spelling, grammar, pronunciation, punctuation, and so forth, rather than the development of language functions. But, the tradeoff of teaching structures in place of language functions is enormous! Structures are additive and developmental but not conceptual. Structures do not help a child think better, problem solve, or use language for academic, social, or behavioral purposes. On the other hand, the emphasis on *language functions positively affects a child's social and cognitive development, and, in turn, improves a child's literacy function.*

With a little understanding of the characteristics of language function, an educator or parent can just as easily assess and intervene for language function rather than for language structures. For example, a first grade teacher, Bonnie Robb, emphasized language function in her classroom (Arwood & Robb, 2008) and her students performed better on reading, math, and writing skills than when she previously had taught language arts as patterns of skills or products. In other words, *language functions assist in developing the child's learning system so that the products or skills (structures) come from the child's improved thinking and learning; that is, the child's language function.*

Increasing a child's language function increases a child's ability to think and problem solve; whereas, increasing a child's number of language structures increases the child's number of products. With the increase of products, an educator can quickly show an increase in the child's ability to regurgitate or imitate what the child sees or hears. This increase in products does not help a child think or conceptualize. For example, emphasis on sounds and letters (English is an alphabetic language) helps a child produce sounds and letters, but there are many children who can read fluently or say the sounds of the letters of print, but not understand what they are reading. Children with good language function can make mental pictures or concepts of what they see on a page; therefore, they understand what they read. When a child is able to make sense of print, reading becomes more enjoyable and the child is more likely to read a variety genre. Increasing a child's use of language function allows a child better to use language as a tool for academic learning and thinking.

A child typically completes the development of structural language at about seven to eight years of age, but the functional part of the language continues to develop into a more complex, linguistic way of *thinking* throughout the lifespan. In other words, language structures develop up to about seven to eight years of age, while language functions continue to refine a person's thinking throughout a person's life. This relationship between language function and thinking can be divided into three stages:

1. Early restricted language development represents ***pre-language function***.
2. Full ***language function*** represents a shared conversational relationship with others about concrete social and cognitive development.
3. Maximum ***linguistic function*** represents formal cognition or linguistic thinking and learning.

Assessment methods and intervention strategies are specific to the three levels: pre-language, language, and linguistic function. Part III emphasizes how to assess and intervene for language function across levels and ages, for neuro-typical as well as atypical learners. The stage of pre-language function is divided between those individuals who are non-verbal or are in a pre-production stage of pre-language function and those who are verbal and use restricted production with pre-language thinking or function. Chapter 7 discusses the characteristics of those individuals who are in the pre-production or silent period of pre-language function. Chapter 8 describes how to intervene or assign meaning to those who are in the pre-language function stage and are either in the pre-production or early verbal stage of development. Chapter 9 provides intervention for verbal but restricted pre-language function. Chapter 10 provides the assessment and intervention strategies for those who are developing language function. Chapter 11 provides the assessment and intervention strategies for those who attempt to share conversation and are learning to develop a linguistic function. Chapter 12 discusses the assessment and intervention strategies for those with linguistic function. Examples of assessment and intervention for individuals at each of the three levels of language function (pre-language, language, and linguistic function) will be provided. Chapter 13 describes how behavior and language communicate about how a person thinks and learns.

Part IV of the book will offer classroom assessment and intervention applications for the various grade levels of language function.

Chapter 7

ASSESSMENT OF PRE-LANGUAGE THINKERS

Pre-Production Function

Learner objectives: Chapter 7

Upon completion of this chapter, the reader should be able to:

1. Define who pre-language thinkers are.
2. Define pre-production or silent period of pre-language function.
3. Explain how neuro-atypical English language learners function in the pre-production period of pre-language function.
4. Explain how neuro-atypical English language learners function in the pre-production period of pre-language function.
5. Demonstrate how to assess pre-language function for individuals with pre-production or limited language structures.

To know the world without words or pictures
Is to possess feelings without concepts…
Wanting to converse but with little shared meaning
Is to perceive without language function.

When a person is able to communicate, but in a very limited or *restricted* form, then the person does not possess a full language system. This restricted form is evidence that the person *thinks* with pre-language function. In other words, the person is learning language but does not have use of full language structures for thinking or learning. Individuals who are within this pre-language stage of functioning may present three different types of characteristics: First, they may not use oral language and therefore be in a ***pre-production*** or ***silent period***; second, they may use ***limited language structure*** representing multiple relationships among people, their actions, and objects but function is still ***restricted***, or third, they may appear to have ***lots of language structures*** but the language function is still *restricted*. Those who are in the silent, pre-production period are non-verbal and those with limited or lots of language structures, but restricted language function, are considered verbal. This chapter will address assessment for those who are in the pre-production or silent period of pre-language function followed by intervention specifying how to assign meaning to non-verbal behavior for increasing language development in Chapter 8.

Pre-production or silent period

Pre-production means that there is virtually no speech. The learner is *not* able to produce the language patterns. This lack of ability can occur under a variety of conditions:

- Neuro-typical babies are in a pre-production period until they have acquired enough speech patterns to represent their acquisition of underlying concepts.
- English language learners may be fluent in another language but will endure a pre-production period of listening and trying to assign English patterns to the underlying concepts of their first language.
- Neuro-atypical learners can remain in a pre-production stage for life, if their learning systems do not allow them to organize sensory patterns into concepts or into language that represents their concepts.

Assessment for each of these types of pre-production language learners is similar in overall purpose—to determine what the child is able to do, under what conditions, and what the adult can do to help the child develop language. However, the answers to these assessment questions will be different for the different types of pre-production children. It is the answers, or results of the assessment, that provide the basis for determining specific interventions. Interventions are different for the three different types of pre-production, pre-language function.

Activity: What is the purpose of assessment for the pre-production, pre-language child?

Neuro-typical pre-production

Pre-production, pre-language function for neuro-typical children occurs between the ages of 0 and two years. The newborn cries and Mom picks up the baby checking to see what the baby needs—food, water, a new diaper, sleep. This very early communication depends on the listener to interpret what the baby needs. And even though the newborn baby communicates, the baby is in the pre-production level of pre-language function. *One of the major characteristics of this pre-language function is that a person, other than the communicator, must* ***interpret*** *the* ***meaning*** *of the pre-language person's communication as well as* ***assign meaning*** *to the* ***communication***.

This characteristic of "dependent communication" pertains to all those individuals who are in the pre-production period. In other words, the newborn baby lacks language, but is able to communicate, because the caregivers are able and willing to *interpret* the baby's motor acts. Although the child, at this stage, does not use language patterns of speech, the child is learning the underlying meaning necessary for language development from those who *assign meaning* to the child's motor acts. The child's motor response, such as crying, tells the parents to do something for the child. The parents do something which assigns meaning to the child's motor act such as crying. Therefore, *the second characteristic of this pre-production or silent period is that the child's behavior tells the adult what the child knows.*

Activity: What are the first two characteristics of the pre-production or silent period of language function?

Neuro-typical babies respond to the sensory input of the baby's world (Chapters 1–3) and those around the child interpret the baby's response. Assessment of a neuro-typical child's learning system begins with medical personnel checking the child's physical integrity of the sensory system. Does the child respond to light, sound, and touch?[1] The newborn's body responds to this sensory stimulation through motor responses such as primitive reflexes. For example, the mother touches around a newborn baby's face and the baby sucks. This sucking response shows that the child is able to receive the touching sensation and process the touch. Or, the medical doctor may check for hearing by making a very loud sound and the newborn will startle. More sophisticated methods are available, but screening is the first step: Is the baby's physical system set up to respond to incoming stimuli?

Activity: How is a child's sensory system usually checked?

Assuming that the baby's system is responding to the world's sensory input, then the baby's neurobiological system is also ready to receive the sensory patterns of the people who assign meaning to the baby's responses. Maybe the child reaches for her bottle or tries to grab Grandma's eye glasses. Through these motor movements, the neuro-typical child shows his or her development of the Neuro-Semantic Language Learning System. *The baby responds to the recognition of sensory input with physical, motor movements.* Therefore, a person assessing this child is able to observe these responses and therefore determine the integrity of a child's early learning system.

Activity: How does a baby show that his or her sensory system is responding to input?

The baby, who is *neuro-typically in the pre-production stage of language* function, responds to people, their actions, and their objects through motor movements. For example, within the first three weeks of development, the baby will move his or her eyes toward familiar sounds and begin to "watch" adult movements signaling the child's recognition of the adult's patterns of action. This type of ***gaze indicates*** that the child is beginning to connect the child's recognition of others to what others do. As the sensory patterns of input increase, the baby's body continues to develop physically with an increase in more sophisticated motor movement. The child begins to use his or her hands along with the eyes to communicate to others what the child needs, wants, or desires. Through these movements of the baby's eyes and body, the infant shows an understanding of people and their actions and objects. Neuro-typical babies show the following development:

1 Remember that the physician is checking the child's learning system. The sensory system must be intact to provide the child with the input for developing perceptual patterns, concepts, and language.

- Physically responds to sensory changes—temperature (wet diaper or cold for example), light (brightness or darkness), touch (holding, rocking, etc.), smell (cooking, baby powder, for example), taste (stops crying to feed), sound (music, Mom's voice, for example)—with reflexes.
- Baby uses gaze by three weeks to track recognized patterns such as Mom's movements during changing or mobile characters about 12–18 inches away.
- Baby responds to familiar voices or sounds by quieting and then becoming noisy (body movements are noise as well as vocalizations) when sounds cease at about four to six weeks.
- Baby imitates facial smiles and open eye movements at about six weeks.
- At four to six months, the baby is babbling with all sounds in a consonant-vowel combination such as ba-da-ka. Baby increases or decreases his or her babbling in response to others' sounds. At this age the baby is able to move his or her hands toward an object in an attempt to bring objects to the baby.
- At four to six months, the baby will watch and imitate others' motor patterns such as hand movements for the use of manual ***signs***. Baby uses the first hand signs to indicate language functions of requesting objects or people (agents) to do something such as giving the baby her bottle (provided family uses signs as a language form) or using the sign, "more," with the hands to indicate "more milk," "another hug" (recurrence), "more ball" (existence), and so forth.
- At six to eight months, the baby can sit up and therefore the baby begins to use his eyes to follow others around the room (12 foot proximity). The baby can easily request adult actions through manual sign or with consonants and vowels that approximate words such as "ba" for bottle.

The most important feature of neuro-typical development during the child's first year is that the baby is using many different body movements and types of vocalizations to connect the adults and their actions to the child. The infant is busy communicating!

Activity: What is the baby's neuro-typical development for communication like?

The baby's non-verbal actions represent cognitive development of functions about people, their actions, and their objects in meaningful or basic semantic relationships. Remember from Chapter 3, the prerequisite for natural language function is the underlying development of the basic semantic relationships between or among a person or agent doing something, an action, and with an object or objects. This development results in the child's acquisition of ***sensori-motor cognition***: *The baby thinks in these semantic relationships and demonstrates such understanding through a motor response to the sensory organization of the child's world.*

Activity: What is the first type of cognition that a child develops? Describe what this type of cognition represents.

As the neuro-typical child is able to recognize the relationship between caregivers and their abilities to provide for the child, the child signals with his or her eyes and body movements what the child needs. The 9–12-month-old baby looks at the bottle, then up to Mom's face, then back to the bottle while reaching toward the bottle. This signals to Mom to look at the bottle and then to do something with the bottle. At the pre-language level of function, Mom interprets the baby's non-verbal gestures and vocalizations, such as, "Oh, baby wants the bottle." So, Mom puts the bottle in the baby's hands and tries to position the nipple for the baby to drink. But the baby also wants to be held. So, the baby moves her arms away from the bottle and begins to cry. Mom picks up the baby and holds the baby while Mom feeds the baby the bottle. The baby's response to being held while fed tells Mom that she has met the child's needs; needs that the baby indicated through non-verbal representation. This sensori-motor acquisition is the child's cognitive language function. Baby is able to think in meaningful, semantic relationships about non-verbal concepts of agents, actions, and objects.

Activity: Describe the first year of neuro-typical language function development.

The neuro-typical child continues with the pre-production period of development by including more and more non-verbal semantic relationships to expand his or her cognition. The second year of neuro-typical language development proceeds as follows:

- At 9–12 months, the baby is now able to produce a speech pattern associated with objects. For example, the child says, "mama" for "mom," or "bata" for "bottle," or "ba-kie" for "blankie" or "blanket."
- Children at 12 months use their vocalizations to ***mark*** or indicate the connection between a sound pattern and the non-verbal semantic relationships. For example, the child says, "Gama" for Grandma and reaches toward Grandma. Grandma picks up the child. The child's vocalization coupled with the child's motor movements indicates the following semantic relationships: Grandma and the child are people who perform actions or agents; the reach by the child is an action followed by Grandma's action of picking up the child. The child is showing how he or she is learning the *concepts of people*, *agents*, and the *concepts of actions*, what the people do. It should be noted that these concepts will continue to grow: Agents grow into concepts of "self" while actions grow into verbs, adverbs, and abstract time concepts. More about these concepts will be discussed in later chapters.
- By 18–24 months, a child is able to imitate many sound patterns for which the child may lack "understanding." For example, the child says, "Go Daddy" and the adult says, "Yes, your Daddy flies a 747." And the child says, "Daddy flies 747." The child really does not know what a 747 is, but the child can imitate the adult's pattern. Because the meaning of the adult's words is in context, the adult interprets the child's vocalizations as if the child does understand some of the meaning. "Oh, you are so smart! Yes, your daddy does fly a 747. See, Charles, baby knows what Daddy flies." The child later answers to an adult prompt of "What does Daddy fly?" with the utterance "Daddy flies 747." Such natural imitation is spontaneous and thus referred to as ***spontaneous imitation***. Spontaneous imitation can last a few days or several weeks. This type of imitation does *not* stay spontaneous for more than six months because the neuro-typical learner uses spontaneous

imitation as a process by which to acquire more meaning. Within six months of the onset of spontaneous imitation, a neuro-typical child's meanings have expanded significantly enough that the child no longer needs to imitate. In fact, by 30–36 months, a child with good language function is able to use natural language structures to represent a lot of thinking. If imitation continues longer than six months, then the development is not typical (see the next chapters for explanations about problems with developing typical language).

- By three years or 36 months, the child is able to share language about concepts in the here-and-now. The child's utterances might sound like this: "Grandma gives me Care Bear." The adult might be confused about the time that Grandma gave the Care Bear; so, the adult says, "When did Grandma give you Care Bear?" The child responds, "I like Care Bear. He's pink. His name is Batly (Barclay)." The child changes the conversation to "here-and-now" concepts about the bear. Although the child's grammar is understandable, the child's ideas are about common, everyday thoughts. At three, the child may show some deviations in sound production (Batly for Barclay) as the full sound system is not developed. And the child may evidence some problems with word usage, sentence structure, and sharing the meaning with complete language structures. The child is moving out of the pre-production silent period.
- The language between three and seven shows exponential growth in structural use. By seven years of age, the child is moving out of the pre-language function of a restricted grammar. The language structures represent the child's increase in thinking based on more acquisition of meaning (Neuro-Semantic Language Learning). *It should be noted that a neuro-typical child will begin to maintain a spoken conversation by three years of age, even if the child does not fully understand the concepts spoken by the adult. But, the adult must still follow the child's lead. With pre-language function, the child is still not able to share with the adult 100 percent of the conversation.*

Activity: What is language development like for a child between one and three years of age?

English language learners (ELLs)

Children who have developed a first language (L1) other than English will also experience a pre-production or silent period when English (L2) is introduced. For example, a child who has Latvian as a first language begins her first school day in an English speaking Kindergarten. She is quiet because she is listening and trying to see or hear what the sounds of the English patterns mean in relationship to what she knows as Latvian concepts. She has acquired concepts for one set of language patterns, Latvian, and now she is trying to use her Latvian concepts to assign meaning to the English patterns. She is an English language learner (ELL), even though she has already acquired the underlying concepts to Latvian and speaks Latvian as her first language. This period of language function for an ELL is sometimes referred to as a *pre-production* or a silent period. This silent period can occur at any age for a person who has acquired a first language and is in the first stage of learning a second language.

A child at this pre-production age of pre-language function needs the patterns of English matched to her underlying concepts. Therefore, an ELL, who uses sophisticated gestures along with sophisticated actions to tell others what she needs or knows, definitely has developed the underlying thinking or concepts necessary for more developed language function. A neuro-typical ELL, in a pre-production period, needs exposure with the L2 to see and hear how the English patterns connect to *previously acquired* knowledge or concepts underlying the L1.

Assessment of pre-production for an ELL includes two issues: Does this person have a complete, grammatical and functional L1 or first language? If the ELL child or adult has developed a functioning first language, then attaching the English patterns to underlying concepts is what the child or adult needs. The underlying conceptual development in L1 provides the basis for a second language or L2.

Activity: If an English language learner has developed a complete L1, then what does the learner need to do to learn the L2?

However, an ELL may also have difficulty with his or her first language learning. Then a second question is pertinent: Does this ELL demonstrate a problem with learning in the first language? Information about how the ELL functions in the first language is usually gathered by informal or formal interviewing of family members. Sometimes, the first language is not intact for the parents either. The parents may have a restricted form or pidgin type of language as well. In any case, the ELL should show non-verbal actions and abilities comparable to age level, with or without English. For example, a family brought their child from Brazil to the US for a language assessment. The nine-year-old child used a variety of consonant-vowel combinations when putting together puzzles and playing with toy cars. The child did not do anything such as draw a picture when given paper and pencil, and his vocalizations did not sound like a language that has endings like Spanish or Portuguese (alphabetic, sound-based, inflectional languages). When given books, the child did not turn the pages or look at the pictures. The child's parents were educated professionals and spoke conversational English. When asked about the child's language, they said the child spoke a lot but they had trouble understanding him. When asked if the child's ideas were typical of a nine-year-old, the parents said they did not know because they were not around nine-year-olds. So, the author phoned a colleague who spoke fluent Portuguese and asked the colleague to sample the child's L1 or Portuguese, using traditional language sampling procedures (see sections on language sampling). Within minutes, the colleague said that the child was not using words, nor was he talking about the picture. He was using jargon, sequences of sounds that did not function as language. Since the child did not have Portuguese as a first language, the child was provided intervention as a ***neuro-atypical learner*** rather than as an English language learner. Intervention consisted of providing drawings or concepts of what they saw in a pictured story, then ***hand-over-hand*** writing of the words, and so forth. As English developed, the child dropped the jargon and eventually recognized that there was another way of saying what he knew. At that point, he began to try to use some Portuguese. His inability to learn English was not because English was a second language; his inability to learn English was because he did not have the grammaticality and function of any language. His inability to draw or play age-appropriate games in any language; suggested that his lack of language was also affecting his cognition. At age seven or eight, a child typically begins to use language to develop more depth to concepts. This child was nine years old and should have had a complete grammar with functional Portuguese, his L1.

Activity: What are the two major questions for deciding how to assess a child who is an English language learner?

When a child does not develop language, like the child from Brazil, then the child's cognition will also be restricted. Therefore, he continued to play much like a seven or eight-year-old child. This was not a neuro-typical ELL. This child was a neuro-atypical language learner.

Activity: What does an ELL typically need to learn English? What is neuro-atypical learning of an L2 like?

On the other hand, another child, Miroff, came to school as a third grader with no English. Her parents were international students at a local university. Even though the parents had an academic command of English, they never spoke English in the home. Miroff and her parents spoke Russian. At nine years of age, Miroff would draw great pictures of what she saw, did, and others did. She would elaborately tell stories with language (Russian) while pointing to the pictures she had drawn. Although shy, when she arrived at school for the first time, she immediately sought out another Russian speaking child in another grade and had great conversations at recess. Obviously, Miroff is a speaker of Russian. Therefore, she is truly learning English as a second language. Miroff is a neuro-typical English language learner. By pairing her with a buddy who was in her classroom and trained to "name" all actions in the classroom with English and to draw and write academics for Miroff, Miroff was able to do her own academic learning in English after six weeks. In this way, her pre-production was related to learning new language patterns for her already acquired concepts. Therefore, once the patterns of English were assigned to her underlying Russian concepts, Miroff quickly (within six weeks) was able to move out of the pre-production or silent period of English. She began to use English words to communicate basic ideas. Her English was still restricted to pre-language function but she was no longer in a pre-production or silent phase. And, more importantly, she could now begin to learn academics in the one language the school offered, English.

Activity: What is pre-production like for a neuro-typical ELL who has acquired another first language?

Neuro-atypical pre-production

In addition to the neuro-typical learners and the English language learners with pre-production function, there are also atypical learners whose learning systems do not acquire concepts through the natural environment. As a result of impairments in learning, these children's verbal and sometimes non-verbal behaviors are often atypical. For example, the child from Brazil did not develop an L1 so his learning of a language was neuro-atypical and he functioned at a pre-production level of learning any language. This neuro-atypical learning can also be seen in observing their behaviors. For example, children diagnosed with autism spectrum disorders (ASD) will often show repetitive behaviors such as spinning or twirling, indicative of their inability to make patterns but not concepts. Or, a child diagnosed with ADHD may show a non-stop flow of motor patterns in an attempt to organize and acquire concepts. Or, another example is an older child, for example, a 12-year-old, who has multiple diagnostic labels and is still in pre-production. She does not speak, read, write, or use any language type of function. She is non-verbal and in the pre-production phase of pre-language functions. Children older than seven or eight who are still in pre-production of pre-language function will not show the social or cognitive development that is age appropriate. Remember language development and cognitive developments are intertwined so that restricting language development affects cognitive development. And restricted cognitive development will be evidenced in restricted language function.

Activity: What are neuro-atypical pre-production children like?

All learners acquire language in the way they process their world for the development of concepts. Therefore, assessment for these atypical learners consists of three questions to be answered:

1. How does the child process the world in order to learn concepts?
2. If the educator provides the opportunity for the child to learn the concepts in the way the child processes the world, what is the sequence of access to learning concepts?
3. What are the gaps in learning and development for the child?

The following section of this chapter will address these three questions used to assess atypical learners who are functioning in the pre-production stage of language development.

Activity: What are the three types of pre-production, pre-language function?

HOW DOES THE CHILD LEARN CONCEPTS?

Remember that learning concepts is part of the Neuro-Semantic Language Learning System, so assessment begins with looking at how well the child's system functions to learn concepts. As previously described, the first level of the system is the sensory level. Sensory function is assessed typically by medical or allied health professionals (eyes, ears, touch, smell, taste). And, the next stage of the learning system is the recognition of patterns. So what patterns does the child show?

Using the previous information on the typical motor representation of semantic relationships, the adult observes the child to see what the child physically does with his motor system to represent what he knows or can do. A typical learner shows a use of the motor system to represent needs, wants, desires—reaches, crawls, uses gaze, takes turns with speech patterns as if talking and listening to the adult. However, an atypical learner may begin with some of these patterns but without being able to use the patterns for conceptual development; atypical motor movements or behaviors will start to emerge. These atypical patterns express the child's cognitive development. For example, children with autism spectrum disorders will often show an increase in repetitive movements such as spinning objects beyond the second birthday (Arwood & Kaulitz, 2007). These repetitive movements indicate the child is increasing his or her development of patterns but that the patterns are not becoming concepts for language representation. The result is that the child gets bigger and the inappropriate repetitive behaviors expand while the language to represent thinking does not improve. Over time, without the language as a cognitive tool, the child shows a cognitive lack of development.

Assessing neuro-atypical children (see Appendix A for the Arwood Neuro-Semantic Pre-Language Assessment or ANSPA) uses the same observation protocol as for the neuro-typical children, but the interpretation of the behavior is different. A completed protocol below shows an assessment of a neuro-atypical 12-year-old female, Samantha, who does not have any oral language, is very aggressive, and is diagnosed with several labels including severely cognitively impaired (SCI), severely impacted by an autism spectrum disorder (ASD), severely language delayed, and pervasive developmental delayed (PDD).[2] Over the years, she has been medicated with a variety of drugs and she has received excellent applied behavioral analysis (ABA) (e.g., Maurice, Green, & Luce, 1996) therapies, including those to develop speech.

The first section of the assessment is set up to allow the educator or parent to record the "productive" motor patterns or functions. The term "productive" is used to cue the adult to look for how the child's motor system functions for learning. In this way, the adult observes the child's use of her motor system as a way to indicate how she is learning. Determining how the child learns also decides what type of assessment will help her change inappropriate behavior to communicate positive, pro-social behavior. This type of assessment is chosen specifically because she is non-verbal (pre-production silent period).

Arwood Neuro-Semantic Pre-Language Assessment (ANSPA)

Section I: Pre-Language Assessment

Name: Samantha Smith **Date of birth:** June 6, 1992 **Assessment date:** September 15, 2004

Pre-Production or Silent Stage—Observe the child during three different activities such as free play, working to do a task with a parent or educator such as winding up a new toy, and during routine activities of daily living like eating. Check for patterns of behavior. Record those patterns of behavior.

	Activity 1: Lunch	**Activity 2: Sorting**	**Activity 3: Bus**
Productive use of hands—e.g., reaches	Uses spoon to hit on table...when food arrives, she holds spoon and eats	Flails arms, hits adults, knocks off objects from table, throws objects; shoves table forward and pushes chair back	Pounds seat in front of her with fist, hits seat, repeats hitting of seat motion, hits adults when close
Productive use of eyes—e.g., gazes to connect people and objects or actions	Looks at food adults bring...not at adults... is seated toward wall... looks at food	Looks at objects, at table, at wall, at objects, looks around but not at people	Looks outside bus and down aisle

2 See DSM-IV-TR for explanation of diagnostic labels (American Psychiatric Association 2000). Samantha was diagnosed with DSM (medical model) as well as IDEA (school) disabilities.

	Activity 1: Lunch	Activity 2: Sorting	Activity 3: Bus
Productive use of feet—e.g., walks, stands	Feet are on the ground under the table, shoes are on	Kicks adults, takes off shoes when sits on floor, walks by using edge of table to get from sorting task to sitting on floor, stands up and fills space while feet move forward (twice)	Takes off shoes, kicks feet, does not walk when asked to get up and leave bus…25 minutes to get off bus
Productive use of body—e.g., sits, orients toward speaker	Body posture is relaxed and she is facing the food she is eating	She throws back head when adults try to help her sort, stands up and falls through space, adults physically redirect her body back to chair but she stands up and falls through space and sits her body on the floor and then physically is redirected to stand and sit—when moving through space she is "filling" the space with her body	Has to be physically moved off the bus…does not move body in response to adult language
Productive use of mouth—e.g., talks, uses C-V-C jargon, imitates	Some use of C-V-C; ba, daga	Non-differentiated vowel sounds—e, e, e, e…	Non-differentiated vowel sounds—e, e, e, e…

Interpretation:

Activity 1: She appears to understand the concepts related to eating…the food is "helicoptered" to her and she eats…food is pureed into thick liquid…she does not have meaning for the texture of food but she sits and eats as if age appropriate which means she has a good learning system…she is able to act as an instrument for food, object.

Activity 2: Sorting is a career task. She does not understand the object of the task or the spoken words for compliance…does not appear to process adult speaking…

Activity 3: She does not get on or off the bus with words, behavior repetition, practice of behavior, rewards, reinforcement with words and/or rewards…she does not appear to make meaning out of adult speech.

Note that in the protocol, only the behaviors Samantha is *able to perform* are recorded, as the question, "How does the child learn concepts?" is based on Samantha's strengths. Assessment of her strengths will result in writing recommendations for using her strengths for intervention.

Activity: What type of behaviors are used to assess a non-verbal learner? Why?

Because Samantha has learned to walk (her body is upright but she fills the space so she looks like she is falling as she "walks"), she is learning basic patterns about semantic relationships, herself as an agent or object. This is further supported during her eating activity where she looks typical for her age. So, to answer the question, "How does she learn concepts?" knowledge about the Neuro-Semantic Language Learning System can be applied to the behaviors recorded on the protocol. The following chart shows how to take the behaviors and put them into a Neuro-Semantic Language Learning paradigm in order to determine how a person uses their learning patterns to form concepts for the development of language as a social and cognitive tool.

Apply the Neuro-Semantic Language Learning Theory to the recorded behaviors			
Sensory input	**Perceptual patterns**	**Concepts**	**Language**
Puts hands over ears when hears band next door, audiologist reports no hearing loss...parent says eyes tested and okay	Atypical: Fills space with body, hands, feet, taps, repeats hitting, repeats pounding, repeats rocking of body (visual-motor[3]) Typical: Uses g-sign for food during rest, brings food to mouth with spoon, sits still with feet on floor while feeding herself	Is not responding to sound of adult voices so visual-motor patterns remain and increase but do not connect to sounds of adults' speech Typical: Shows semantic relationship between object (food) and action (eating) and food (sign) and action	None...does not read, write, sign, or speak
Interpretation: Senses okay	Interpretation: Uses motor patterns meaningfully attached to vision—eating	Interpretation: Learns concepts through motor acts for (eating) meaning...sound and sight alone do not work	Interpretation: Must teach concepts with motor overlap of patterns to create concepts for language to develop

The question of "How does Samantha learn concepts best?" can now be answered. Samantha can use motor patterns such as the use of her hands (eating), the shape of people's mouths when talking, hand-over-hand writing of words, physical motor assistance to point, reach, pick up and so forth for actions, and pictures that she crosses off or points to, that represent semantic relationships.

Activity: How do you assess for how a child who is a neuro-atypical learner acquires concepts?

3 Within the neurobiological learning system, there are three primary pattern options for the development of concepts: acoustic patterns overlapped with acoustic patterns; acoustic and simultaneous visual patterns, or visual patterns overlapped with visual patterns. Acoustic patterns form no concepts (see Chapters 2 and 3 for explanation). Overlapping acoustic and visual patterns, in a culture that uses an auditory language like English, will result in spoken language that represents auditory concepts. Since Samantha was raised in an auditory culture but has no language, then she also does not have the ability to make auditory concepts from overlapping what she hears and sees in her world. Samantha does not use sound and sight or auditory patterns to form auditory or spoken English or she would be speaking. She would not be "hitting" if she matched visual patterns to form concepts so she is also not using visual patterns to see what she should look like.

WHAT DOES THE CHILD NEED FROM THE ADULT?

Once the child's ability to use patterns to learn concepts has been assessed then intervention pathways are determined. To determine what the adult must do for the child to learn concepts, the adult must assess the different types of patterns Samantha uses to develop concepts (agents, actions, objects for example). From assessing her "productive behavior" it was determined that she is able to make meaning out of the motor patterns such as eating the food she sees or watching the movement of the adults bringing her food to her. So, she was able to learn the concepts of how to eat which consists of motor patterns. Samantha is able to use motor patterns to form concepts. Motor patterns can neurologically form shapes of ideas, a form of visual language function.[4]

As motor patterns are a strength, looking to produce speech may be desirable but not realistic. As she does not speak or use the basic speech patterns of English (consonant-vowel-consonant) or complicated gestures to indicate what she wants, imitating speech sounds to develop oral language is not an option. In other words, if she were able to imitate speech patterns, she would be producing those basic patterns whether or not she had the concepts for the patterns to create language. Therefore, working on speech patterns is not useful for her or any student like her (for more information see Arwood & Kaulitz, 2007) until she has developed language to produce as speech.

Activity: What types of motor patterns are useful or productive for Samantha? Why is working on speech patterns not productive?

Knowing how Samantha is learning patterns helps determine how she might be learning concepts. Knowledge about how Samantha learns concepts can be used to establish intervention. Adults can use movements such as hand-over-hand support of Samantha's hands to develop tasks as mental shapes of meaning. For example, with the adult's hands on Samantha's hands, they can make a bed together. In this way, Samantha learns the motor patterns of the concepts about making a bed. Additional forms of hand-over-hand motor shapes were created by assisting her in activities of daily living such as making her own food, using hand-over-hand pointing to pictures of stick figures of Samantha riding on the bus, putting on shoes, making a bed, etc. (for more examples of what these stick figures might look like, see Arwood & Brown, 1999; Arwood & Kaulitz, 2007; Arwood *et al.*, 2009).

Once Samantha's non-verbal motor patterns were turned into productive, functional ways to learn, Samantha's behavior immediately began to change. She began to look at the speaker's mouth to see the movement make oral mouth shapes, she watched others' hands and then looked at their faces, she used appropriate hand movements to reject objects and appropriately pointed to what she wanted, and so forth. Note: Samantha was not told to look at faces or watch hands but her change in behavior was the result in the development of cognition. She was given meaning through hand-over-hand motor patterns which helped her learn the concepts in her environment. Since Samantha learns concepts with motor patterns, this intervention quickly (six weeks) showed a change in her behavior.

In six weeks of motor-pattern intervention to create a visual way of thinking through an overlap of motor patterns to create mental visual shapes, Samantha's behavior changed

4 Sadato (1996) discovered that people reading Braille record these motor movements in the visual cortex.

dramatically. Her change in behavior represented an increase in cognition. She was able to learn to be an agent, a person who acts in response to or with others. Samantha learned to maintain relationships non-verbally during multiple activities including making her own food, collecting attendance sheets at the middle school, crossing off pictured events as she completed them, and so forth. Giving Samantha more meaning in the way that she learns concepts (overlap of motor patterns) resulted in Samantha gaining much higher functioning. She could act like an agent and no longer functioned in response to sensory input by filling her space (hitting, sitting on the floor, rocking, falling through space like she is bolting, etc.).

Activity: Explain how to assess a pre-production neuro-atypical learner's way of forming concepts? Why did the intervention that matched the assessment findings result in such quick improvement in functioning?

ARE THERE GAPS IN DEVELOPMENT?

Even though Samantha showed an increase from the sensori-motor cognition to acting more like an agent who non-verbally maintains with the adults through non-verbal semantic relationships, Samantha still functions at the pre-production or silent level of language function. Her development of language is restricted because she learns concepts through the motor overlap of patterns to form concepts but she lives in an auditory culture. The second question had to do with what does Samantha need from the adult? She needs motor overlap of motor patterns to learn the concepts in her immediate environment. The next question to answer is whether or not there are developmental gaps that would indicate that she is neuro-atypical in development. This question is easy to answer for Samantha. Because she is 12 years old and is not talking, not toilet trained, not able to use typical forms of non-speech communication prior to the motor language intervention, she obviously has some huge gaps in her learning. The fact that the macro-culture uses an auditory language, English, in an auditory way to teach behavior, compliance, concepts, language, and so forth, and the fact that Samantha does not learn auditory concepts nor can she cope with learning visual concepts through watching what she sees others model, mean that she has not learned the meaning of the basic world around her. She has not learned about agents, their actions, and their objects. She has not learned the basic semantic relationships that are required for language to develop. Her development of language function is restricted to a pre-production or silent period of pre-language function.

Activity: What does Samantha need to be able to learn concepts? What are her gaps? Explain how culture affects her development.

Restricted pre-language function with limited language structures

The first type of development within the pre-language function is a pre-production or silent period basically characterized by limited, if any, oral or signed language as exhibited by

Samantha. The second period of development within the pre-language function is restricted use of limited language structures. In other words, some children do acquire lots of patterns, and therefore they express some basic language structures, but their language function is still restricted, so they are at a pre-language level of function.

During this period of pre-language function, if the child develops language structures, the structures are still dependent on others for interpretation; so, the child's language function remains restricted. For assessment purposes, the pre-production assessment protocol (ANSPA) is used to see if the child is developing semantic relationships. But, the assessor will want to add a language sample, as the child has developed some language structures. The following example is from a child who is no longer in a silent period of pre-language function but whose language is still restricted to pre-language function.

Arwood Neuro-Semantic Pre-Language Assessment (ANSPA)

Section I: Pre-Language Assessment

Name: Jeremy Smith **Date of birth:** June 17, 2002 **Assessment date:** October 5, 2008

Pre-Production or Silent Stage—Observe the child during three different activities such as free play, working to do a task with a parent or educator such as winding up a new toy, and during routine activities of daily living like eating. Check for patterns of behavior. Record those patterns.

	Activity 1: Table play	**Activity 2: Waiting for Mom**	**Activity 3: Interacting with sister**
Productive use of hands—e.g., reaches	Age-appropriate handling of materials, puzzles, scribbles with pencil	Turns the pages of books, pulls on Mom's coat, spins some toys	Does not use reciprocal play but does use hands to get sister to help with toys
Productive use of eyes—e.g., gazes to connect people and objects or actions	Watches people do things, watches faces, watches hands, tracks well	Looks around room, looks at objects and pictures focusing on different parts of pictures	Signals basic semantic relationships with sister—to do, to reject, again, etc.
Productive use of feet—e.g., walks, stands	Walks and sits in age-appropriate ways, climbs up into large chairs, etc.	Walks around the room, sits and stays busy, stands by door to leave, opens and closes door with balance	Sits on the floor and plays with the objects, stands up, throws ball overhand, reaches down and picks up ball while still moving
Productive use of body—e.g., sits, orients toward speaker	Always appears ready and willing to engage with others, orientation is toward speakers or doers	Body is natural and in alignment with feet, balance is good, waits on one foot and then the other, pulling and closing door	For gross motor activities, his body movements are typical; for drawing and pointing to pictures in a book, he tends to finish quickly and move on
Productive use of mouth—e.g., talks, uses C-V-C jargon, imitates	Limited talking (see sample)	Limited talking	Limited talking

Interpretation: *Activity 1*: Typical non-verbals for a young child in all three activities. *Activity 2*: *Activity 3*:			
How does this child learn best? Apply the Neuro-Semantic Language Learning Theory to the recorded behaviors.			
Sensory input	**Perceptual patterns**	**Concepts**	**Language**
Checked at doctor… okay	Child shows responses to sound but does not comply to spoken language	Child shows through body use semantic relationships of basic agents, actions, and objects that he sees	Limited talking: "more go" "hold this" "my piece" "momma more" "me too play" "some more please"
Interpretation: Sensory input okay	Interpretation: Can do visual-motor patterns	Interpretation: Learns concepts from what he sees	Interpretation: Telegraphic utter-ances…shows semantic relationships verbally

Jeremy shows an ability to maintain non-verbally with the people, objects, and actions in the child's environment. This means that the child has developed a basic set of concepts (cognition) related to what he sees others do in his environment. This child is functioning higher than Samantha. Jeremy is cognitively developing concepts to relate himself to and with others socially. His language is restricted to that of a younger child, more like a two or three-year-old. He learns visual-motor patterns such as turning pages, throwing balls but he is not learning the sound of the words for oral language. His language functioning is limited to basic semantic relationships such as the throwing the ball to his sister but he did not initiate a game with shared rules or roles. This restricted language function also restricts his thinking. Until his language functions at a higher level, his socio-cognitive development will remain restricted. Even though this child has developed some language structures, his language function is restricted for his age. He is still basically non-verbal, in a pre-production level of pre-language function. He is limited in his language structures and functions. He needs more visual-motor intervention from the adults to provide for him what the spoken words look like, such as hand-over-hand writing. More about the intervention will be found in Chapters 8 and 9. He also shows a gap that is between what he shows non-verbally and what he produces verbally. He has not learned what the spoken language looks like even though he has been able to acquire age-appropriate non-verbal behavior that represents age-appropriate concept development.

Activity: How does a child who shows typical non-verbal semantic relationships also show restricted limited language?

Pre-language function with lots of language structures

Samantha had no language development and had to learn about who people were, what they did as agents in her environment in order to participate as an agent. Jeremy could relate to others with lots of appropriate non-verbal semantic relationships but his language structures were restricted to basic two-word, telegraphic utterances. The third type of pre-language function is the child who shows the development of lots of language structures, but language function is still restricted. In the previous case, Jeremy's language was limited and so collecting his few utterances during the observation period was adequate. But if the child uses a lot of language structures then a more formal language sampling (see language sampling in Chapter 9) with analysis becomes imperative. The child with lots of language structures is no longer in the silent or pre-production stage of pre-language function. Chapter 8 will discuss how to intervene for children with limited language structures who are in the pre-language thinking period. Chapter 9 will provide the assessment and intervention methods for those children and adults who have restricted thinking but use lots of structures.

Summary

There are three different types of pre-language functioning: those who are in the pre-production or silent period with either atypical or neuro-typical development (Chapters 7 and 8); those who function with limited language structures that are restricted in function (Chapters 7 and 8); and those who function with lots of language structures but are still restricted in thinking (Chapter 9).

Neuro-typical children between the ages of 0 and two develop concepts followed by language structures that represent the beginning of understanding of concepts and therefore are limited in function. Increased language structures indicate that the child is no longer in the silent pre-production period of pre-language function. The second period of pre-language function is telegraphic (around two to three years) but is still restricted to pre-language function. As a child's understanding of concepts increases, the language structures continue to expand in complexity and increase in number. The telegraphic period expands to an inter-language function between three and seven years of age. The adult maintains with the child's talking so that the child's ability to converse is still restricted to the adult's interpretation. This means that the neuro-typical child's language development is restricted in function. Neuro-typical learners continue to acquire parallel social and cognitive development to their language function so that by seven to eight years of age they are sharing their use of adult language structures in meaningfully shared conversation and are no longer in the pre-language function stage of development. Their language functions in a shared, reciprocal fashion.

A second type of pre-production, pre-language functioning person is an English language learner. A child or adult who possesses a first language and who is then exposed to a second language, for example English, also experiences a pre-production or silent period of pre-language function followed by the development of language structures that function to represent the speaker's typical development of underlying semantic relationships (agents, actions, and objects). If the ELL has acquired a first language, then learning English is learning the meaning of tags or words that represent their already acquired concepts.

A third type of pre-production, pre-language functioning person may be a neuro-atypical learner. Neuro-atypical learners may remain in the pre-production period or develop limited language structures for years or even a lifetime because they lack the development of the underlying semantic relationships to develop a full language function. Further samples will showcase how some older children are thought to have adequate language function but lack the social function of their structures. Remember: *Language functioning is a way of thinking. Language represents thinking and mediates more advanced thinking. Because thinking is a socio-cognitive function of the learning system, a person who lacks cognitive or social or socio-cognitive development also will exhibit a lack of typical language functioning.* Chapter 8 describes how to assign meaning to those who are in the pre-production or non-verbal period of pre-language function while Chapter 9 describes how to assess and establish intervention for those who are restricted in thinking but use lots of language structures.

Applications

- Use an ANSPA protocol for assessment of pre-production, pre-language function for at least one person.
- Assess a pre-production ELL for whether or not he or she has developed age-appropriate concepts in an L1.

Chapter 8

INTERVENTION FOR PRE-PRODUCTION, PRE-LANGUAGE THINKERS

Learner objectives: Chapter 8

Upon completion of this chapter, the reader should be able to:

1. Assign meaning to a child's activities of daily living.
2. Use an event-based picture to set up the intervention for a child with pre-language thinking.
3. Explain why event-based materials assist in developing the preoperational thinking of a child.
4. Use hand-over-hand methods to assign patterns to drawn concepts for language function.
5. Explain the different type of learners who might need event-based assignment of meaning to acquire language for reading, writing, and thinking at a preoperational, pre-language function.

I see, I hear
I know not what I think or do
I need you…
To assign meaning to what I do!

Children who are pre-language thinkers exhibit a wide range of abilities from being silent, having no language, to being very talkative with lots of language structures. Individuals who function at this pre-language level have one common characteristic: They exhibit *restricted language function* that requires the listener to interpret their non-verbal or verbal communication. *Intervention is based on the premise that the adult must assign meaning to the child in the way that the child learns concepts so that the child can begin to make progress.*

The intervention for those who are non-verbal or in the silent period of pre-production, pre-language function like Samantha, a 12-year-old female, who lacked language development, and Jeremy, a six-year-old male, who exhibited some limited language structures, necessitates an intervention designed to develop their thinking or cognition for how they, as agents, function in their sensory world. Each of these individuals was introduced to the reader in Chapter 7.

This chapter describes how to develop assessment-based intervention for those who are non-verbal and who are in the pre-production or silent period of language function like Samantha or who are very limited in their language development like Jeremy. This chapter also addresses intervention for those pre-production individuals who are neuro-typical English language learners. Chapter 9 provides intervention methods for those who exhibit pre-language thinking but who have developed a lot of language structures. Chapter 10 provides the assessment and intervention strategies for those who are developing a reciprocal, rather than restricted, function of language. Chapter 11 provides the assessment and intervention strategies for those who are trying to function linguistically with maximum levels of displacement, semanticity, productivity, flexibility, and efficiency (limited redundancy). Chapter 12 describes how behavior and language communicate about how a person thinks and learns.

Foundation to intervention for pre-production, pre-language thinkers

The basis to intervention for the pre-production (silent period), pre-language thinker comes from the knowledge about how children learn to think at this early, sensori-motor level of cognition. According to the Neuro-Semantic Language Learning Theory, neuro-typical learners develop their social and cognitive being from other people assigning meaning to children's motor responses to sensory input. In this way, the child's learning system receives sensory input and then responds. For example, the child's tummy is empty and the child cries in response. The mother picks up the child and feeds the child. The child's neurological system recognizes the mother's actions as previous patterns and so the child responds in a typical way. But, the input is always new and so the mother feeding the baby creates another ***layer*** of input to the child. The more the child does, the more meaning the caregivers assign. So, patterns ***overlap*** and the meaning between the child and others creates a ***scaffold*** of layers of meaning called ***concepts***. These concepts continue to develop across the lifespan. This acquisition of meaning occurs in the way that the child's patterns will form concepts, auditory or visual (shapes or pictures) movement. In an auditory culture, children with auditory systems have a match between the input of the adults and the way the children learn, so, with adequate input, they do not have difficulty acquiring their language learning system. As long as the child's neurological system is able to recognize the input of patterns, then the child will develop concepts.

Activity: What is the knowledge needed to set up intervention for children with pre-production, pre-language thinking?

From the input of patterns, the first concepts learned are the basic semantic relationships—agents, their actions, and their objects. Therefore, the first goals of intervention at this level are for the learner to acquire concepts of agency, actions, and objects in non-verbal relationships. For the pre-production child, who is in the silent period of pre-language function, the educator or parent *assigns meaning* to what the child *can do.* The child does something, the educator or parent assigns meaning. In this way, the meaning scaffolds to develop layers of patterns necessary to form basic concepts. The parent or educator must be able to do the following: First, assign meaning in the way the child learns concepts; second, assign meaning through the use of the child's body so the child is the agent (pointer, drawer, writer, speaker, etc.); and third, recognize that every little non-verbal movement (sigh, shrug of shoulder, a scratch, point, hand twitch, and so forth) communicates. The foundation, the initial goals, and methods will be explained in the following sections.

Activity: What is the first goal based on for a child who is at the pre-production, pre-language level of sensori-motor cognition? What are the three components necessary for the educator or parent to be able to do for intervening at this level?

Assigning meaning to atypical pre-language, pre-production learners

Atypical pre-language learners who function in the silent period of pre-production often remain at this level for years, sometimes for life. The key to intervention rests with providing the meaning of concepts in the way that the learner acquires concepts. In this way, the learner acquires the concepts that support a higher level of thinking. The higher conceptual level will support the development of social skills and communication.

Case 8.1: Darin

Darin is a five-year-old male who is diagnosed with autism. He has been referred by his parents because Darin is not making progress in his special education program at school. He is growing older and bigger, but his behavior is becoming more aggressive; he does not speak, read, or write. His parents report that he has limited understanding of their language.

From the parents' description summarized above, it is apparent that Darin is in the pre-production stage of pre-language function much like Jeremy and Samantha (Chapter 7). Darin does not yet produce language in any form. So, before seeing Darin the first time, the educator makes some assumptions based on Darin's case history. What is "known" about Darin provides for an opportunity to decide what questions must be answered during the assessment. These answers become the basis for intervention. In essence, assessment is ongoing and becomes the intervention.

- *Knowledge*: If Darin were able to imitate the sounds of a language, he would have already done so because his parents probably use a lot of good oral language, as they are educated professionals. *If he used an auditory system or could use the sounds of speech with his mental visual concepts, he would have attached sound to what he knows and he would have developed oral, spoken language, but it is reported that he uses limited, if any, natural language.*

Assessment question: How does Darin communicate if he does not use sound? And what information in his world does he understand, as he is able to walk, a learned set of skills?

- *Knowledge*: There are limited ways that the neurobiological system can create concepts from sensory patterns (see Chapters 1–3); and, sound patterns do not work for Darin because *he hasn't developed any sound usage for speech, etc. and, yet, his environment is full of spoken language so using any type of sound input may not be effective.*

  Assessment question: Since sound patterns do not work, then he is not auditory in thinking (sound and visual), which means he uses the visual-motor language system.[1] Can he imitate visual patterns such as copying manual signs, written words, drawings, etc.?

- *Knowledge*: Darin's behavior does not follow what he sees others do or he would sit when others sit; but, it was reported his behavior was becoming more aggressive which means he does not learn from the visual patterns of what he sees alone.

  Assessment question: If he is drawn into a cartoon of what he looks like during a behavior like sitting, will he change his behavior to match the behavior of the cartoon? Can he see himself drawn into a picture?

- *Knowledge*: Darin has had therapy for speech that includes imitation of sounds and he has had behavior therapy for how to sit. Darin's behavior has not generalized from deliberate scheduling of rewards and punishers in his therapy to natural settings; so, he must not understand the concepts of the rewards and punishers. *He needs to learn the basic concepts of an agent, in relationship to his actions with and to objects or other agents so that he can begin to think about his world.*

  Assessment question: If rewards and punishers do not work, then what does Darin need to learn conceptually to be able to choose to behave differently? What layers of intervention will the adult need to offer Darin so he can learn a new concept, like a behavioral concept? (Learning means not only to produce but also to remember the concept for later retrieval.)

Activity: What knowledge does the person have before the first meeting? How will this knowledge help define what Darin will need from the educator during the first meeting? What do we know about Darin?

Given the aforementioned knowledge for the parents' information, Darin is functioning at the pre-production or silent period of pre-language function. Furthermore, the educator knows before Darin arrives for his assessment that Darin's behavior is difficult to handle. To assist Darin in being able to understand what is expected of him in the assessment, the

1 Most children who are diagnosed with autism use a motor access to their visual thinking (Arwood & Kaulitz, 2007; Arwood *et al.*, 2009)—*so, Darin probably uses a visual-motor system for learning concepts.*

educator put some effort in developing a *visual* way for Darin to see himself and how he was to act when he was in the assessment. Figure 8.1 shows a cartoon drawing that the educator developed before Darin arrived to help Darin participate. The cartoon puts the child into a series of pictures that shows him what he looks like when his behavior matches with expectations.

4:00
Darin
looks
chair
picture
sits
table
At 4:00 Darin sits down on his chair at the table and begins to think about the people he sees in the picture.
4:05
Darin
puts finger
picture
Darin puts his finger on the person in the picture who he will draw about today.
4:15
Darin
draws
Darin draws what he sees the person do. Darin tells Mabel about his drawing so she can label it.
4:30
boy
The boy picks up.
Darin writes about what the person does. He puts a bubble around each word. He puts a picture above each word.
4:45
can
can
boy
bubble
Darin writes, bubbles and pictures new words in a picture dictionary. Darin reads the words he wrote.
5:00
Bye
Darin copies his work papers on the copier and then waves and says, "Good-bye." to Mabel.

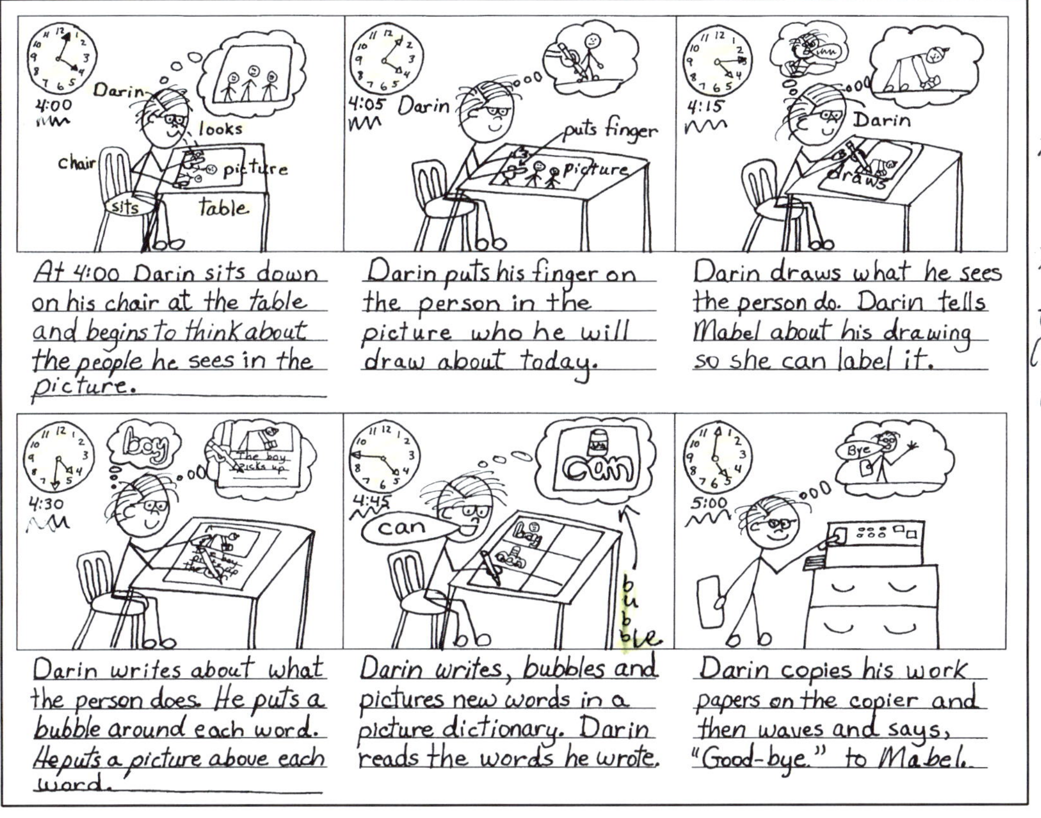

Figure 8.1 Darin sees the expectations

However, prior to the assessment, the educator does not know what patterns of overlapping motor acts Darin needs to learn.[2] The educator does not know which concepts Darin has acquired or if he can see the ideas within the cartoon. Depending on the answer to these first questions, the educator will know, first, what the educator needs to provide Darin so that he can learn concepts, and second, what level of concept development Darin possesses.

> ***Activity:*** What does the educator need to determine during the first meeting?

2 There are several motor pattern types: hand-over-hand (H/H) finger spelling, H/H signing, H/H doing of a task such as making a bed, watching the mouth move, watching the hand write, H/H writing, H/H bubbling of the letters to create a shape of a word, H/H pointing, H/H drawing, H/H cartooning, and so forth. Most individuals with ASD learn concepts from developing some form of overlapping motor patterns.

Remember that concepts underlie a person's language so to develop Darin's language for behavior or academics or speech or social thoughts, he must be able to acquire concepts in a way that works for him to learn concepts; that is, in a way that his neurobiological system allows. Instead of completing an ANSPA for three settings, the educator was using the tasks in Figure 8.1 to create the three settings: drawing, writing, and speaking within the assessment. This type of assessment also provides the first level of intervention.

Sometimes, educators will possess a lot of testing information but must still meet with the student in order to determine how to intervene. This first meeting is an assessment meeting to determine intervention.

When Darin came to the first meeting, he was *not* able to follow the cartoon in Figure 8.1. Even though the educator drew Darin into his picture so he could see himself do the tasks, Darin did not recognize the meaning of the drawing. He did not have enough conceptualization to understand the visual representations in the cartoon. However, the first meeting did provide additional information: Darin did not use any speech or any other conventional forms of communication. He did communicate through the following behaviors: kicking, crying, screaming, trying to bite, hitting, and trying to leave. Notice in Figure 8.1, the educator expected Darin to be able to sit, point to the picture, talk upon imitation, and engage in the task. Based on the assessment, it was apparent that Darin did not use a visual input either by watching another person's gestures, etc., or by looking at pictures and the written words to learn concepts. His excessive motor acts tell the educator that Darin has to use movement to be able to learn a concept. *Remember: There are limited ways to learn a concept. These ways include the following*:

- An overlap of acoustic and visual input for auditory language learning, English is an auditory (sounds-letters) type of language; but, since Darrin does not learn English, he does not have an auditory learning system for concept acquisition.
- A second option would be to overlap visual with visual input which means that he would make his body look like those he sees around him. He sees what others do and he makes a visual mental image of what he looks like that matches others' behavior. As Darrin does not match what he does with those he sees around him, he does not use seeing to create visual concepts.
- He did use his body to hit, cry, scream, move and so his learning system must use movements to create the shapes of ideas—visual thinking through motor movements to form shapes. Intervention based on how children learn at the sensori-motor level is always based on what the child *can do. And this child can do a lot of motor acts.*
- There are no other options for language learning. Acoustic overlapping data will not form concepts. And, the non-distance senses like taste, touch, and smell will not form concepts that refer to concepts for most oral language concepts.

Activity: How does Darin learn concepts the best (acoustic-acoustic, visual-visual, acoustic-visual, or motor to create visual concepts)?[3] And why do you know this?

As Darin could not use the visual cartoon, the words with the cartoon either spoken or written or visually modeled, the educator redid the cartoon to emphasize Darin's motor

3 Remember that these options are not learning styles but the options that the neurobiological system possesses for forming patterns into concepts.

overlap of patterns as a way to ***access*** his learning of concepts. Figure 8.2 shows the second cartoon. This cartoon includes the motor hand-over-hand steps of intervention that will be used to help Darin learn concepts for language, written, signed, and spoken…and in that order of acquisition.

At 4:00 Darin sits down on his chair at the table and begins to think about the people he sees in the picture.
As Darin points to the drawn picture, Mabel tells him what the people are doing.
boy
boy
boy
boy
Darin looks at a word on the P.D. H/H Darin and Mabel fingerspell, write, bubble, pictograph and then 'sign' and say the word.
boy
H/H Darin and Mabel write the word on the line as Mabel fingerspells the word. After bubbling and pictographing the word, Darin points, 'signs' and says the word.
H/H Darin moves his finger under his written ideas and 'reads' back the words by saying what he sees.
At 5:00 Darin copies his work on the copier and then says, "Good-bye" to Mabel before leaving.

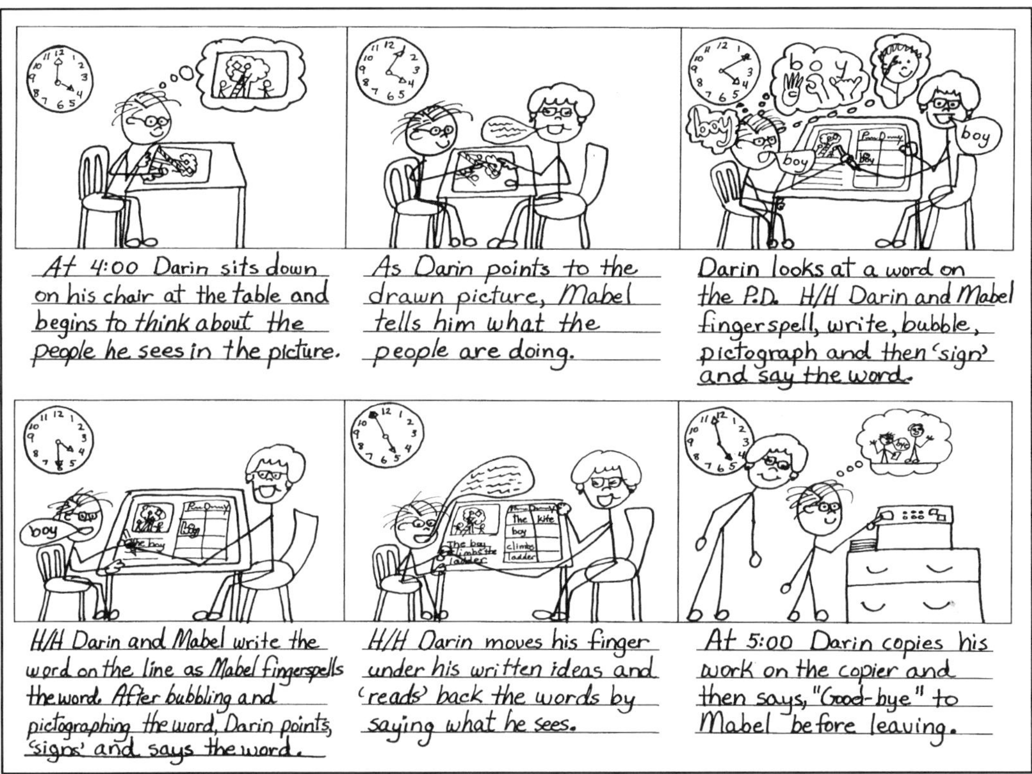

Figure 8.2 Darin learns the concepts

This cartoon worked for Darin. Intervention required no visual or acoustic imitation or production, only assisted motor acts such as pointing or the educator taking Darin's hand and using his hand as an instrument in a "hand-over-hand" (H/H or HOH) act. Because this cartoon worked, intervention based on H/H motor overlaps will work. Hand-over-hand work by the adult puts Darin into his picture as an agent and makes his hand a visual-motor instrument that records the shape of the hand movements to create concepts that are visual in nature. It should be noted that at Darin's level of learning, the hand-over-hand method is designed to be a tool where his hand is an instrument and his body creates the movements so he is the agent. In this way, he learns agency patterns to begin to develop the semantic relationships. *Darin will learn from overlapping the movement of the hands with the movement of the mouth to create concepts.*[4]

Activity: Look at the second cartoon (Figure 8.2) and determine how many layers (different types) of input it takes to have Darin begin to learn a concept.

4 This same understanding of Darin's learning system would not have happened with norm-referenced testing, criterion-referenced testing, or formal or standardized testing.

Assessment-based intervention

There are three basic questions that should be answered with all of the cases similar to Darin:

1. *What does the educator know about the case that can be interpreted according to knowledge of the Neuro-Semantic Language Learning Theory*? For example, Darin uses limited oral language and his parents use a lot of language. This knowledge was applied to the theory and it was determined that Darin did not use sound for learning concepts. By answering this question, the educator can speed up the assessment process. For example, one first grade teacher has 22–26 students yearly and she assesses each child on the first day so she knows how they learn concepts. She does this without any testing.
2. *How does the child learn concepts the best?* This is answered based on the Neuro-Semantic Language Learning Theory that indicates concepts are only learned with specific types of input. By answering this question, the educator will know what input the child needs for learning concepts.
3. *What does the child demonstrate about conceptual learning?* There are three different developmental domains that can be assessed: language, cognitive, and social development. Darin did not use any conventional language forms (manual signs, speech, reading, writing, drawing, etc.). Cognitively, he cannot follow another person's rules so he acts on the world around him. Therefore, his cognition is in the sensori-motor or preoperational levels. Because he can walk and because he acts on his environment by crying, screaming, and so on to *get others* to change the environment for him, he is above the sensori-motor level which means he is preoperational in the way he thinks. Socially, he uses his body and others' bodies as objects which means he also lacks the concept development of being a person who does something or an agent. Preoperational thinking means that he is able to be in the center of his universe and that all agents, actions, objects, activities are about him. He is egocentric as an agent.

Activity: What are Darin's developmental levels for social, cognitive, and language development? How do you know this?

There are three basic ongoing questions about intervention:

1. *If the educator presents the child a task using the sensory input that the child requires for developing concepts, is the child able to perform the task?* For example, if Darin is shown, by hand-over-hand movements (visual-motor patterns of shapes), how to point to the different people in the picture, is Darin able to do this task without hand-over-hand prompting? If he needs prompts, what are those prompts? The prompts are motor acts that help Darin learn the patterns needed for the development of concepts. Once he can do a task, is he able to do the task when presented a new, but similar, activity? Therefore, once Darin shows he can perform a task in response to a specific type of input, then a new event is offered. More about the event used to help develop concepts follows.

Activity: What is the first basic question that must be addressed to develop intervention based on assessment?

2. *Does the same input continue to work?* For example, sometimes a low-functioning child is able to write the words for a story, but, later, the child is not able to read the words that the child wrote. This means that the child is able to follow the input but that the input is not forming enough meaning to develop his own concepts for the writing to be language based. Unless a task is language based, the learning will not go into long term memory. The child is probably imitating patterns but not learning concepts for long term storage and retrieval. In order to increase the learning over time, an increase of meaning has to happen. To increase meaning, more information is added in more layers. Often educators try to take away information to simply a task. Taking away information makes the task more difficult (Arwood *et al.*, 2009) because the learner does not have enough information to form concepts. For example, Darin was able to come to therapy on the second visit and do the tasks in Figure 8.2 because there were plenty of motor movements that overlapped to create meaning for Darin. But, Darin did not have enough conceptual information to continue doing these tasks at later sessions. So, he began the crying, kicking, etc., again. Once he began crying, he could continue crying for hours. This behavior communicated that Darin did not have enough meaning to understand the purpose of the task. So, the educator had to add more meaning. Remember the goal to develop semantic relationships so there has to be more meaning about agents, actions, and objects to help him learn.

Activity: What does Darin's behavior mean? What are layers of meaning? What type of meaningful layers does Darin need to learn concepts?

The crying and kicking (and other inappropriate social behaviors) indicate that he did not see himself as the person or agent doing the task. He could not do a task as an agent until he knew he was an agent. To be an agent, Darin had to see himself performing his acts throughout the day, not just during therapy. Since he learns his concepts through motor access, his parents were encouraged to draw him as an agent in his environment with therapy as one of the objects of Darin's actions in a day. In this way, he was watching the parent create meaning for him through drawing and the drawing showed Darin as an agent going through his day where therapy was a part of his day. Figure 8.3 shows the drawing that Darin's parents produced.

Because both the educator and Darin's parents were willing to draw Darin as an agent, he began to see the movement of their hands make patterns of shape that occurred in multiple places. Darin began to develop the concept of himself as an agent, a person who could perform acts in therapy as well as at home. Multiple uses of the concept of Darin helped him learn who he was and how to behave in multiple places. *Remember: Learning the basic semantic relationships of agent-action-object is necessary to the acquisition of language. And, if the concepts of these relationships are learned, then the meaningfulness of the concepts becomes language-based or semantic in nature. Conceptual, semantic, learning is long term in nature because it represents cognitive and language development.*

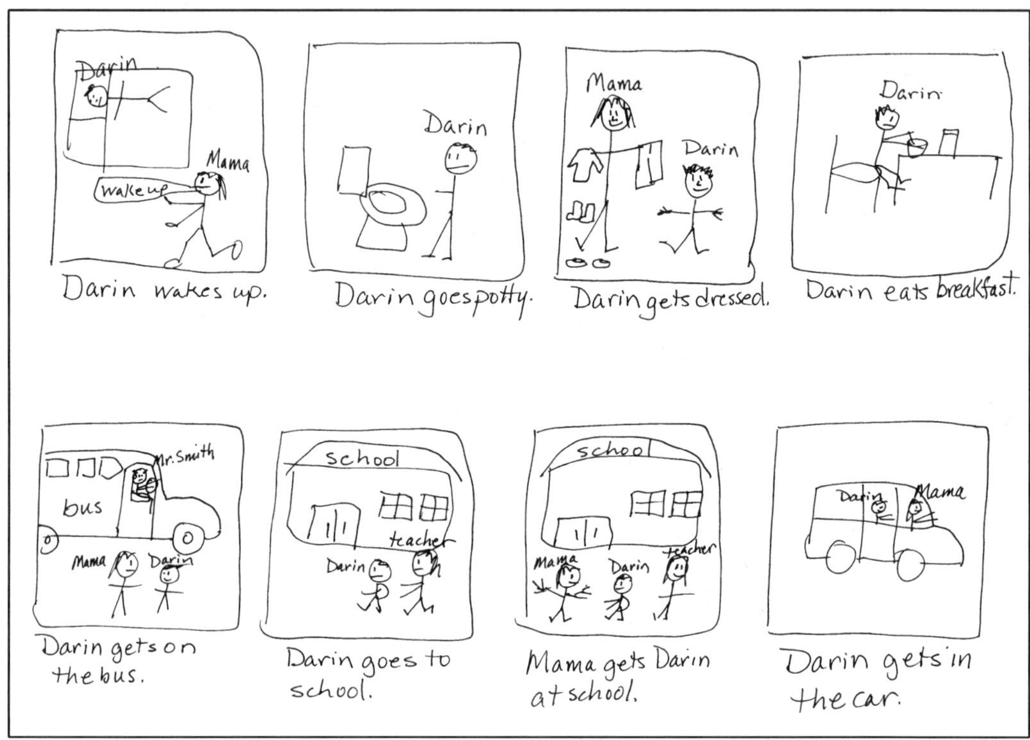

Figure 8.3 Darin is an agent in his day of actions

Activity: Why does Figure 8.3 help Darin learn the concept of being an agent?

3. *Is the intervention changing to meet Darin's changes in learning?* As soon as Darin could match what he did to what his mom and the educator drew about Darin acted like an agent. Darin began to be able to follow the cartoon of actions within the therapy session. His mother drew to get him into his day and the educator drew to help Darin learn how to look during the therapy session. Darin began to learn concepts for writing hand-over-hand (H/H) and he began to be able to "say" back what he wrote which means he began to develop speech (Arwood & Kaulitz, 2007; Arwood *et al.*, 2009). The layers of presentation consisted of the following: (1) showing him visual concepts of people doing actions within a picture while talking about the concepts and pointing to the concepts,[5] (2) visually labeling the concepts by writing the labels on the picture from the story, (3) writing the labels into a picture dictionary, (4 and 5) two types of finger spelling—both writing with the physical finger held and also using the manual alphabet to create a shape in his hand, (6) hand-over-hand writing the concepts or labels that are in the picture dictionary, (7) adding hand-over-hand pictographs to

5 These pictures are event based and simple because they show the entire set of agents, their actions, and their objects. For an understanding of the developmental levels of visuals like pictures refer to *Visual thinking for individuals with autism spectrum disorders: The language of pictures* by Arwood *et al.* (2009).

the hand-over-hand picture dictionary entries to the hand-over-hand written words, (8) more finger spelling in his hand along with encouraging mouth watching, (9) hand-over-hand pointing to what he wrote hand-over-hand on the page while educator pointed to the words that were hand-over-hand written, and (10) he says back what he wrote while pointing (hand-over-hand, if needed). Darin's speech, in addition to his reading and writing, began to emerge from this layered development of motor shapes.

Activity: Why does Darin's learning process of acquiring the meaning of new concepts always stay the same even though he might need less information or fewer layers for old concepts?

Case 8.2: Samantha

The reader was introduced to Samantha in Chapter 7. Samantha needs the same type of assigned meaning as Darin needed even though Samantha is much older. Both children are functioning at a pre-production, pre-language level of functioning. When intervention was provided to Darin, it began as an hour a week with a therapist that helped the parents carry out helping Darin become an agent in his home and at school. With Samantha, the therapy began at school throughout the day so instead of working with pictures cartooned into a single activity or event, the hand-over-hand (H/H) motor assists occurred throughout the day for all activities for Samantha: H/H schedule of the activities of her day to which she pointed to the naming of the activity and she eventually could cross off the activity as they finished it; H/H preparing her own food with pictures to be able to ask for what she wanted to eat and drink; H/H putting her socks, shoes, coat, etc. on as needed to take walks, etc.; H/H making of a bed to take a nap; H/H chores such as collecting school attendance sheets, filling bags for work assignment, and wiping off tables in the cafeteria; H/H pointing to the pictured cartoons in a book to indicate the beginning of a task, activities within a task, and end of a task.

Activity: How are Darin's and Samantha's learning systems alike? What do they each need to learn concepts?

All of these activities provide for motor overlapping of patterns through H/H assigning of meaning or motor imitation to produce concepts that are basic to the early development of semantic relationships to acquire language. In this way, both Darin and Samantha are able to acquire concepts because they receive the appropriate motor shapes from movements of the hands to create the appropriate behavior of doing a task like making the bed or writing an idea as with Darin.

Activity: What are the layers of input provided for Samantha? Why did these work when years of therapy designed to work on products of the learning system such as speech therapy to produce sounds and behavior therapy to act appropriately had failed?

Case 8.3: Jeremy

The reader was introduced to Jeremy in Chapter 7. Jeremy had typical non-verbal semantic relationships. For example, he played like a child typically plays for his age, but he lacked the language to share in the play as an initiator of games or a provider of rules. His language was restricted to telegraphic utterances—two or three-word utterances that require interpretation from the listener. Jeremy has some utterances so he is not in the pre-production, silent period of pre-language function, he is in the telegraphic period of the pre-language function. His utterances represent basic semantic relationships—agents, actions, objects—but it is the listener's responsibility to interpret which relationships are being expressed. For example, when Jeremy said, "Mommy more," did he mean: (1) I want more snack; (2) I want to play more with the toys we just put away; (3) We just put away these toys, so I want more toys, different toys; or (4) I don't want any more toys or snack or other activities...I want to go home. Obviously, the possibilities of interpretation are endless. Even with the very best interpretation based on the context and the child, the child could have a different meaning or intention.

Activity: What type of meaning does Jeremy need to be able to learn concepts for better language development?

A child's pre-language intention (Dore, 1975; Halliday as reported in Maybin, 2003; Halliday, 1975) is based on the interpretation of the adult. The adult interprets the child's intention with the hopes that if the child means something else, the child will begin to refine his thinking and therefore his expression to represent a meaning that is closer to the child's intention. For example, a child says, "No toys." The adult interprets the child's meaning and says, "Oh, you don't want any more toys" and starts to put away the bag of toys. The child begins to emphatically reach for the bag of toys and shakes his head and says, "No, more toys." The child takes the bag and opens the bag to reach for the toys. The child is trying to express his intention that he wants more toys because he does not have any toys. The child's verbal refinement, coupled with his non-verbal acts, help the adult narrow down the child's intention. However, there still exists some interpretation: Does the child mean "I want to play more" or "I want some more toys from the bag" or "I want to see if there are more toys that I haven't played with" or "I want to know what these toys do" and so on. Again, there are many more interpretations, but the adult knows that the child wants to do something with the bag of toys. The adult follows the child's lead and assigns meaning accordingly. This is the basis for intervention for Jeremy.

Activity: What is the basis of intervention for children with limited structures and functioning at the pre-language, pre-production level like Jeremy?

To every activity of the day, meaning is assigned in the way that Jeremy learns concepts. He is not able to use the auditory system of integrating what he hears (sound) to what he sees or he would have developed more language in an auditory culture. So, he does not use an auditory way of creating concepts but he does learn from visual-motor patterns (see assessment in Chapter 7). So, an activity such as going to the store is followed by drawing and writing about the activity. Again, the drawing and writing may need some H/H assistance to help assign the visual-motor patterns to form concepts, as Jeremy is young and has not acquired reading and writing skills. Figure 8.4 shows a typical way to assign meaning to concepts about Jeremy shopping at the store. This example shows the hand-over-hand (H/H) drawing to a picture, H/H bubbling of ideas into a dictionary, H/H writing, and H/H bubbling of the shapes along with the drawings of the meaning to go with the writing.

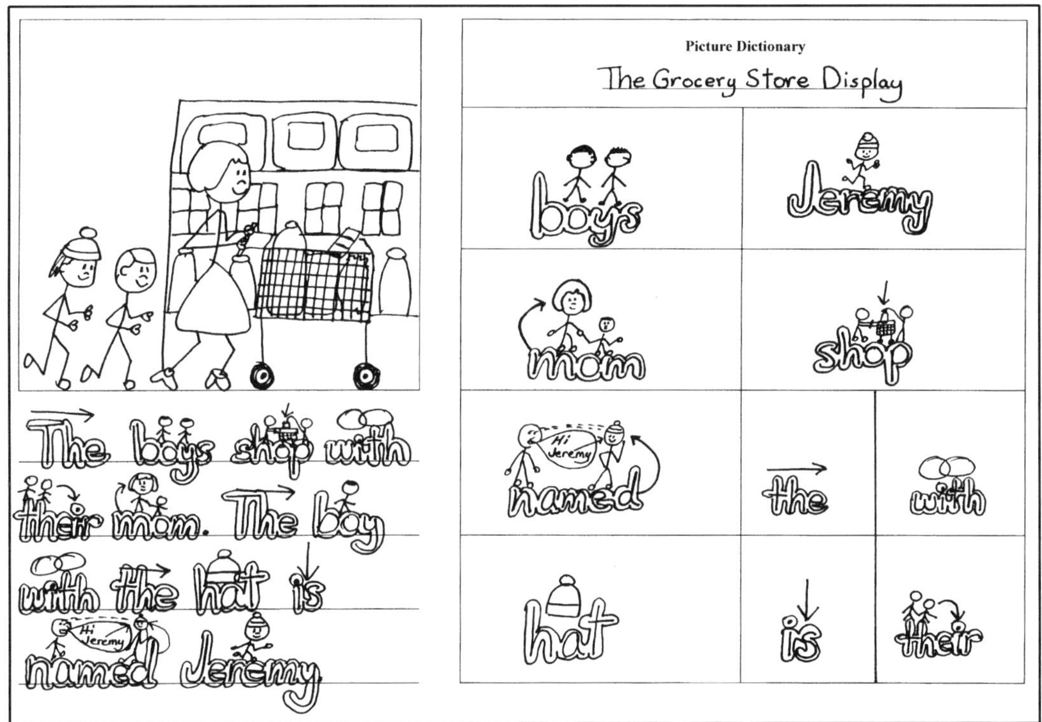

Figure 8.4 Jeremy is learning a visual-motor way to read, write, and speak

Activity: How is Jeremy learning to think for reading, writing, and speaking?

The picture dictionary provides the visual-motor patterns of what English looks like while the drawing shows the concepts that go with the patterns. The writing below the drawing provides the language.[6] When these patterns and concepts are attached to multiple experiences, pictures, and activities, then Jeremy acquires the function of language. He learns the way the oral language *looks* from seeing the visual-motor patterns of the speaker's mouth and hand movements, overlapped with the printed vocabulary words. He learns the spoken and written patterns because they are connected to the concepts which are the drawings. In this way, Jeremy's concepts about himself related to other agents increases. Jeremy begins to develop language that represents his cognitive development. Likewise, as he sees himself in a picture of what he looks like when he works on these tasks; so, he begins to see how he socially relates to others as his language develops. Figure 8.5 shows a cartoon of Jeremy going to the store and then writing about the activity.

6 When patterns and concepts are connected, then language functions.

Bread
Grocery Store
Jeremy and his mom walk into the grocery store to shop for the groceries that are on their grocery list.
Jeremy waits while his mom selects a grocery cart for carrying the groceries that they will pick up.
Bread
Sometimes Mom asks Jeremy to take a food item from the shelf and then hand it to his mom to set in the cart.
5
When all the foods from the grocery list are in the cart, Jeremy and his mom push the cart to the check-out area.
5
After the clerk has finished scanning all the foods, she tells Jeremy's mom how much money she owes for the groceries.
Thank you Good-bye
Bye
Jeremy's mom pays the clerk before they leave the store with their bags of groceries.

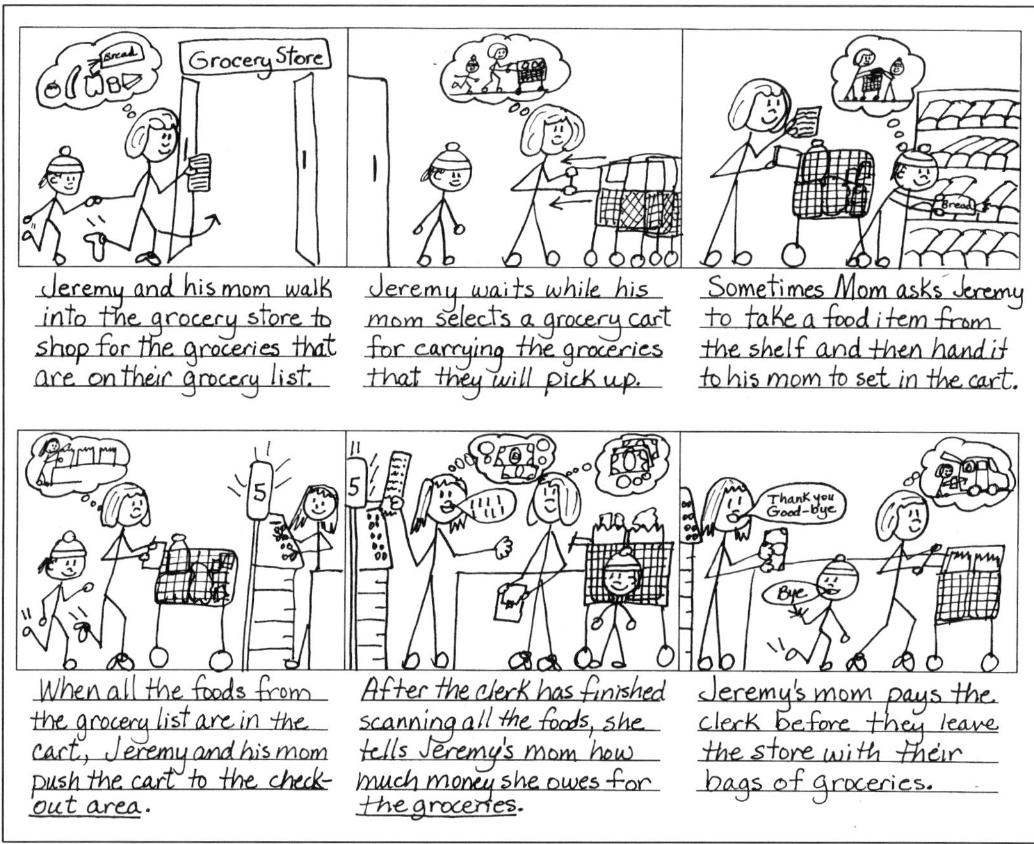

Figure 8.5 Jeremy grocery shops with his mom

This cartoon puts Jeremy into his own picture and helps him develop the visual-motor written patterns of the language structures that assign meaning to his everyday thinking concepts. In this way, Jeremy is also learning to read and write. He is learning to become literate in the way that his learning system develops language. Instead of drills on sounds and phonics and phonemics and phonetic rules, he is learning what the words look like as visual concepts for what he sees and does. He is learning in a visual way that allows his thinking for better language development. His writing allows him to become a good academic learner, as the written language shares the meaning among all types of learners of English.[7]

Activity: How can assigning meaning to what a child does, in the way a child learns concepts, help children learn language? What does the intervention for Jeremy look like?

7 The reader should be reminded that the author is referring to how concepts are learned through the Neuro-Semantic Language Learning Theory, not to learning styles which are educational preferences.

Assigning meaning to neuro-typical English language learners

English language learners (ELLs) experience a silent period when they are introduced to English as a second or third or fourth language. This silent period of time allows for ELLs to listen to the lexical tags,[8] or words being used in English to represent the ELLs' already acquired underlying concepts associated with their first language (L1). English, like all languages, represents the concepts the ELL has already culturally and linguistically acquired in another language (L1).

Intervention for ELLs works incredibly well when speakers of English willingly assign meaning to the concepts previously acquired by ELLs. In other words, a neuro-typical ELL needs to learn the English tags for his or her previously acquired concepts to be able to move out of the silent period and into English language production. In this way, the productions in English represent what the ELL knows from his or her previous conceptual development. The ELL possesses underlying concepts but needs the English structures to represent those underlying concepts.

Activity: What do English language learners need to develop if they already have concepts underlying their first language (L1)?

Imitation and practice of vocabulary and grammar in English or any other language provides the speaker with the structures necessary to represent underlying concepts. As long as the ELL is able to make the structures and vocabulary function to represent underlying concepts, then assigning meaning with English as an L2 or L3 works well. Remember that in the four-tier model of Neuro-Semantic Language Learning, the patterns or language structures must form concepts that the language represents. So, learning more patterns or language structures without conceptual thinking or function will result in imitation and production without comprehension.

Activity: What does imitation of patterns or structures provide?

Case 8.4: Eliza

Eliza is a first grade student who has two first languages spoken at home: Spanish and Vietnamese. English is not typically spoken. She entered first grade with little English. Her sample shows that she has some word-like productions or jargon and a few short, *telegraphic* (two or three words) utterances, typical of the silent, pre-production period of pre-language function. Because children in this developmental level of thinking and learning language are restricted to their use of basic semantic relationships, they are given materials that provide the language and the social-cognitive development that matches the ability to think about themselves as agents in relationship to others and others' actions.

8 Lexical tags refer to the precise words that an individual uses to represent a specific meaning. For example, one person refers to the shiny hanging decorations on a Christmas tree as "tinsel" whereas another person calls those decorations "silver rain." Both tinsel and silver rain are lexical tags for the same concept. Because all people have different experiences, all people have their own *lexicon* consisting of lexical tags, specific to their individual backgrounds.

This age of thinking typically goes from three to seven years and is referred to as preoperational thinking. Pictures that provide these relationships are ***event based*** in nature. By using a picture with all of the language in the picture, the child is given the concepts while the educator provides the patterns that go with the concepts, either through writing, drawing, speaking, signing, and/or finger spelling. This way the educator is giving the child both the thinking and the language. Together the child is learning to think with language and learning language to be able to think.

Activity: How does an event-based picture help a child with language learning?

To an ***event-based*** picture[9] (Arwood, 1985; Arwood & Unruh, 1997) about some men picking up the garbage cans when suddenly a kitten jumps out of one of the garbage cans and scares one of the garbage collectors, Eliza says: "um…uh…um…put. kitty, him." Fortunately, Eliza is in a language-based classroom where the teacher does not teach the parts of language or language structures but emphasizes language functions (Arwood *et al.*, 2005; Arwood & Robb, 2008; Arwood & Young, 2000). Her teacher draws concepts, labels them with English patterns or words so that Eliza can see what the English word looks like that goes with the drawn concept; and then the teacher gives Eliza the opportunity to draw her own ideas that go with the classroom story.

Activity: What does an event provide a child for learning?

In this way, Eliza learns to write the patterns, say the patterns, read the patterns of the English words (lexical tags) that represent the concepts that Eliza knows in her first language. In four months, Eliza's English changed dramatically. To an event-based picture about a family working in a garden plot, Eliza says:

> They are working in the garden. The dad, what's this called (rake)…rakes the dirt. The boy pick the lettuce. There is a Grandma that peel the corn. She gives the corn to this boy. This boy and his dad grow a big garden and Grandma helps them with the corn. Then they go inside and cook the corn and eat it.

She also is at grade level with her English speaking peers for academic subjects; reading, writing, and calculating.

By the end of the year, this ELL student, as well as 11 other ELL students in this general education classroom (26 total students), perform at grade level or up to three years ahead of peers on district tests. The teacher is providing Eliza and her peers with the lexical tags or language patterns with concepts so that Eliza is able to transform her knowledge she has acquired in Spanish and Vietnamese into English forms of expression. She and the other 11 students are no longer in the silent period of pre-production of language function.

Activity: Why did this type of classroom work for Eliza? What was the basis to the intervention that moved her out of the silent, pre-production period of pre-language function?

---

9 Events are people or agents doing their actions with objects in a shared context.

Older students and adults are able to perform with similar success with English as an L2 or L3 or L4 or L5, as long as they receive the English lexical tags for their already acquired concepts. Emphasis on memorization of language structures such as vocabulary and grammar for English will not provide them with language function. For example, the author once worked in an elementary school where a buddy system was used. Many students arrived at the school with no English but they came from rich language environments of a first language. Children with excellent English function volunteered and were trained as buddies. Each buddy was assigned to mentor an ELL for six weeks. During the six weeks, it was the buddy's responsibility to assign meaning to all academic and social tasks that the buddy could talk about, point out, show, demonstrate, draw, etc. The buddy was to provide the English tags for everyday (including academic tasks) activities. The ELL could see the concepts as long as the buddy pointed out which concept went with which English word. In six weeks, the ELLs were able to do their own academic tasks in English at grade level expectations.

Activity: Why does the buddy system work for assigning meaning to an ELL?

Adults also come to the US without any English. Again, if they have acquired and have used a rich first language, then they just need the tags. Often after a week or two of English designed to assign meaning to their knowledge, they are able to move out of the silent pre-production period and into more language function. How effective these programs are for ELLs depends on three criteria:

1. Does the ELL have an intact first language that functions at a grammatical level of complete language function (shared reciprocal conversation in the L1)?
2. Does the program provide the ELL with the opportunity to see the concepts (drawing, pointing, doing an activity) that look like the ones in the L1 and then show the word (print and spoken overlapped) to go with the concepts?
3. Does the program provide for the ELLs to use their own drawings or representations for their conceptualization to be assigned meaning in English to ***retag*** concepts?

Activity: What are the necessary intervention characteristics of an English language learning environment?

It is important to realize that if the English language learner does not have a complete, grammatical first language, then the assigning of meaning will need to be more like the neuro-atypical language learner. Meaning will need to be assigned using an overlap of layers of a different type of input such as drawing with hand-over-hand writing and signing (e.g., Darin) or with pointing to sequenced pictures (e.g., Samantha) or with drawing and writing (e.g., Jeremy). An English language learner who is not successful in quickly learning the English tags when given the opportunity to see what the English tags and structures (patterns) look like matched to concepts (drawings) has other difficulties than just learning English.

Summary

Intervention for pre-production, silent pre-language thinkers is based on how to assign meaning. Meaning is assigned based on how the child learns concepts. If the child learns the concepts by overlapping motor patterns, the adult can use hand-over-hand motor patterns with activities of daily living to reading and writing and drawing to develop language. Goals at this level should be to move the child from the silent, pre-production period of cognitive thinking to the telegraphic period and eventually to the inter-language period (Chapters 9 and 10).

Goals and objectives should reflect the type of layers used to create patterns that will form concepts. Darin, for example, requires nine to ten different layers of motor patterns to create enough meaning for him to form concepts. But, an ELL student like Eliza with a grammatical first language will need only an overlap of spoken and written language to form the patterns or language structures to go with the concepts of the L1. How many layers a child requires will depend on how the child's learning system acquires concepts and how quickly the child can use those layers to form concepts. Of course, this is all based on the notion that the adult is providing the input in the way the child learns concepts.

Concepts at the pre-production, pre-language function stage are restricted to the development of basic semantic relationships of agents, their actions, and their objects within an event or context. So, as soon as a child develops sufficient conceptual development to use language in a written or spoken form then, the child is moving out of the silent period into the telegraphic period. These telegraphic utterances also refine to include more semantic relationships in complex language structures. The child then shows a verbal pre-language way of thinking. Chapter 9 discusses how to assess children who are very verbal but still exhibit a pre-language restricted way of thinking.

Applications

- Try to cartoon at least one set of activities for a session with a pre-production, limited language thinker.
- Try to assign meaning for a child without language by using hand-over-hand methods.

Chapter 9

INTERVENTION FOR VERBAL, PRODUCTION-LEVEL, PRE-LANGUAGE THINKERS

Learner objectives: Chapter 9

Upon completion of this chapter, the reader should be able to:

1. Explain how to assess and evaluate the language of a verbal, pre-language thinker.
2. Assess and evaluate a verbal, pre-language thinker.
3. Explain the types of Viconic Language Methods™ to help a verbal, pre-language thinker become literate.
4. Explain how language function affects the seven processes of literacy: speaking, thinking, viewing, listening, reading, writing, and calculating.
5. Explain how to teach reading and writing as a visual-motor way of thinking rather than as a sound-based, alphabetic property of oral English.

I see some of what you know,
I view some of what the world knows.
But, my abilities are restricted,
I am in my own picture.

Children learn language. If there is a disruption in the learning process (Part I), then there is a breakdown in a child's language. Assessment of a child's language function will provide information about how a child is learning (Chapters 7 and 8) and subsequently, the assessment results provide knowledge about how to intervene to help the child learn to be literate. The overall purpose of intervention for individuals with restricted language function has two different types of emphasis: First, assign meaning to develop the learning of basic concepts such as agency for those with pre-production or limited structural development (Chapters 7 and 8), and second, provide literacy options to increase cognition and language function. Chapter 8 offered suggestions for how to intervene with those who are in a pre-production or limited production period (Chapter 7) of pre-language thinking by assigning meaning to activities of daily living as well as to basic events of agents, their actions, and objects.

The purpose of this chapter is to discuss intervention for those individuals who function as pre-language thinkers, but who possess lots of language structures. Two cases showcase the different ways to intervene to help verbal children, youth, and adults who function at this pre-language level. Upon completion of this chapter, the reader should be able to plan intervention for individuals with lots of language structures but who think in a restricted, pre-language manner.

Case 9.1: Charley

What is known about Charley? He is a six-year-old male who is referred for a language evaluation by his grandmother. His grandmother reports that Charley doesn't "sound like other children" and he never stops talking. Charley has no other siblings and the non-stop talking bothers his parents, but they do not know what children at six years of age are supposed to sound like. Charley received a formal speech and language evaluation at a university speech and hearing clinic. His "receptive vocabulary" was above age level. He could perform at age level to a picture type of test that measured grammatical forms such as "Which picture shows the boy carrying the elephant?" He passed speech tests that evaluated articulation and fluency. Based on a language sample, the clinicians determined that Charley was capable of producing speech at age level along with complete grammatical sentences. The university clinical personnel indicated that Charley had no speech or language problem.

The people at the university speech clinic referred Charley and his family to a psychologist at the same university. The psychologist completed a battery of tests on Charley. He found more than a 50 point discrepancy between Charley's performance and verbal IQ scores on a test where 13 points is considered statistically significant. Furthermore, the psychologist realized that there was something different about Charley's communication. The child was then referred to the author, who evaluated Charley's language by assessing his *function of language*, rather than his development of language structures.

Activity: What did the speech and language tests tell about Charley's language development?

Assessment

The assessment questions for a child like Charley are similar to those asked about Darin, a pre-production, pre-language child. But there are also some differences in questions for a pre-language thinker who uses a lot of language like Charley. Because the educator knows from the grandmother's referral that Charley talks "all the time," it can be assumed that he has a lot of language structure, but how his language functions is unknown. So, a sample of his language structures must be collected to evaluate how his structures function.

LANGUAGE SAMPLING

For a child younger than seven or eight, a picture that shows the complete event of agents, actions, and objects provides the meaning for a child to tell his story of what he knows.

To assist the child in understanding that the evaluator wants a story told about the picture, the adult uses an event-based picture to tell a story. As the adult tells a story, the adult uses very complex language that the child cannot imitate. And then the adult puts out some new pictures and encourages the child to select a picture to tell his or her story: "Okay, it is your turn to tell a story. You pick a picture to tell your story." The child is supposed to pick a picture and the adult asks the child, "Okay, tell me your story about this picture."

Sometimes, the adult must cue the child with a verbal prompt such as, "You can begin your story with 'Once-upon-a-time…'" In sampling Charley's language, he chose to talk about the Berenstain Bears (1962) book, *The big honey hunt.*

Charley looked through the pages and told his story. He turned the pages as he talked. Charley's words were audio recorded and then transcribed to be sure that his words were written exactly the way he spoke them. The utterances were numbered according to the child's natural pausing between ideas.

Activity: What is the process of language sampling?

Note that Charley's utterances are all consecutive. Any comments by the adult are in square brackets.

1. "Who's in the tree?"
2. "Oh, oh! He water!"
3. "Who fall in that?"
4. "That's his coppee."
5. "He…(pause)…he's pouring coppee in the cup, more gone."
6. "Boy…(pause)…eats the coppee."
7. "A house…(pause)…light."
8. "Who's…(pause)…he's run."
9. "Who's that doing?"
10. "Honey."
11. "Boys put the foots and his toe, see."
12. "Oh he's…put his tree foots."
13. "He's sawn the butterfly." ["Bees."]
14. "He flowed away and its butterfly."
15. "See, de, de, de." (The child pointed to the three bees.)
16. "He's taking the hand."
17. "Oops! He's sweet the butterfly."
18. "Climbing."
19. "He's climbing the ground."
20. "Who's on the match?"
21. "A match!" ["That's a flower."]
22. "Flower?"
23. "See."

24. "Flying the tree?"
25. "Who's fall the bee?"
26. "Who's fall?"
27. "Wait! That's an owl!"
28. "He's tryin to go bye bye."
29. "He's go bye bye."
30. "See go bye bye."
31. "See, that's trees."
32. "Goed away."
33. "He took a mouth and climbs."
34. "He's took a teeth and he bites…over the key."
35. "Where's the flies?" ["Where's the what?"]
36. "Butterflies in the door."
37. "Who's bumped it?"
38. "Who's bumped?"
39. "That's a tree."
40. "He's go away in the butterfly."
41. "He's bye bye."
42. "Boy bye."
43. "Boy."
44. "He's giving the hand and bang."
45. "Wait! He falled the lap."
46. "Look butterfly!"
47. "Goes in the bucket and the tree."
48. "Who's in the coppee? Huh?"
49. "In the coppee."

The first time the child was referred to the university speech and language clinic, in addition to testing his language, his oral language was analyzed for structures: average morphemes per utterance, number of different words, and intelligibility. The results of the structural analysis suggested that his language was adequate for a child his age. When Charley was sent back by the psychologist to the university speech and language clinic, the author collected a new sample (Berenstain Bears sample) and analyzed it for language function. This is the second sample. For example, in the first two utterances the child uses a complete grammatical sentence, "Who's in the tree?" and also an incomplete sentence, "Oh, oh! He water!"

From a structural standpoint, he is able to produce complete sentences. However, from a functional perspective, Charley omitted critical components of meaning in the sample. For example, in the utterance, "Oh, oh! He water!" there is information that is missing: Who is in the water? What is the person or bear doing with the water? Why is Charley referring to water when the picture is about a dark substance like coffee or tea being poured into a cup? Where is the act taking place? When does the act occur? In other words, from a functional language perspective, Charley's thinking is restricted.

Activity: How is Charley's language functioning? Is it restricted?

Evaluation of assessment

Charley's language structures were ascertained to be okay through language sampling and formal tests, but, according to the second language sample, his language function was restricted to another person's willingness to complete Charley's intended meaning. If a child has a lot of language structures but still appears limited in his or her ability to converse with others, there are some questions to add to the pre-language function, ANSPA, protocol (Appendix A) to assess a child's pre-language function (see Appendix B). Box 9.1 shows these questions followed by an analysis of Charley's language function.

Box 9.1 Assessment for restricted language function

Pre-language functions of restricted language:

1. Does the child address others and expect others to respond? This assesses the function of the child (agent) in *relationship* to others (relational function).
2. Are the child's utterances appropriate for the *context*? This assesses the function of whether the child's language *refers* to the topic (referential function).
3. Does the child use the utterances to *share* the meaning of the context? This assesses the child's *shared-referent* function (shared function).
4. Does the child use *consistent* age-appropriate forms? This assesses the child's ability to use different forms for different meanings (*productivity function*).
5. Does the listener have to interpret the child's *intent* or *specific meaning*? This assesses the child's ability to develop a variety of meanings (*semanticity function*).
6. Does the child talk about the "*here and now*?" This assesses how well the child can talk about ideas that the child cannot see or touch or may be in time or place that is at a distance from the child (*displacement function*).
7. Does the child talk about a *variety* of different topics? This assesses the child's ability to use a variety of different types of utterances (*flexibility function*).

8. Are the child's utterances semantically *accurate* in meaning? This assesses another aspect of how well the child is acquiring concepts (*semanticity function*).
9. Are the child's utterances succinct in meaning or *redundant*? This assesses how well the child can use the English language to mean exactly what is intended—who, what, where, when, why, how?
10. Does the listener understand the speaker's meaning without having to take on more than a "shared" level of understanding? This assesses whether or not the language functions in a concrete way of sharing meaning.

Answering the questions in Box 9.1 for Charley helps provide data for establishing goals for intervention.

1. Does the child address others and expect others to respond? Even though this child has lots of language, he asked several questions that he did not expect anyone to answer. He would continue to talk after asking a question. This means that the child does not have a good conceptual understanding of himself as a person who does something (agent) with others (agents). This suggests that he is struggling to become an agent. A problem in developing agency restricts his ability to function in relationship to others. He is in his own thoughts, but is he thinking about anyone else? At his age of six years, he should be at the end of the preoperational level, which means he should see himself as an agent and see others as agents. In other words, when he asks a question, he should be directing the question to someone else, and then he should wait to have the other person answer.

Activity: What does not responding to others mean?

2. Are the child's utterances appropriate for the *context*? The context was provided by giving him a story book. He talked about the story. This suggests that he has lots of information about this context, information that a six-year-old would typically have. The child talks or refers to the general meaning in the book. But there are times when he does not recognize the different ways that the bears or their actions or their objects look. In other words, there are times that his utterances do not represent what most six-year-olds would say; for example, when he saw the flower as a match. Or, when he recognized the bears at one point but not at another time. This means that he is learning certain types of ***semantic features*** of the concepts, but he is having trouble putting all of the features together as a concept that does not change meaning just because of the way the concept looks or is illustrated.

Activity: Why do you think that Charley is seeing parts but not the whole?

3. Does the child use the utterances (language structures) to *share* the meaning of the context? No, he really did not expect others to engage in the story. In fact, he ignored or refuted what the clinician did say. For example, when she tried to tell him the butterflies were bees, he said, "No…" This means that his language structures do not function for the purpose of sharing meaning between two or more people. It also may mean that he cannot utilize the sound of a person's voice in order to add meaning to some of his thinking. For example, Charley could not use the clinician's spoken words to refine his understanding when the clinician tried to provide him meaning with her oral language.

Activity: Why does Charley not maintain a conversation with the adult?

4. Does the child use *consistent* age-appropriate forms? No. He sometimes uses grammatical forms and sometimes he does not. He does not show products that are at the same developmental level. If the language develops at a consistent rate, then the structures will demonstrate consistent development. Since Charley is six years old, almost seven years old, his language structures should be in grammatical forms that are similar to adult sentence structures. Remember from Part I, most children possess a complete, grammatical set of adult language structures by seven to eight years of age. Most adults, without any language training, are able to report intuitively whether or not language structures are grammatical in their native language. So, look at the child's or adult's utterances and determine whether or not the utterances are grammatical. Notice that for Charley, the first utterance is the only fully grammatical utterance of the first five utterances.

Activity: At what age should a child show a consistent grammatical use of language?

1. Who's in the tree?
2. Oh, oh! He water.
3. Who fall in that?
4. That's his coppee.
5. He…(pause)…he's pouring the coppee in the cup, more gone.

Because utterances 2, 3, and 4 are not grammatical, Charley's oral language is not grammatically complete which would be expected for his age. And, notice that utterances 2 and 3 are only telegraphic utterances, approximately two-word utterances that would be more typical of a two-year-old child. A six-year-old, like Charley, should be able to tell a story with grammatical structures that the listener would understand. There are several places where he does not tell a complete story. This means that even though he passed formal language tests at age level, his lack of age-appropriate language utterances in a context like this suggests that he is having difficulty acquiring the meaning necessary to support the language structures. Even though he "talks a lot," his language is not very productive. Productivity is an important language function. *When inconsistent development is present in language structures, the underlying development of meaning or semantics is not fully developed. In other words, the underlying semantic meaning is limited by restricted function and so is his productivity. Charley is missing some of the essential meaning needed to support grammatical structures.*

Activity: Using the answers to questions 1–4, why does the analysis of Charley's language sample show that Charley has a problem acquiring semantic development underlying the structure of language?

5. Does the listener have to interpret the child's *intent* or *specific meaning*? Yes. In fact the listener lost track of the number of different meanings the child assigned to the bees—butterflies, bees, flies, and several places he wanted to know what the "bees" were. This suggests that the child's learning system restricts the way he is able to acquire meaning. In other words, he is not learning meaning from the auditory way the dominant culture assigns meaning. His development of meaning (semanticity) is restricted to the specific way this child's learning system functions to bring information into the patterns that form concepts.

Activity: What is the problem with Charley not using the same "word" for bees?

6. Does the child talk about the "*here-and-now*"? Yes. In the pre-language stage of language function, the language operates only in a restricted form so it is in the here-and-now. Charley should be showing signs that he is beginning to talk about ideas that are removed from the here-and-now; that is, ideas that are more displaced. When the bees change shapes and move from one place to another, Charley should be able to recognize that they are still bees.

Activity: In what way is telling this story not like Charley's own life?

7. Does the child talk about a *variety* of different topics? He does talk about a lot of different ideas but he is not able to refer to specific ideas to show how ideas connect to form topics. To be flexible, an important language function, Charley's utterances would have to be able to stand alone and provide adequate meaning to the listener to understand. For example, when the child says, "He water," the child is referring to the Bear pouring coffee…there is no water. When the child said, "Who's on the match?" there is no match but a flower that has the shape and color like a match. His flexibility is very restricted for a child his age, even though he talks about different ideas; the ideas restrict the meaning of the topics. So, he is acquiring some meaning but there are gaps in his development of concepts as part of a whole story.

Activity: Which language functions are restricted (e.g., displacement)?

8. Are the child's utterances semantically *accurate* in meaning? Again, the answer is no. He struggles with putting the meaning of what he sees with the words he knows; he says "who" when he means "what" and he does not recognize agents like bears or bees when they change actions or visual features, such as resting instead of flying or flapping wings. This means that he is acquiring meaning but not by the sound of what others say (argues about the clinician's words) and not by just seeing the objects or people and what they look like when they perform an action. Charley uses the two utterances of "Boys put the foots and his toe, see" and "Oh he's…put his tree foots," probably to refer to the footprints that the author illustrates for the reader. And, "Who's on the match?" refers to "Who is on the flower?" as he does not understand that when the "butterflies" are no longer flying he does not recognize them. And, when the bees are no longer in the hive, Charley no longer recognizes the bees. Charley is able to use movements such as flying or not flying to give him meaning about what defines the insects. His development of meaning (semanticity) is restricted to what he sees move and the features of movement that characterize the meaning of a concept. Charley's ability to create meaning from the movements suggests that these movements form shapes for him in a way that develops his concepts. But this also means that sound and some visual features do not create conceptual meaning.

Activity: Charley does not have an auditory language learning system. What type of input does he appear to understand?

9. Are the child's utterances succinct in meaning or *redundant*? The utterances do not stand alone, and do not share meaning with another person without the other person interpreting from other cues or information; so the child's utterances are not functioning in a reciprocal way. In fact, the utterances are not succinct to the point that there is also some unnatural redundancy. For example, it takes Charley the first five utterances to process a basic agent, action, and object utterance. "Who's in the tree?" means who is the agent? "Oh, oh! He water" names the object. "Who fall in that?" refers to the action, pour. "That's his coppee" is a renaming of the object, coffee, which he has recorded as a word, coppee. And, finally he says "He's pouring coppee in the cup, more gone." He uses "more gone" for the past tense. There is redundancy elsewhere as well…by the end of the story, his own processing of the story with oral language has not helped his utterances become succinct. Instead, he asks the same questions he did at the beginning, "Who's in the coppee?" English is designed to have the words as the unit of analysis and therefore words can stand alone. For this child, the words are relative to what he sees as features of meaning such as "flying" being a specific characteristic of action. Therefore his function of English is not succinct.

Activity: What type of properties of English help make English succinct?

10. Does the listener understand the speaker's meaning without having to take on more than a "shared" level of understanding? This assesses whether or not the language functions in a concrete way of sharing meaning as part of a conversation.

The simple answer is "No, the listener does not know what Charley is intending to mean in many of his utterances." More about this lack of "shared meaning" follows later in this chapter.

Activity: Using the answers to questions 5-10, in what ways is Charley's language restricted in language function?

SUMMARY OF ASSESSMENT

Charley's language is restricted in function (not necessarily in structure) because he does not possess the underlying semantic relationships fully to support grammatical language for which the listener does not have to infer. In other words, he can produce language structures such as present tense, present progressive tense, a variety of vocabulary words, appropriate sounds for the most part, questions, declaratives, and so forth. But, Charley does not create shared meaning between himself and the listener. The listener must follow along and infer or guess at Charley's meaning. This sample is a classic, restricted example of function which means that Charley is able to produce utterances; but, Charley's thinking is restricted to the here-and-now in relationship to what he is acquiring as meaningful information. Therefore, he is a verbal, production-level, pre-language thinker.

Activity: This sample shows a number of concerns related to the child's language function. What are the concerns?

Planning intervention

The previous questions provide the educator with information for intervention. Charley needs more help with his meaning. If the assessment stops at this point, then intervention may focus on vocabulary. But vocabulary is a product of learning, and Charley passed a vocabulary test at age level. His products are okay. Charley has a lot to say and a lot of language structures. More assessment about how Charley is *learning* to function or think with his language is needed to provide intervention that is based on function, not structures. The following questions must be answered to plan intervention:

1. Is this language function neuro-typical, for a child of Charley's age? This question helps determine if intervention is warranted.
2. Does the listener have to interpret the meaning for Charley by using pictures, visuals, context cues, and so forth? This question helps provide information about how Charley learns concepts.
3. How does Charley learn the words he uses? How does he learn concepts the best? This question helps determine how to provide material for Charley so he can learn.
4. What is Charley able to learn? This question helps focus intervention on strengths, not deficits.

The chapter now answers the aforementioned questions.

1. Is this language function neuro-typical, for a child of Charley's age?[1]

Language structures and language functions should be at the same level of development. Charley should show all utterances at the same grammatical level (previous question 4) but he does not. This means that there is uneven learning. Some features of input are becoming patterns for concept development and some features of sensory input are not. Furthermore, his development of agency by the time he is about three should show that he recognizes that there are others to whom he talks while they listen and so forth. This exchange stems from those basic semantic relationship functions (Chapters 3–6) that are the foundation to all language. Basic semantic relationships (agents to agents performing shared actions in a story) provide the basis for conversation. He should have those semantic relationships functioning as agents to other agents at around three years of age. This language function increases in a neuro-typical learning system and meaning becomes shared for a reciprocal conversational quality by about four years of age. The speaker says something to which the listener responds or refers. In this way the listener becomes the speaker and the first speaker is now the listener. Because Charley does not have that type of shared semantic relationships (agents to agents) and is six years old, it is apparent that he does not have the basis for conversation. With restricted development of meaning, he will be restricted in the most important functions of auditory language: displacement, semanticity, productivity, flexibility, and redundancy.[2] In fact, since his language is restricted to utterances about concepts in the "here-and-now" then he shows limited displacement, flexibility, productivity, and explicit meaning (semanticity). He is thinking in the preoperational level of thinking where no one else is in his picture and where his ideas relate to himself and to his needs. Because he talks a lot about a lot of ideas, he is able to acquire lots of meaning but is not able to refine his meaning with the sound of his voice or someone else's voice. His learning system must not be using the sound of others' voices or his own voice to refine his thinking. In turn, his thinking will not refine his language.

At Charley's age, which is comparable to preoperational thinking, his ability to be an agent speaking to another agent suggests that not only is his language restricted but his ability to think or function with his language is not typical of a child his age. Intervention is warranted even though he is of a preoperational age. *If language function is restricted then the speaker's language represents pre-language thinking. Pre-language function represents preoperational thinking at any age. However, with Charley who chronologically is at a preoperational age, his inability to relate his thinking to others is not typical.*

Activity: Why is Charley's language function, even though he is of a preoperational age, not neuro-typical?

1 This question is very important because Charley is only six and still developing structures. Beyond seven to eight years of age, the question is not related to age. In other words, the question is: Is this speaker's language function neuro-typical in nature?

2 A book about animals was chosen by the clinician. Note that personification, where animals are agents, is more difficult, but with as much language structure as Charley possesses, he should not have difficulty recognizing the animals as agents in relationship to himself. Most three-year-olds are able to handle some personification. By five years of age, simple personification where the animal does everyday tasks such as pouring a liquid is easy for most thinkers.

2. Does the listener have to interpret the meaning for Charley by using pictures, visuals, context cues, and so forth? Does the listener understand what the child means by interpreting just the speaker's oral language? Or does the listener need pictures, additional cues, answers to additional questions to understand clearly what the speaker means?

For example, look at the first five utterances:

1. Who's in the tree?
2. Oh, oh! He water.
3. Who fall in that?
4. That's his coppee.
5. He...(pause)...he's pouring coppee in the cup, more gone.

If the reader needs the pictures to understand these utterances fully, then Charley's words do not stand alone. The words by themselves should tell a story to someone who is listening. If Charley is telling a story and is therefore talking to someone, his questions require a response. Charley is *not* waiting for responses to his questions. Charley is not talking to another agent or listener. Charley's words are not telling a story to anyone. Children with really good language are able to tell excellent stories by five years of age. Charley is six. The lack of clarity of meaning between Charley and an intended listener means that Charley's language function is *restricted* in meaning at a level lower than his chronological age. Restricted language function suggests that the language structures do not stand alone without additional interpretation, cues, gestures, pictures, and so forth. Without additional cues or additional information, the listener cannot determine intended meaning.

Activity: Why does a lack of clarity indicate that English is not developing the way the language typically does?

Remember that the words should stand alone in this story. But, there are many times that the listener does not understand what Charley means by his words. For example, what does Charley mean by "he water" or "that's his coppee?" The adult has to interpret the meaning of the words by using the pictures or the adult has to understand the picture book, not Charley's words. For example, these words could mean that the liquid pours like water or that Charley does not know what coffee is or that the Bear is thirsty and wants more water. The options for interpretation are many. On the other hand, if the reader thinks that there is only one interpretation, the reader is assuming the meaning for Charley. The reader is the speaker and the listener.

It is important in analyzing language function that the evaluator not take on the responsibility of the conversational roles. Language functions establish the shared meaning between a speaker and a listener. Being able to listen and to speak in a shared conversation is a part of becoming literate. Literacy includes speaking, listening, thinking, viewing, reading, writing, and calculating. Without the ability to share the speaking, listening, thinking, and viewing aspects of literacy, teaching a child like Charley how to read and write utilizing sound-based properties of English will not be very effective. Charley will need some other approach to his literacy since he does not develop sound-based semantic relationships for shared meaning. He does not learn meaning from the sound of others speaking.

Activity: Why is it important not to interpret the meaning for the speaker?

3. How does Charley learn the words he uses? How does he learn concepts the best?

In the Neuro-Semantic Language Learning model, each level of acquisition is a semantic or meaningful level. The sensory input is *meaningful to the receptors* (first level). Then the sensory input becomes organized into recognizable or *meaningful patterns* of perception. These perceptual patterns become concepts if the learner is able to turn the patterns into concepts. Concepts are ideas or cognition and so they are *meaningful* and underlie the development of language. And, at the fourth level, language patterns or structures represent the concepts. So, natural language *meaningfully* represents the underlying concepts.

An educator is able to evaluate the child's language for what the child knows about the concepts in his world, concepts like bees or butterflies. By determining what information Charley has acquired and what information he is lacking, the educator can determine how Charley is learning concepts; in other words, which patterns in Charley's learning system form which kind of concepts? For Charley, semantic acquisition is very different than might be expected. Neuro-typical concept development allows meaning to be additive. When a speaker uses one concept like "butterfly" and someone corrects the meaning by saying "bee" then the neuro-typical speaker integrates his thinking with the semantic correction. Charley is not able to integrate all of the input that he receives to form concepts. For example, even when the educator corrects the use of butterflies or flies for bees, Charley does not integrate the meaning from the educator. *This suggests that Charley does not use the sound of the educator's voice for adding meaning to his conceptualization.*

So how does Charley learn concepts the best? Remember that concepts are only acquired in the way that a learner can process the sensory input into patterns that will form concepts. And, there are neurobiologically limited ways that sensory input can form concepts: acoustic-visual overlapping patterns form auditory concepts (English); visual-visual overlapping patterns will form visual concepts such as seeing others' actions and being able to imitate those actions; or a motor access to developing the shapes forms visual concepts. Because Charley's oral language shows that he does not have typical English use of concepts, he does not develop concepts the *assumed* way that most people learn an auditory language like English, by the speech of others. Charley is well behaved and imitates what he sees others do so he is able to imitate some visual overlapping patterns into concepts. So, what does he see that others do or don't see?

In the sample, he sees something flying so it is a butterfly because in his mind he knows that butterflies fly. When he is corrected, he argues by saying, "He flowed away and its butterfly." He is not learning concepts through the integration of speech or sound and sight (what he sees) which means that his own corrections of what he speaks also do not help him build concepts. For example, notice that in the first utterance he wants to know who is pouring the coffee and in the last utterance he wants to know who is pouring the coffee, even though he eventually identified the character as a bear. He did not learn from the spoken utterances of the adult or from his own spoken utterances.

Charley processes the visual features of what he sees into patterns but not concepts. He has trouble labeling anything that changes visual patterns. It should be noted that children really do not learn to label and Charley is a good example of that notion. He is able to say the name of the object but Charley does not have the underlying meaning of the concept, bee, at a high enough level to understand all of the visual features that a bee might have. Charley relies on the movement of the visual features to give him more information to form concepts that he cannot see, touch, or feel. For example, he sees the bees as flying so they are butterflies. When they rest on a flower, he confuses the shape of the flower for a match and does not see the bee move so he does not know what it is. When the flying critter arrives at the hole (bucket) in the tree, then he sees the insect as a bee because bees "make" honey. He notices the movements or actions but he cannot create a concept from "seeing." Later when the flying bees approach the door of the tree house and bounce off the door, he *sees* the bees as flies because he has seen flies come into a house. Charley uses movement to identify different insects rather than using a word to represent the visual features he *sees*. This means that Charley uses his motor system for helping him gather information to form concepts that he can mentally see.

Activity: Why is Charley having difficulty "labeling" a bee?

Another example of Charley's thinking or language function which determines how he learns best can be seen in utterance 11: "Boys put the foots and his toe, see." This utterance refers to "walking"...the act of seeing one foot move up and then put down; and, then another foot move forward and put down. Charley is able to "see" the actions of the feet as still photographs. Each picture frame shows a movement. Multiple frames of the feet up and then down is how Charley sees the feet move. But, Charley is not able to take the sound of the word "walking" and attach that sound word to what he sees in the still photographs of the feet being up and then down. So, Charley learns object vocabulary easily. Objects like tables don't move. This is why he uses vocabulary such as "match," "owl" (not moving), "coffee," and "ground," and he performs well on picture vocabulary tests. The ball always looks like a ball so he seldom confuses its image with other objects. But people, insects, mouths, feet... anything that moves creates multiple mental pictures for Charley. He is not able to see how one sound word refers to all the different mental pictures he possesses for the actions of something or someone that moves.

Activity: When does Charley have trouble learning some "word names" but not other word names?

4. What is Charley able to learn?

Charley thinks in *what he sees that moves.* So, Charley has a literal interpretation of his world. If an object is constant, he can put the language label to what he sees. But, semantics includes not only the literal concepts of what a person sees but also an expansion of meaning for concepts that do not remain constant; concepts one cannot see, touch, and feel. Because people or agents move or perform actions, Charley has difficulty relating to people. He struggles with the meaning of ***social interactions***. For example, notice that he uses "who" (agent) for "what" (object) interchangeably as in utterance 3 "Who fall in that?" for "What is he pouring?" or possibly in place of a "who" question, "Who is pouring that?" In utterance 25 he also confuses the who and the what: "Who's fall the bee?" for "Who is reaching into the tree?" or possibly for a what question, "What is he reaching for?" Charley also has trouble recognizing personified animals, the bears, because they too move into different positions as agents.

Activity: Why does Charley have trouble identifying people or personified animals?

Charley is learning to put a *tag*, his vocabulary word, onto his mental picture. But insects and people and personified animals all move and create numerous pictures for Charley. So, Charley thinks every time he has a different mental picture, there should be a different lexical tag (word name). Because the bees are seen in this story performing different actions, Charley creates different tags (names for what he sees). For example, a butterfly flies, a bee makes honey, and a fly is in the house so he calls the bees, butterflies, flies, and at one point asks what they are. Literally, Charley is attaching lexical tags (word names) to every mentally still picture. For example, if the artist shows the legs of the bears going high off the ground, then the bear is climbing even though the bear is walking. Or, if the arm is extended out, that position of the arm is called "fall" whether it is for pouring coffee in the cup or reaching into a bee hive in a tree. When the author was trying to talk with Charley's mom and he was running around the waiting room, she told him to "take a seat" and so he squeezed his body in behind a large chair and put his arms around the back of the chair… he took a seat! When a clinician told him to "get on his coat" he stood on his coat with a puzzled look on his face. Charley's world consists of single still pictures.

Activity: Why is Charley viewed as being very literal?

Because Charley is not seeing how sound refers to multiple single picture frames, such as how the word "walking" refers to the act of putting the feet up and down, Charley is having difficulty using sound for learning language. For him to be able to see how words name actions that occur over space and time, Charley needs to be able to develop the basic semantic concepts of agents, their actions, and objects. He must be able to *see* the words that go with what he sees people do. For example, he needs to see the written language that goes with the picture of a "bear running." Currently, Charley is using multiple utterances in a slide show to create the semantic relationships. For example, in utterances 1–5, he builds the underlying meaning orally:

1. "Who's in the tree?" refers to the agent, the bear.
2. "Oh, oh! He water" refers to the object, a dark liquid like coffee.
3. "Who fall in that?" refers to the action of the bear.
4. "That's his coppee" remarks or renames the liquid object. Coppee is not an error in articulation of sounds but a ***misperception***. He has coded this word with this pronunciation.
5. "He…(pause)…he's pouring coppee in the cup, more gone" refers to the entire agent, action, object relationship that he built in utterances 1–4.

Charley is working through the individual pictures and the individual utterances eventually to say the whole sentence, "He's pouring coppee in the cup." *Charley uses the movement of his mouth to create the meaning that goes with his mental pictures eventually to create the sentence*. It should be noted that Charley's need to use his mouth constantly to work through the pieces of what he sees results in constant talking.

Activity: Why does Charley use several utterances to say what he wants to say? Analyze utterances 28–32.

Summary of assessment for planning intervention

Charley learns concepts from what he sees and he sees every movement. If an object does not move, he can put a label to the object but if the object moves and therefore changes visual features he cannot tell what the object is. This is also true for agents who are always changing the way they look such as their hair, facial postures, and their clothes. Furthermore, as agents are people who perform actions, then Charley also struggles with recognizing people's actions or personified animals. For example, Charley said, "He took a mouth and climbs" in utterance 33. To understand Charley's semantic development, eliminate all inferred meaning and think literally of what a person would look like if a person "took a mouth." As mouths don't exist visually on the outside of the body, to see a mouth, the lips would have to be open. In the picture in the book, the artist drew the bear's mouth open because he was running and trying to catch his breath. So, the bear's open lips mean that the bear literally "took a mouth." The rest of the utterance, "and climbs" refers to Charley seeing that the bear's knees are high up so he thinks the meaning is that the bear climbs. The artist was trying to show that the bear was hurrying so the bear's legs went faster and so the bear's knees would be higher. Then in utterance 34, Charley says, "He's took a teeth and he bites…over the key." Again, the visual literal meaning (without inference) is that the bear (he) is now drawn with his teeth showing because his mouth is bigger for more air. When teeth show, they "bite" and the bear has a key in his hand to open the door so his teeth bite over the key. In 44, Charley says, "He's giving the hand and bang." Literally, the daddy bear who is in the tree house holds out his hand to the baby bear, who is still running from the bees and "gives" his hand to the baby bear. As he pulls back his hand, the bear is pulled inside and so the daddy bear shuts (bangs) the door.

Activity: What does it mean to "take a mouth?"

To help Charley learn concepts that do not remain still, he will need to see the written words matched to the pictures such as cartooning out a person walking. In this way, Charley will need to *see* the print words that go with the pictures or concepts. Drawing the concepts with writing the language that goes with the drawings will help Charley understand the spoken words. Figure 9.1 shows an example of a picture that helps Charley learn the language for what he mentally sees.

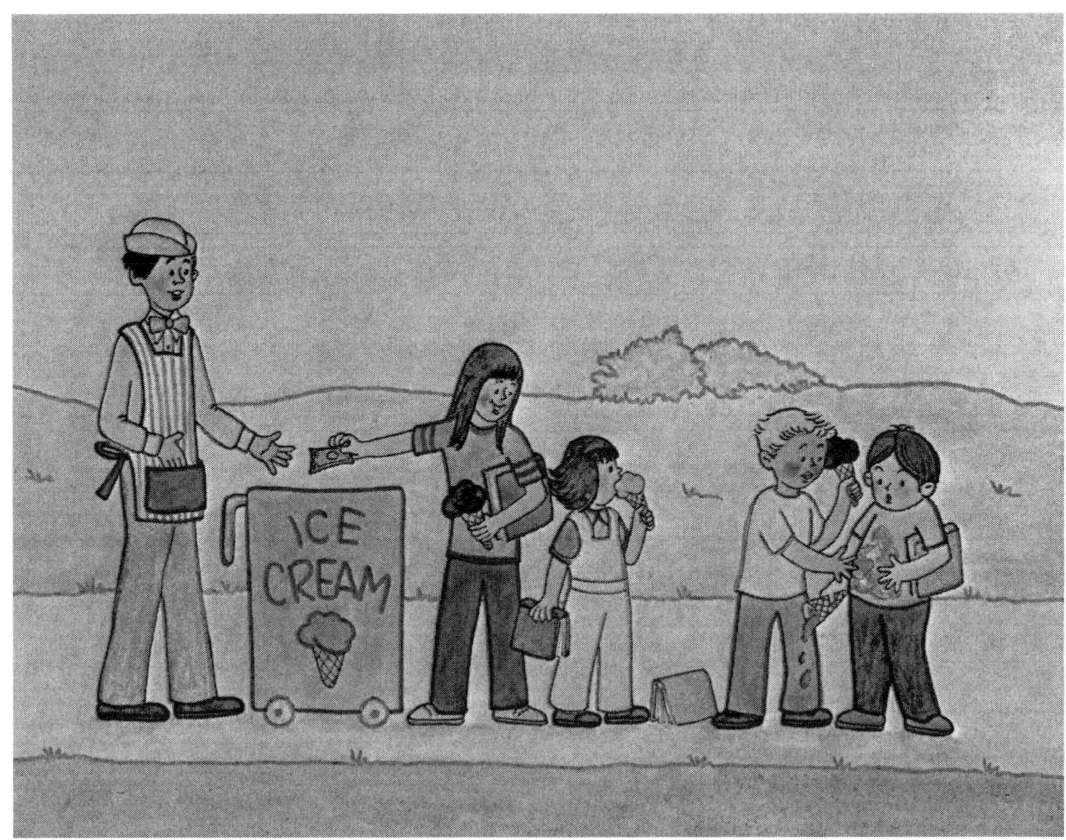

Figure 9.1 An event-based picture

Activity: What type of input does Charley need to be able to learn more advanced concepts?

Intervention

To provide intervention based on an assessment of Charley's language function, the following two questions are asked and answered.

1. What is the most basic thing that Charley needs to learn to make language function better?

As the meaning of Charley's utterances is not always clear, the child's conceptual knowledge needs development. Remember that early concepts revolve around agents, actions, and their objects. Charley struggles to talk about basic agents, actions, and object story. Because Charley does not have a basic agent, action, object type of conceptual knowledge based on what he sees in a picture, the first goal of intervention is to provide Charley with an event-based (agent, action, object) picture so that he can develop these concepts. Then, intervention will involve helping Charley develop these semantic relationships into concepts that language will represent with expanded grammatical structures.

Activity: Why is an event-based picture used for Charley?

2. What does Charley's language show about how he learns the concepts?[3]

This question addresses how to teach Charley the agents, actions, and objects that will form grammatical utterances. This addresses the first question under the interpretation of the language sample (see Appendix B: How does the child learn concepts?).

Charley is not able to integrate all of the input that he receives to form concepts; so, his use of the language structures varies according to what he knows or understands. For example, even when the educator corrects Charley's use of "butterflies" or "flies" for bees, Charley does not integrate the spoken correction into his knowledge. Therefore, he does not use the sound of the educator's assigned meaning to correct his conceptual knowledge. This suggests that Charley does not use the sound of the educator's voice for adding meaning to his conceptualization. Because Charley is also not able to "see" differences in features of movement, the remaining option about Charley's learning system is that he learns best with what he sees as shapes of movement...wings moving, hands pouring, legs running, and so forth.

Charley processes the visual features of what he sees into patterns but he does not process the visual patterns of what he sees into concepts. He has trouble labeling anything that changes visual patterns. It should be noted that children really do not learn to label and Charley is a good example of that notion. He is able to say the name of the object but Charley does not have the underlying meaning of the concept, bee, at a high enough level to understand all of the visual features that a "bee" might possess. Charley relies on the movement of the visual features to give him more information to form concepts that he cannot see, touch, or feel. For example, he sees the bees as "flying" so he names the bees "butterflies" because he knows that butterflies fly. When the bees rest on a flower, Charley confuses the shape of the flower for a match and does not see the bee move, so he does not recognize the features of what he sees as "bees" or "butterflies." When the flying insect reaches the hole (hive) in the tree, Charley sees the insect as a bee because bees "make" honey. He notices the movements or actions but he cannot create a concept from "seeing" the patterns. Later when the flying bees approach the door of the tree house and bounce off the door, he *sees* the bees as flies because he uses movement to think about ideas. So flies come into a house, so when the bees fly into the door, he thinks they are trying to come into his house. Therefore, Charley thinks the bees are flies.

If Charley cannot use sound for acquiring new concepts, then he is not an auditory thinker. If he cannot use the sight of what he sees as patterns to form concepts then he also does not use visual patterns alone to form new concepts. This means that Charley uses his motor system for helping him gather information to form concepts that he can mentally see. He is able to see the shape of the movements as concepts. So, *the first goal is to help Charley learn agents, actions, and objects that are expanded, extended, and modulated into grammatical language structures through his visual-motor way of learning.*

3 Agents, actions, and objects are modulated through the correct use of tenses, adverbs, prepositions, etc. and are expanded through the addition of more complex structures, and are extended in meaning through adding more conceptual depth or meaning.

> ***Activity:*** Which types of sensory patterns is Charley not able to use for learning concepts? Which patterns is Charley able to use for learning concepts? If a strength-based approach to intervention is wanted, then which type of patterns should be emphasized?

Based on how Charley learns concepts, the intervention plan must provide Charley with motor acts that form shapes such as through learning to write the patterns of the shapes of words that visually assign meaning to the drawings. Charley's intervention plan includes the following steps:

1. Provide an event-based picture. Help Charley name the people, their actions, and objects. Then write the names of those ideas on the picture (Figure 9.1).
2. Charley then draws his picture (Figure 9.2) and the adult helps Charley put the labeled words into his picture dictionary. Charley does not yet write, so writing will be a visual-motor way for him to learn to see the refinement of meaning (motor shapes). Writing will be accomplished by hand-over-hand.

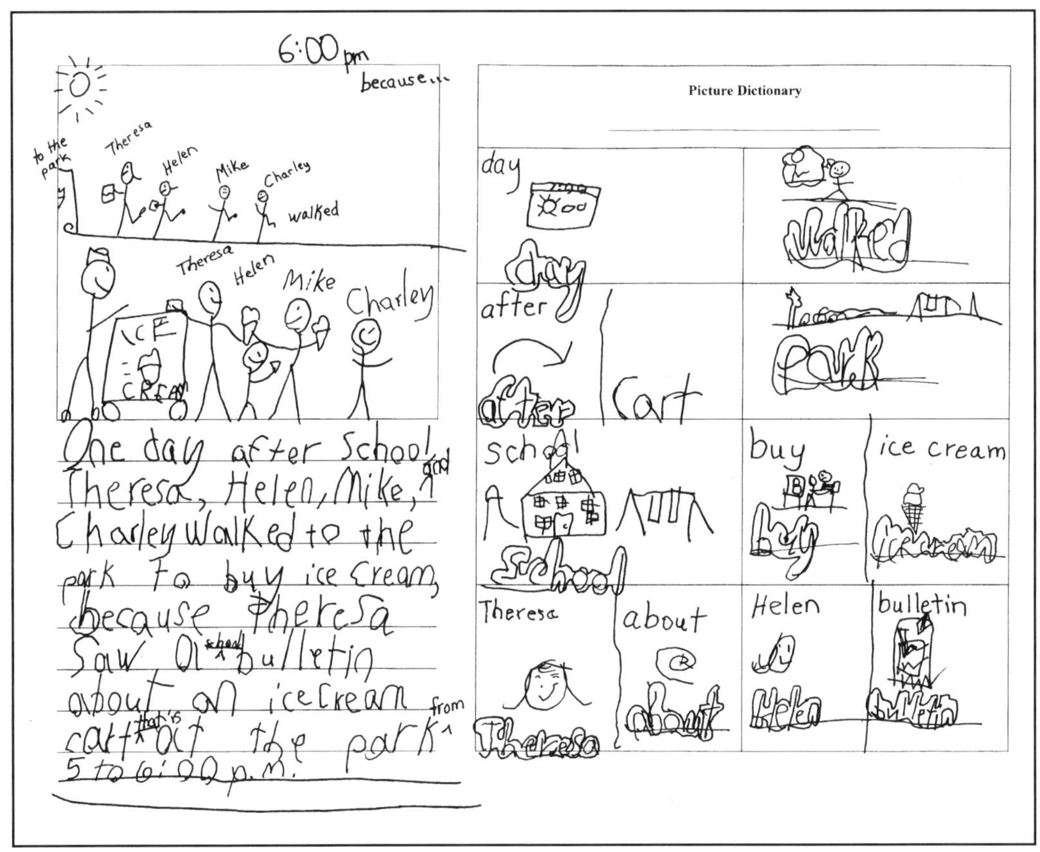

Figure 9.2 Charley hand-over-hand draws, writes, bubbles to learn the motor patterns

3. Bubble the words and put pictures with the bubbled words in the picture dictionary. Bubbling provides shapes.

4. Help Charley write the words to the drawn picture using the picture dictionary. Then he tells the words back (reads). The educator points or he points and says.
5. Refine the story with who, what, where, when, why, and how questions and answers. This refinement will take many lessons, lots of paper, and lots of redrawing and writing to create a final complete story with all of the age-appropriate language functions. Figure 9.3 shows an example of a final story about another picture. This also answers the last question on the interpretation of the assessment (see Appendix B: How does the child's behavior change in response to what the adult provides in the way that the child learns concepts?) Obviously, the process is working. Charley is able to engage with others in conversations more appropriate for his age level.

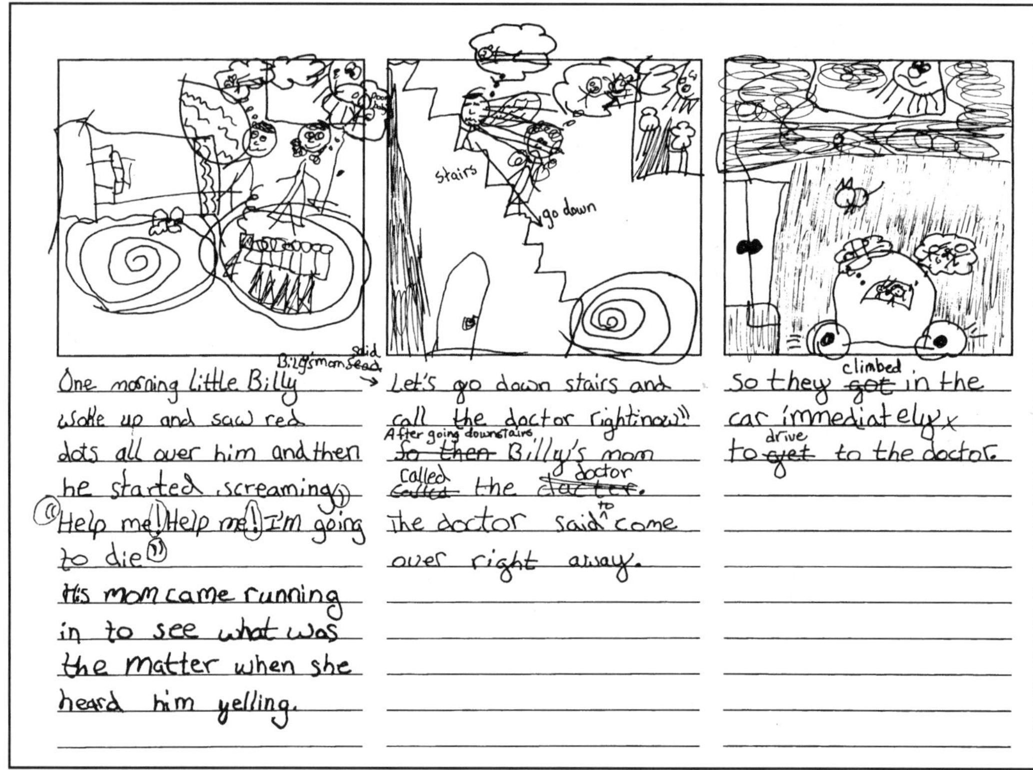

Figure 9.3 Charley is able to draw and then write

Activity: What is the plan of intervention for Charley?

The second question under interpretation in Appendix B was: What does the adult need to provide the child to meet the child's learning of concepts? Charley thinks in *what he sees that moves.* So, Charley has a literal interpretation of his world. If an object does not change the way it looks, he can put the language label to what he sees because the shape of the object does not change. But, semantics includes not only the literal concepts of what a person sees but also an expansion of meaning for concepts that do not remain constant and concepts one cannot see, touch, and feel. Because people or agents move or perform actions, Charley has difficulty relating to people. People's shapes change constantly. Their hair, faces, clothes, body postures, and positions constantly change. *A second goal for Charley is based on developing a higher understanding of agency where Charley is able to share talking with other agents (concrete cognition) because he is able to learn from them.* By refining his thinking with this process of drawing and writing and then retelling or reading what is written, Charley will add layers of meaning to his concepts so that he begins to think more like a concrete person with language function instead of a preoperational thinker with pre-language function.

Activity: Why does Charley have trouble identifying people or personified animals? What is the second goal about agency? Why do the adults want Charley to have more conceptual understanding?

As Charley is learning the concepts for his language to function better, he is also learning to become literate as long as the intervention is provided for him in the way he learns concepts. Because learning is a socio-cognitive process, in addition to learning about the social components of how he relates to agents, Charley needs to learn strategies for academics such as being able to see the shapes of lexical tags (written words that go with drawn pictures or concepts) as mental concepts. Writing words creates the pattern of a word which does not change. The written word "bee" always looks like "bee." To make the words into shapes that match the way Charley acquires concepts, he will be introduced to bubbling the shapes of concepts within a picture dictionary. Figure 9.2 shows the bubbling.

As Charley learns these shapes of patterns, he is learning more meaning about the concepts through his visual-motor system and these concepts will form the basis for his reading, writing, and spelling. The more Charley writes, the more he will learn the underlying meaning of concepts he sees. Learning to write is the key to successful intervention for Charley. But, writing must be a task of motor development of shapes of words. Hand-over-hand layers (like used with the pre-production cases in Chapters 7 and 8) can also be used with individuals who function at this level. Emphasis on sound for letters, sound for spelling, and sound for reading and sounding out words to write were replaced with visual shapes of motor movements of the mouth and hand because Charley was not able to use sound, but he was able to use visual-motor types of patterns for concept development (refer back to Figure 9.3).

Activity: What type of strategy can be used to help Charley see the shape of concepts?

Case 9.2: Laquatia

Laquatia, a nine-year-old female, was referred to a speech and hearing clinic for language problems related to math or numeracy, often called dyscalculia. She had undergone comprehensive testing by a multidisciplinary team of medical and allied professionals of a medical rehabilitation center. Based on their testing, Laquatia's language was "delayed in expressive and receptive" areas. Her strengths from the intelligence testing were described as in the "visual-motor area" and in "verbal reasoning." Standard age scores ranged from 65 to 84 (100 is average). Laquatia was diagnosed as having an "anxiety disorder with obsessive features" and routines as well as a course of medication were prescribed in addition to chromosomic testing for possible genetic disorders and further follow-up for educational testing. It was noted in the report that Laquatia did not know "her addition or subtraction." Even though Laquatia had had considerable testing, the parents were not convinced that a course of medication or further educational testing would resolve the language and anxiety issues, so they sought an assessment related to how Laquatia learns.

Assessment and evaluation

For assessment, the first question is: What is known about Laquatia based on the anecdotal history that can be connected to what is known about learning and language?

- Laquatia is in third grade and is nine years old. Because it is reported that she has trouble with numbers, the assumption that she talks can be made, as learning numbers is traditionally added to oral language learning.
- A child Laquatia's age should be in the language level of function, have concrete cognitive development, and think of others in relationship to her and her actions in relationship to others' rules.
- Because Laquatia is over eight years of age, she should have developed adult-like grammatical structures of oral language. But, since the report said she was delayed in language, it can be assumed that her underlying conceptual development is also delayed.[4]
- Adult grammatical structures of English are temporal or time based which means that Laquatia's oral language can be sampled for her ability to use "time"-based properties of English...this relates to all of the complex language functions: displacement, productivity, flexibility, semanticity, and efficiency or limited surface redundancy.

In order to decide how well her language functioned for learning, a sample of Laquatia's language was collected by asking her "What do you do on a typical day?" Her answer was audio-recorded and then the educator transcribed Laquatia's language from listening to the recording. This specific question, "What do you do on a typical day?" (see Arwood & Beggs, 1989) works well for determining how language functions, as it is a time-based question and English is a time-based language (Arwood, 1991a). A *Temporal Analysis of Propositions* (*TEMPRO*: Arwood & Beggs, 1989) was also completed to determine how Laquatia's language functions with concept development.

4 Remember that the surface forms of language are patterns and that when they function meaningfully, then the surface patterns represent the underlying development of conceptual meaning (concepts).

Laquatia's oral language response to the question consisted of one utterance, "Play with my dog." Because she did not answer the typical part of the question, the question was simplified to "What do you do at school?" Laquatia said, "Read," which indicates that she still did not understand the whole task. So, the question was made easier, "What do you do from the time you get up out of bed in the morning until you go to bed at night?" She said, "I get up and mow the lawn, that's it." Laquatia was trying to be a part of the language conversation but she lacked enough language to understand the meaning of all the words used by the educator. It should be noted that most children, who have good language, are able to answer the last question with story type of language. Most children who are seven to eight years old are able to answer the first question, "What do you do on a typical day?" with complete language function of grammatical utterances.

So, the educator began to draw out a cartoon strip of what Laquatia does and she immediately jumped in and began to describe what she does, "Oh, I get up, brush my teeth here (points to cartoon frame), then I go eat breakfast...and my bed would be here and the bathroom is over here (pointing)," and so forth. From this language sample, it is apparent that Laquatia understands the semantic relationships of a pictured idea with her in it. Being able to sequence from the pictures is a preoperational (3–7 years old) level of language and socio-cognitive development. But, when Laquatia was talking about where her bed and other aspects of her room would be in relationship to the cartooned picture, she was showing concrete socio-cognitive learning (age appropriate for 7–11 years old). Her cognition is concrete because she is able to understand the concepts that are not in the here-and-now in relationship to one another or to rules. This also means that Laquatia is able to use the pictures or visual input at a much higher level than she is either able to talk about the topic or understand the spoken words of the adult. This means that Laquatia is not able to use the sound of the oral language of the adult for forming her concepts but when she *sees* what others do or what is in the picture then she is able to assign meaning. This means that she is able to use the visual material better than the spoken message.

Activity: What type of input can Laquatia learn from?

The educator then gave Laquatia an age-appropriate reading passage that lacked pictures or headings for predicting the passage. Laquatia struggled with reading the passage out loud but she could draw and could answer questions after drawing about what she read. This suggested that she could understand more than she was pronouncing, again an indication that reading aloud, an auditory task for learning, does not match with the way that Laquatia learns concepts. In other words, the sounds were not providing meaning but looking at the words was providing meaning for Laquatia. This matches with how she performed on the testing which indicated that Laquatia has a strength in visual-motor learning. In other words, Laquatia can learn from seeing ideas, typically through a visual-motor means like writing but she does not do well with learning concepts from sound. Figure 9.4 shows an example of her drawing and writing.

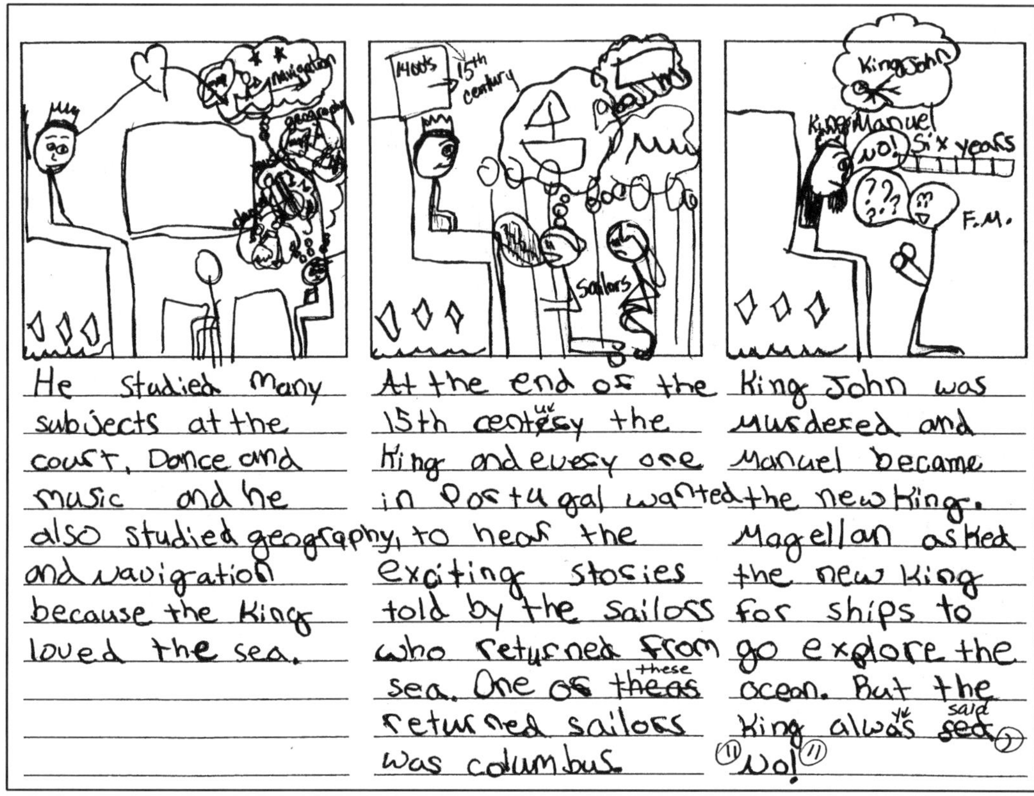

Figure 9.4 Laquatia can draw and see the concepts

Summary of assessment

Laquatia did not go on a medication course of action but she did receive language therapy, stayed in regular education, and became an honors student. She graduated from a regular high school and is now in college. Effective intervention for Laquatia followed five basic steps:

1. Draw out all new concepts (see Figure 9.4).
2. Add the written words to the drawn concepts. When this was applied to math, she learned the meaning of the number concepts and there was no longer any anxiety. Figure 9.5 shows her vocabulary dictionary for science words.
3. Use the shapes of concepts with pictographs to create the meaning of sound-based vocabulary and concepts (see Figure 9.6) even for science, math, social studies, etc.
4. Cartoon out any concepts that relate to what Laquatia needs to perform as an agent, scientist, author, etc. (see Figure 9.7).
5. Turn spoken language (teacher's voice, oral reading, spoken directions) into drawn concepts with written language explanations (see Figure 9.8).

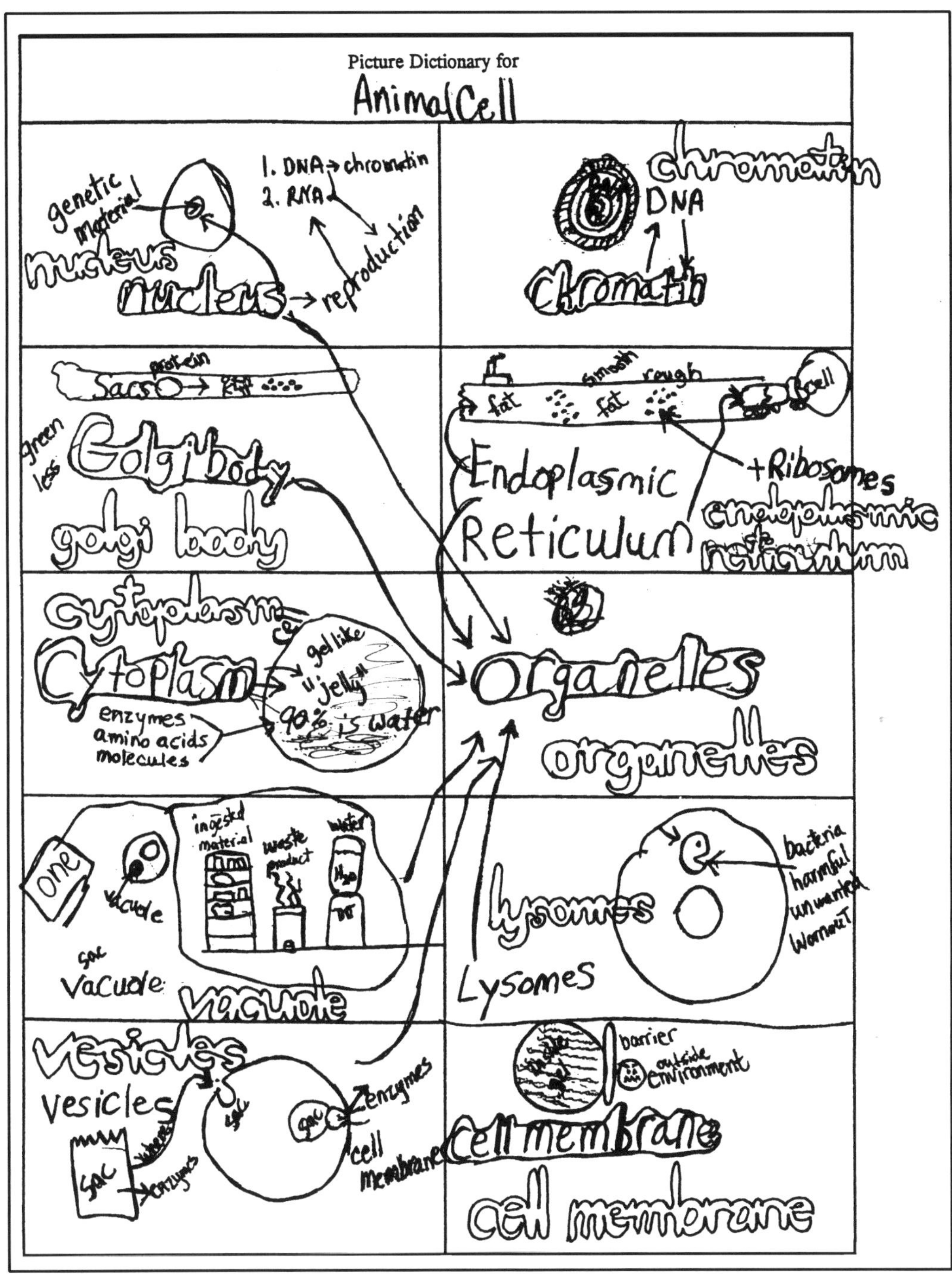

Figure 9.5 Draw out meanings of words

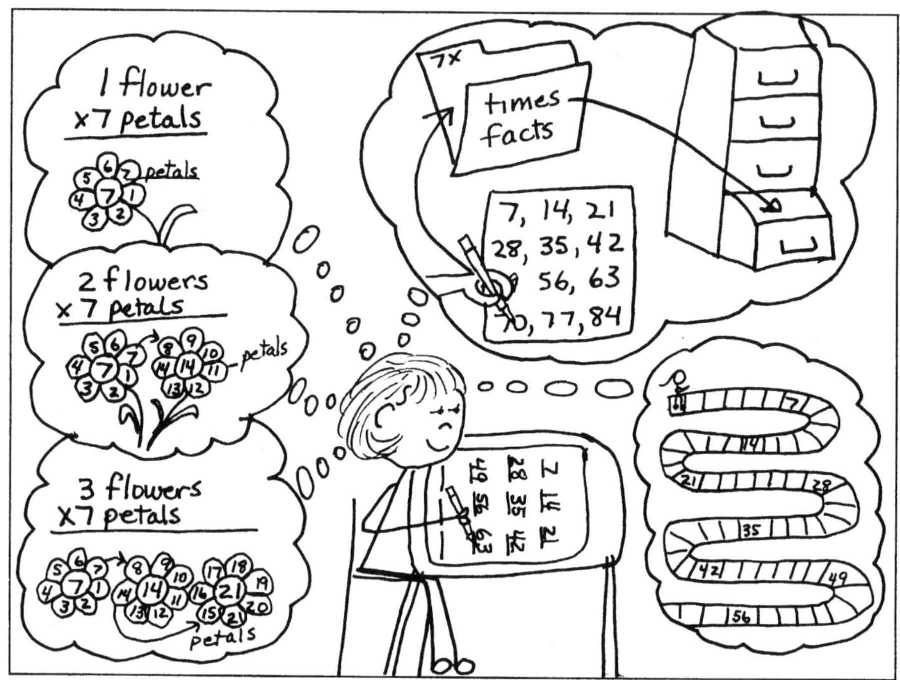

Figure 9.6 Laquatia learns about math concepts

Laquatia thinks about her Harry Potter book.
Laquatia wonders how the author created the characters.
Laquatia draws herself thinking about her characters.
Laquatia cartoons out the story about her characters.
Laquatia writes the words that go with her pictures.
Laquatia edits her writing by answering who, what, where, when, why and how questions.
who
what
where
when
why
how

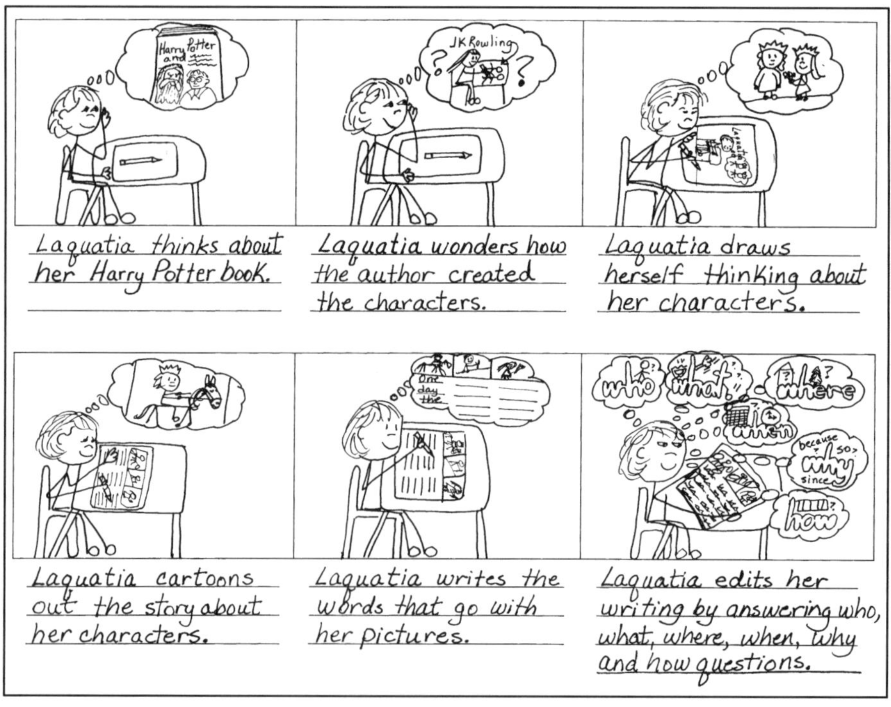

Figure 9.7 Laquatia cartoons out her book report

Listen up class it is now time for math...
p.131
So please take out your math book and then turn to page 131.

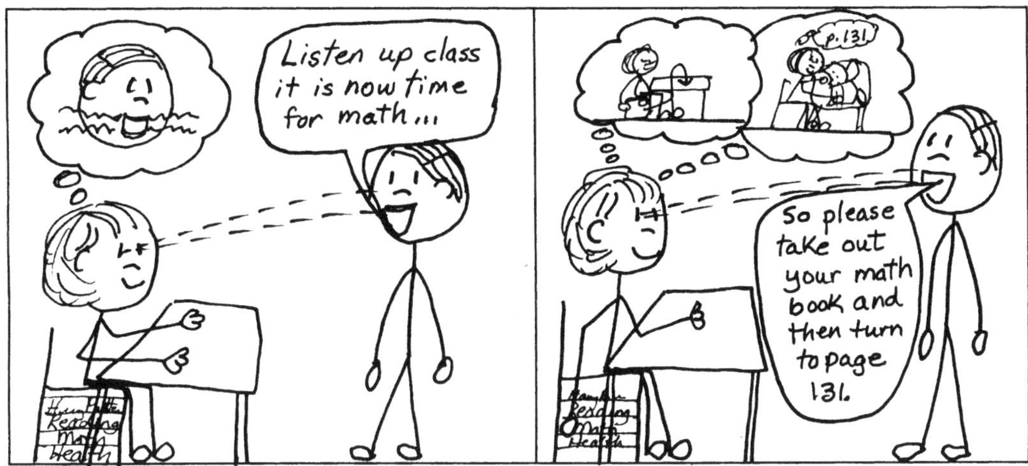

Figure 9.8 Laquatia watches the teacher's mouth move

It should be noted that over time, Laquatia moved from the pre-language function of learning language to the language level and finally the linguistic function of learning. See subsequent chapters for recognizing how pre-language thinking is so different from language and linguistic thinking.

> ***Activity:*** How does Laquatia learn concepts the best? What type of intervention worked for her? Why does language intervention help her with her thinking as well as math and other academic subjects?

Summary

Children who are very talkative so that their motor movements of their mouths and face help to "move" their mental pictures are typically in the pre-language level of thinking. Their motor movements are for their own processing. They do not expect others to respond (Charley) to their talking and they most likely do not realize that others are hearing their mouths move; they don't process the sound of their own voices. This means that therapy for language learning and for literacy or academics based on the sound of oral language is not effective for these children or adults to learn conceptually. The most effective intervention should match the way they learn the concepts: motor movements that form shapes that will create visual mental cognition. ***Viconic Language Methods***™ *(VLMs) for these children and adults include drawing, writing in context by either using a modeling or hand-over-hand approach for the learner to create his or her own hand and mouth movements to see the print and its meaning. Viconic Language Methods*™ (Arwood & Brown, 2002; Arwood & Kaulitz, 2007; Arwood *et al.*, 2009) use what is known about visual languages imposed upon auditory English so as to help a visual thinker translate visual cognition into auditory English. For example, writing helps create the shapes of ideas from motor movements.

The language of children who are very verbal but who possess pre-language functioning is restricted in nature because their thinking (cognition) is limited to the here-and-now. They are thinking of being in their own pictures. And, they put themselves in any pictures used with them. They don't think about others, except in relationship to what others do for them or in blaming others for what others do in relationship to them (see Chapter 13). Language at this level functions as well as the individual is able to learn the concepts from the environment. If the environment provides the learning of concepts in the way that the learner acquires concepts (visual-motor), their thinking improves as do their products as measured by standardized or formalized measures such as vocabulary tests, academic tests, intelligence tests, and so forth. Intervention for these individuals must include motor ways such as writing to see what is in the printed form.

Restricted, pre-language function is not limited to children. Adults may also function at this level when they possess certain disabilities. Chapter 10 discusses the next level of language functioning.

Applications

- Write out the steps of intervention for a verbal, pre-language thinker.
- Explain how Viconic Language Methods™ use how the learner thinks to construct a plan of intervention.

Chapter 10

LANGUAGE THINKERS

Learner objectives: Chapter 10

Upon completion of this chapter, the reader should be able to:

1. Explain what a language thinker is able to talk about.
2. Explain how language function relates to areas of literacy.
3. Assess and plan intervention for someone who thinks about others as part of their world but does not have the language function for conversation.
4. Describe Viconic Language Methods™ for expanding pre-language thinking into language thinking.
5. Explain the relationship of time and thinking.

I talk a lot about what I know,
I share with you what I know.
I think about what you know,
But I can't always talk about what you know.

At the pre-language level of function, learners think about themselves as central to any communication, and they either possess limited, if any, language structures, like Samantha (Chapters 7 and 8); or, they may possess a lot of structures that function in the here-and-now, like Charley and Laquatia (Chapter 9). In essence, *pre-language* thinkers possess *restricted* language *function.* This chapter is about those individuals who try to use language for conversational purposes—those who are language thinkers.

Language thinkers talk about ideas that are not in the present. They use grammatical, adult language structures to relate to what others say and do, and they maintain a conversation with others. At this level, language becomes a tool for accessing literacy. Literacy is operationally defined as the ability to use language function for the processes of reading, writing, thinking, viewing, listening, speaking, and calculating (Cooper, 2006). This chapter discusses how to assess language at this level and what the interventions might look like.

Neuro-typical language function

By seven to eight years of age, children with neuro-typical development begin to exhibit an adult grammatical system. They are able to use these adult language structures for acquiring more meaning about their world, academics, and self. As these children with adult language structures begin to think about what others say and do, they begin to use language that is not just in the here-and-now. No longer are they in the pre-language level of restricted function, but they are in a *language level of function.*

For children with neuro-typical language function, the development of an adult grammatical set of structures allows the language thinker to use the ***conventions*** or structures of an adult system to engage and maintain conversation.

Christy

The following conversational sample is from an eight-year-old female, Christy, who is telling an adult about a picture she drew:

> "My mother took me and the kids to the Montevilla Park."
>
> "Is this your drawing about it?"
>
> "Yes, this is my mother and my sister, me and my brother."
>
> "What did you do at the park?"
>
> "Uh, well, we went to the swimming pool at the park and went swimming, 'cept for my brother. He is too little."
>
> "How old is your brother?"
>
> "He is, um, he is about 14 months, a little over a year, so he is too little to swim in the big pool."
>
> "Oh, is there a little pool at the park?"
>
> "Well, it is not a swimming pool. It is a, walking, um, what do you call it?"
>
> "Do you mean a wading pool?"
>
> "Yes, he can walk in it but he can't swim. My mother walks in the pool too…she wades in the pool with my brother. And, the life guard watches my sister and me swim. Then we all get ice cream…um, after we got dressed, of course. And we had to dry off too and then get dress and then go get the ice cream."
>
> "I don't see the ice cream in your picture. Where did you go to get the ice cream and what kind of ice cream did you get?"
>
> "Well, at the pool, outside the pool, (points to outside the picture) there is this wagon, like an ice cream truck but it doesn't have wheels like a truck, the kind that comes around our house. Anyway, this, the ice cream is right there outside the place where we got dressed (points outside the picture and looks up at the adult who nods her head). And, I got a creamsicle. Do you know what a creamsicle is?"
>
> "I think so. Is a creamsicle the ice cream that has orange and vanilla together?"

"Yes, but it is on a stick like a popsicle. Have you had a creamsicle?"

"No, I haven't it…I bet it is good."

She looks at the adult and says, "Do you swim at Montevilla Park?"

"No, I don't live near Montevilla."

"Where do you live?" She continues on finding out about the adult.

Notice that in this conversation, there is a shared point of view. Each speaker listens to the other speaker, and then talks about something (***referring function***) that the other speaker said. For example, if the child talks about the park, then the adult asks something about the park. On the other hand, this child has a shared language function level, so the child listens to the adult and then ***refers*** to something the adult says. For example, the adult asked about the type of ice cream the child had and the child told the adult what type of ice cream and then asked the adult if the adult knew what a "creamsicle" was. This natural way to listen and speak about a shared topic is indicative of the ***conversational function*** that occurs at the language level. The speaker at this level is thinking about others and about what others are thinking (concrete cognition). From a visual meta-cognitive viewpoint, the child is in the picture with others and their thoughts are shared through language.

Activity: What characterizes the language function?

It is also at this language level that the child's thinking emerges from asking many questions to that of a speaker who is able to use language for literacy development. In other words, *language functions as a tool at this level of language thinking.* For example, language is now complete enough to use as a tool to understand the ideas of other writers who have something to say. And the child has enough language to understand that someone else is saying the words printed on the page. The emerging reader at the language function level is able to use his or her meta-cognition to think about what he or she sees printed on the page that someone else wrote. Likewise, the child *now* has the thinking and the language to understand that the writing process is between two or more people. Therefore, the child at this level wants to answer questions about who, what, where, when, why, and how as part of academic tasks such as reading about what others write and writing for others to read.

Activity: What characterizes the thinking of the language function?

In addition to being able to use language in a conversation that has shared referents, speakers at this level are able to talk about ideas that are defined in terms of examples or rules. For example, in telling the teacher about riding to school on a new type of bus, a 7–11-year-old might tell the teacher that the bus used propane instead of gasoline for fuel. By *referring* to the use of propane, the child is providing an example of why the bus is different. Or, the child at this level might say, "The new buses don't smell any more." When asked why the buses don't smell, the child at this level might say, "I think it is because they don't use gasoline." When probed how not using gasoline doesn't make the buses smell, the child might say, "There's no gasoline." The child can give an example and a rule (there's no gasoline is the rule for not smelling) but the child does not explain the relationship between gasoline and propane in terms of combustion, exhaust, etc. These latter language functions occur at the next level of the child's neuro-typical development (over 11 years old), the formal linguistic level of function. *At the language level of function, children and adults use examples and rules instead of formal definitions.*

Activity: How does a language level thinker use rules?

The language level is characterized by concrete thinking in examples and rules that are shared among speakers about people and their events that take place now, in the past, or in the future. The most important aspect of language function is that individuals are able to *share* their thinking, using the culture's rules or expectations. With this amount of language, individuals do not need others to interpret their meanings or help them resource or clearly use language for communicating.

Thinkers at this level are able to live independently in a rule-governed, law-determined, society. With language function, individuals are able to ask the who, what, where, when, why, and how types of constituent questions which allow a person to resource, hold a job, problem solve with concrete rule-based solutions, and to acquire the skills necessary for becoming literate. Persons with concrete English language function are able to deal with events of the *past, present, and future*.

Activity: What characterizes concrete language thinking?

Neuro-atypical language function

At the pre-language or lower level of function, it is possible to have social, cognitive, and language development at the same level. However, with language function, the thinker is no longer restricted in language structures and limited in cognitive development and therefore can use both their language and cognition to be socially developed at the language level. Furthermore, the dominant culture of society does not expect more of its citizens than the following of laws or rules, characteristic of language function. So, individuals who have true language function fit well into society. They do not possess learning problems related to the development of English for academic or social purposes.

Activity: If a person used a language function indicative of concrete thinking, why would the person not show a learning problem?

However, not all learners develop equally well in all areas and therefore a person can be capable of thinking at a concrete or higher level for specific topics and still not have language function. If language function is not typical, speakers will demonstrate a number of atypical structures in their oral language which represents atypical language function. Furthermore, the atypical learner will show "developmental gaps" among social, cognitive, and language development. The rest of this chapter will discuss these developmental gaps as well as some of the possible language problems exhibited by structures and functions that either influence social and/or cognitive development and/or are affected by the differences in social and cognitive development.

Activity: Is it possible for a person with language function to experience problems with learning in a society that expects language function to be the norm?

Language functions

Remember from earlier chapters that there are five linguistic principles of expanded language function: displacement, semanticity, flexibility, productivity, and redundancy. A person who has expanded language function is able to displace to the past, present, or future, is able to use concepts (semanticity) at a concrete level, is able to use language in a variety of places for a variety of purposes (flexibility), and is able to apply the rules of phonology, syntax, morphology, and basic semantics to produce a variety of grammatical, adult-like structures with limited external redundancy. For example, in the sample with the eight-year-old, Christy was able to talk about a past event, wonder and ask the adult about the adult's past experiences, inquire about something not in the present such as whether or not the adult had ever eaten a "creamsicle," and engage succinctly with the adult about specific activities within and outside the shared event.

Activity: Why is Christy's thinking at a language level of function?

Language and literacy

This eight-year-old is able to use the same language function to find out about school homework, to follow through with the teacher's instructions, and to obey classroom and home rules. Christy is also able to use her language for figuring out how the literacy tasks in the classroom pertain to her learning needs. In other words, she has enough language to think about how to use her learning system to do her personal best for someone else's requests. For example, even though this eight-year-old possesses a visual way of thinking in an auditory culture, she is able to use her mental pictures or concepts at a high enough level to understand that the teacher's rules for spelling don't pertain to her learning system. Christy knows she cannot do the sounds and letters for spelling, and she anxiously awaits the day when her classroom teacher or parent introduces a new way for her to write words in a conventional way that meets her visual way of thinking. If the school and family continue to expect Christy to think in someone else's learning system, the dominant culture will repeatedly punish Christy for not being able to use sounds and letters for writing words in a conventional form. Eventually, Christy will feel the failure of not being able to "fit in" with the spellers in the classroom. If the school teaches her to write the words she can spell only as an auditory pattern of letters and sounds, she will also fail as a writer. Christy has enough language to know what she can and cannot do.

Activity: How does language function help Christy to understand her learning system?

Language thinking

Even though Christy is only eight years old, she has the ability to function with concrete language. Her social skills are fine. Her cognitive level is age appropriate and so is her language. As long as Christy is allowed to develop her visual way of thinking to access academic tasks, not only will she do well in school, but also she is on her way to a successful life as a member of society. She does not have gaps in development at this time; but Christy will begin to show these gaps if she is not provided her academic and higher order thinking tasks in the way she learns concepts.

Activity: What will Christy need to be able to continue her development? Why?

Lavar

Another child, Lavar, has just had a birthday. He is now 11. At this age, he should have language function that is moving him from being in the concrete level of thinking to becoming more formal. He has struggled with multiple academic subjects from the time he entered school. He repeated Kindergarten and he repeated first grade. So as an 11-year-old, he is in third grade instead of fifth grade. He has very conscientious parents who have sought out help and continue to seek out help. Mom drops Lavar off at school every day. And now Lavar is starting to walk into the front door of school, down the hall, and then out the back door. He spends time outside the school and then comes back into school so Mom can pick him up at the end of the day. School is too painful for Lavar to stay in his classroom. A sample of his language was collected to see how he was learning to think, view, read, write, and do the other components of becoming literate. A small section of the sample is included below. The transcriber wrote what he thought Lavar was meaning and he also wrote Lavar's actual speech using the International Phonetic Alphabet (IPA) symbols where each sound has a corresponding symbol. By the time this sample was obtained, Lavar had had three years of intensive speech therapy to improve his speech sounds and he had an additional two more years of intensive phonological therapy by a university speech and hearing center program. The adult is holding a story book about Santa Claus that Lavar chose to read and talk about. Lavar is looking at the pictures and telling about the pictures. The book is written at a second grade level but Lavar does not read the words, he tells a story to the pictures. The following is a consecutive set of utterances that are taken after Lavar gets comfortable talking:

Then Rudolph a-watching Santa Claus.

/dɛn wʊdɑlf ə-wɑ-ɪn sænə kɑ/

Then Rudolph the reindeer in Santa Claus sled.

/dɛn wʊdɑf də wɛndɪr ɪn Sænə kɑ slɛd/

Then the other deer gettin' ready to fly and off they go.

/dɛn di ədɚ diɚ gɛt ɚ wɛdi tʊ fɑɪ æn ɑ de go/

The educator says, "This is interesting." And Lavar answers:

So had I.

/So hæ ɑɪ/

I don't believe in Santa Claus.

/ɑɪ don biliv ɪn Sænə kɑ/

Cuz it ain't true, just your mama and your dad.

/kɑ ɪt ɛn twʊ dʒə jo mɑmɑ æn jor dæd/

Just your mother and your dad.

/ʒəs joɚ mədɚ æn joɚ dæd/

The educator says, "You don't?" And Lavar says:

I don't.

/ɑɪ don/

The educator changes the topic and asks Lavar how he is doing in school. Lavar says:

Not very good.

/nɑt vɛri gʊd/

Then Lavar changes the topic.

I have six brothers.

/ɑɪ hæv sɪ brʌdɚz/

I mess up.

/ɑɪ mɛ ʌp/

I made three bad grade, Fs.

/ɑɪ med θri bæ grad, ɛfs/

And I make, well, I make, As and Bs.

/æn ɑɪ mɛk, wɛ, ɑɪ mek az æn biz/

He knock me down when I get home from school.

/hi nɑk mi daʊn wɛn ɑɪ gɛt hom frʌm kʊl/

This one time, I make a sled and tie him up to it and he pull me.

/dɪs wən taɪm ɑɪ mɛk ə lɛd æn taɪ hɪm ʌp tʊ ɪt æn hi pʊl mi/

Knowing how learning language occurs (Chapters 1–3) and knowing how language functions (Chapters 4 and 5), some specific questions can be addressed upon analysis of Lavar's language sample:

1. How does Lavar learn language?
2. What is his rate of learning concepts?
3. What can adults do to help him learn his academics (reading, writing, spelling, etc.)?

First, the acquisition of language takes two primary routes, either auditory development of sound-based thinking from sound being connected with sight. Or visual development of visually based thinking from the overlap of visual or shape (motor) based ideas. Since

Lavar's speech is not age appropriate, he obviously cannot use the sound system to develop auditory concepts, as he lives in an auditory culture that speaks an auditory language. Furthermore, his sound patterns are so bad that his speech is affected which means he is not thinking in clear sound patterns. Therefore, he has a visual way of thinking.

Activity: Why does the evaluator know that Lavar has a visual way of thinking?

Second, he has learned to be concretely resourceful. For example, there are rules about school and about staying in class. He knows the rules well enough to know how to walk in one door and out another door so that his mom thinks he is at school; and then he knows when to return to school so that Mom does not know he was not in school. However, he is not high enough to take the school officials' perspectives so he is not at a formal level. Since Lavar can understand the rules, he is able to do concrete thinking (7–11). As a result, the administrators know he is leaving school and they tell Mom. Furthermore, during the sample and testing, Lavar really tried to engage with the adult and to maintain a conversation. Notice, he leaves the topic of grades but returns to the topic. This shows that he is cognitively capable of doing age level concrete thinking about a topic raised by someone else. So, his rate of learning is okay, but he is failing school or school is failing him.

Activity: Why is Lavar viewed as being at age level in terms of cognition or rate of learning?

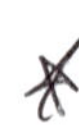

Finally, to determine what to do to help Lavar, the educator must know how to present the visual concepts in the way that Lavar thinks. Educators must present Lavar the visual concepts so he can *see* what others "say." Since Lavar has not learned to match what he sees others do or say with what he says or does, he must need to have the visual concepts given to him in a way that he can make the shapes of ideas from overlapping motor patterns. Is school presenting the processes of literacy in the way that Lavar learns best? Are they presenting to him how to read with the shapes of ideas, not sounds? Are they helping him practice seeing what is on the page and making mental pictures of the content, or, are they practicing oral reading fluency? Are they teaching him the visual concepts in the way he processes what he sees? The answer to these questions is the same: The school emphasizes phonemic awareness, phonetic rules, and sound-based oral fluency for testing whether he is learning to read.

Activity: Why does Lavar need to have the movements of visual ideas and not just a visual presentation of ideas to develop concepts?

Lavar thinks with a visual system, and he is not able to match letters to the sounds to *see* ideas. Therefore, he must need to see the shapes of movements such as the mouth or the hand when writing. Schools need to provide a process of allowing Lavar to see the shapes of movements such as with print or with the mouth just as described in Chapter 9. When Lavar prints words, his hand movements provide the shape of the print. At the same time, he is also able to see the shape of the mouth when someone speaks or reads the printed word. By overlapping the shape of the printed word with the shape of the spoken word, Lavar can begin to see the motor patterns as a concept. With the shapes of print remaining exactly the same (no spelling errors), then Lavar can also begin to make his mouth shapes match the speakers' shapes. For example, the word "kitty" is always produced with the same mouth movements just like the printed word, "kitty," is always written with the same shape. The shape of "kitty" on the mouth is always the same shape; and, the printed word, "kitty," is always the same shape. In this way, Lavar is able to match movements or shapes of print and mouths to form visual concepts. By seeing what the movements look like, Lavar learns to read the ideas on the page, speak with consistent conventions of English, and write ideas as conventional shapes on the page. Lavar is a successful academic student when he learns academics the way he is able to learn concepts for language.

Activity: What does Lavar need from the adults to become a successful learner at school?

The three assessment and intervention questions have been addressed, but what about Lavar's language function at the time the sample was collected? Any time one of the rule systems of language structures is limited or restricted, then the other language structural systems are also impaired. One language set of structures cannot function without affecting the other areas of language development. In Lavar's case, the most noticeable system of impairment is phonology. But closer examination of Lavar's language shows that he is restricted in his use of language. For example, in the second utterance "Then Rudolph the reindeer in Santa Claus sled" omits some of the functor words, little words that connect the time and meaning of the other words. Without these functors, the listener really does not know if Lavar means that Rudolph is riding in the sled or if Rudolph is in the lineup of reindeer pulling the sled or if Rudolph is painted on the side of the sled, and so forth. The adult must guess. As described in Chapter 9, if the listener must guess or interpret the meaning because the words do not stand alone, language is restricted to a pre-language function. Without all the grammatical morphemes included, Lavar's language is restricted in function which means that he exhibits pre-language function even though he cognitively should be able to use language at the concrete level. So, there exists a gap between his cognitive and language function.

Activity: What is the gap between Lavar's cognitive and language levels?

Lavar exhibits concrete cognition but pre-language function. As there exists interdependence among social, cognitive, and language development, how does this gap between Lavar's cognition and language affect his social development?

One of Lavar's concerns is friends. He does not know how to have friends. The students at school do not choose him for their teams because he cannot communicate the rules or sometimes even understand the spoken rules. Parents are concerned about Lavar having friends because he tends to "hang out" with younger children, but parents and the school have him enrolled in classes with students two years younger so he has little opportunity to spend time with other students his age. Lavar has expressed interest in sport activities out of school, but his language is not good enough to follow the rules of the team sports. In the sample, when Lavar switched from grades to his brothers, his next utterance sounded like a brother knocked him down one day after school. But, on the next segment of the sample, it becomes clear that he has changed from grades to his brothers to his dog and it is his dog that knocks him down. Without language that functions to share meaning with others, Lavar marginalizes himself by riding his bicycle a lot and playing a lot with his dog which matches with younger neighborhood children's interests.

> ***Activity:*** How does a gap between thinking and language function result in affecting social development?

Lavar should be moving into social skills of independence as a late pre-teen, but he is still trying to fit in socially with children between 7 and 11. Lavar's inability to be successful at school has prevented him from fitting in with peers (school or home), a social requirement of the concrete age of development. As a result of this restriction in being able to fit in, Lavar is not moving on to the next level of social development. And, Lavar's lack of success at learning how to use language to maintain conversations (language function for 7–11-year-olds) has resulted in him not being able to do some of the social activities he wants to do, which further damages his self-esteem. (Self-esteem refers to how well one achieves.)

> ***Activity:*** Lavar's social development is affected by his lack of language development. How does the lack of language development affect his social and academic learning?

Because social, cognitive, and language development are intertwined, working on helping Lavar access visual mental shapes of people's mouths and of people's writing can also help develop his social thinking. Figure 10.1 is a cartoon that interconnects thinking (cognitive thought bubbles) with the writing (language patterns of shapes of words) with speaking (language patterns of the mouth).

Do you want to play ball?
Lavar is thinking about playing baseball. He asks Chuck if he wants to play ball.
Yes
Chuck thinks about playing kickball. Chuck says, "Yes."
So Lavar runs to find a baseball and bat while Chuck runs to find a kickball.
The boys run in opposite directions.
When Lavar gets to the baseball field he turns around and Chuck is not there. When Chuck arrives at the kickball field, Lavar is not there.
... want to play?
... runs away
you're not my friend
Lavar thinks Chuck does not want to be a friend. Chuck is angry that Lavar asked him to play but ran away.

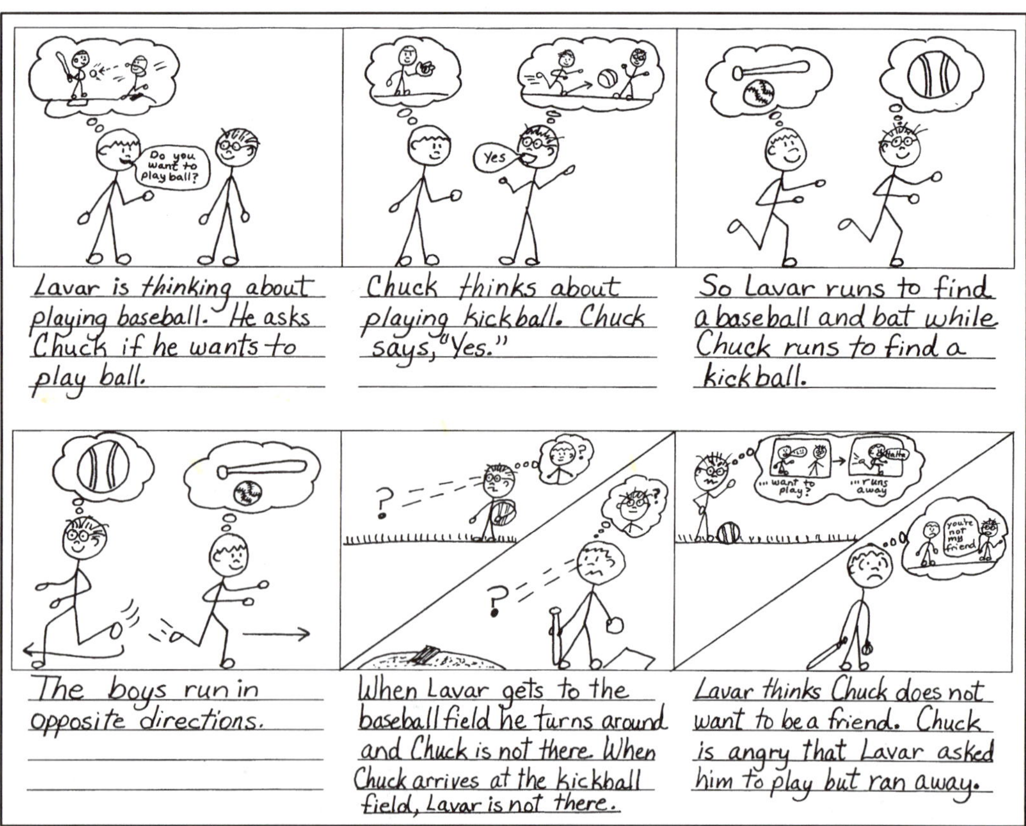

Figure 10.1 Thinking to write

The above cartoon also has a picture dictionary (Figure 10.2) with it so that Lavar is learning how to shape the written words into bubbles that are easy to recall by attaching a pictograph. In this way, the picture dictionary provides visual patterns or shapes (bubbles of words) as patterns that connect to the concepts or pictures. When patterns and concepts interconnect, then language is developed.

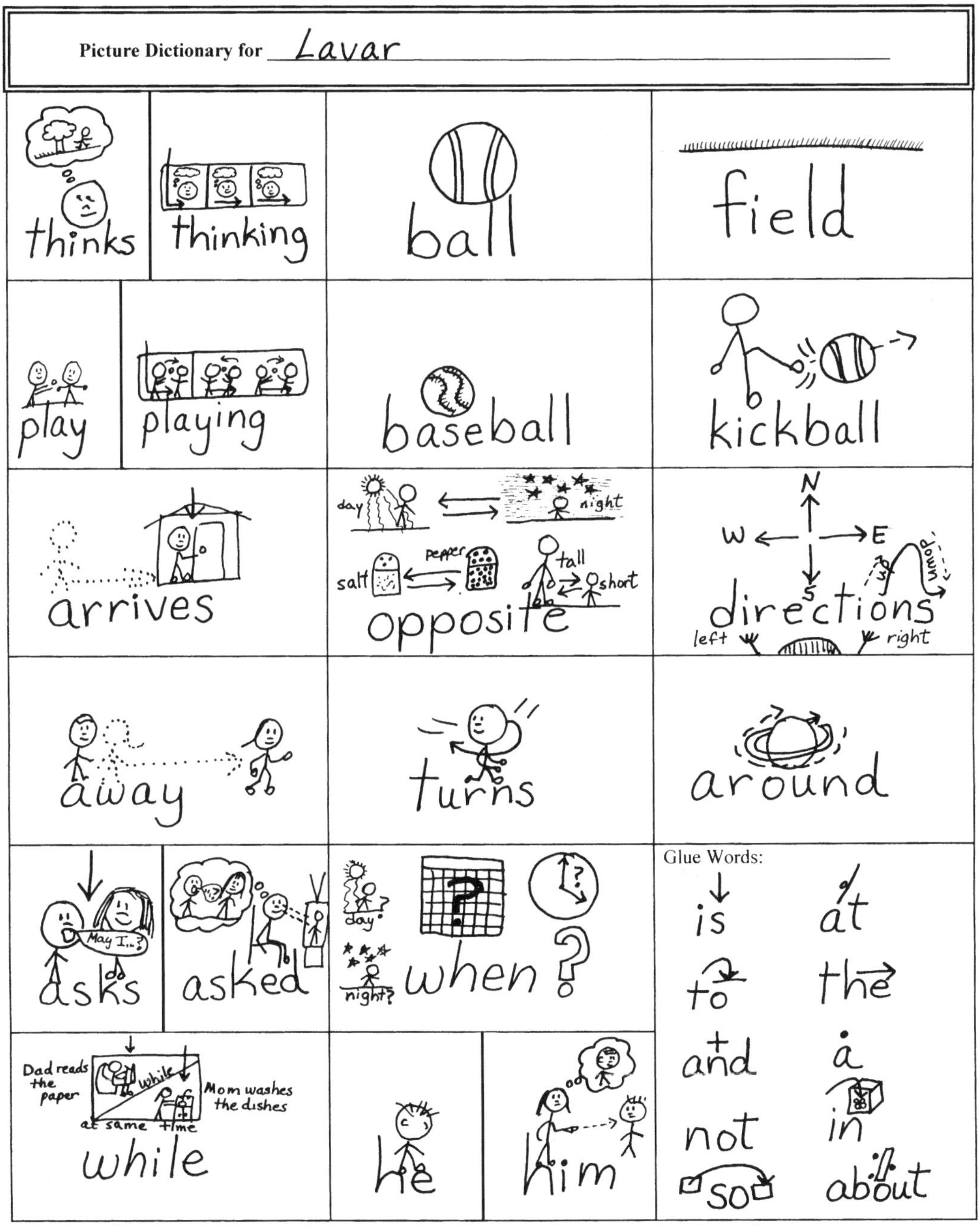

Figure 10.2 Lavar's picture dictionary

When language is attached to the concepts, the opportunity for semantic memory or long term memory occurs. Lavar is learning to use his visual thinking for language learning. As Lavar increases his language, he begins to move from a restricted level of language to a conversational language level. This interconnection between social development and his thinking system for improved language function removes the gaps in Lavar's development. Improved language function occurs through learning to be visually literate—a speaker, reader, writer, viewer, thinker, listener, and calculator with a visual language function.

As Lavar is able to improve his visual concepts, his language function improves. When the language function improves, Lavar is also able to think socially about his performance or achievement in relationship to others. This means that Lavar is able to understand what others expect in social situations such as playing a sport; and peers are able to understand his improved speech. Note: Lavar's improved speech is the result of his ability to see the printed word as a shape instead of a sound. This matches with the way his learning system acquires concepts from the shapes of patterns.

Activity: How does Lavar learn best? Why is his speech a language function issue? What does the educator need to do to help Lavar's thinking function at the language level?

Juan

Juan is also an 11-year-old male. Like Lavar, he should be moving from the concrete level of thinking and using language to the formal level of thinking with maximum language function. Juan is often late to school. His father, a single parent, has trouble getting Juan to school on time. Sometimes, Juan is more than an hour late to his fifth grade classroom. The school is trying to figure out if Juan's lack of academic success is a result of his lateness, his lack of turning in homework that he has completed, his lack of doing some of the homework, or a learning-language problem. An informal interview with Juan provided the following sample:

EDUCATOR: "Juan, how are you this morning?"

JUAN: "Fine, just about."

EDUCATOR: "What do you mean when you say 'just about'?"

JUAN: "Well, like it is an everyday."

EDUCATOR: "I see. Were you on time to school today?"

JUAN: "Not sure. I, well, maybe."

EDUCATOR: "Explain what you mean by that."

JUAN: "Um, well, the first time, the first thing I did today, was, um, well, the first thing, well today, the first thing I was sent out to my first recess. Not the first recess, it wasn't, uh, it wasn't a school recess, it was just right before school started, cause of it was the first recess then I would have been tremendously late. Um, and so it started from that and we came up and, and then, well it was not the first recess, you know? Well, it was right before school, so I would be late but not late, you know. Well, it wasn't the first recess, it was right before school started, cause it was not the first recess. Different-like we come, well, one things we do is we came up and said thinks like, oh yes what was the next discussion on?"

EDUCATOR: "Are you asking me about what we started talking about?"

JUAN: "Well, uh, the first things I do, well it wasn't the first recess."

EDUCATOR: "I think I understand. Let me check my understanding with you. You are not sure if you were on time today because you do not know whether or not you were late?"

JUAN: "Yes, I know I was not at the first recess."

EDUCATOR: "Did you come before school and the students were outside playing, like they play at recess?"

JUAN: "Yes. I get up at seven o'clock."

EDUCATOR: "Why is seven o'clock important for me to know?"

JUAN: "Well, it was before school, right before I come, came to school. Today is 9:00 and sometimes it is 6:00."

EDUCATOR: "You get up at seven o'clock, right?"

JUAN: "Normally, I don't get up at seven o'clock, but I did get up this morning."

EDUCATOR: "What did you do after you got up?"

JUAN: "Let's see for the last few days, I got up at…" (educator interrupts)

EDUCATOR: "What did you do *after* you got up?"

JUAN: "Well, let's see it was right after I got up. I brush my teeth but not at seven o'clock cuz it was this morning, um, well, right after I got up. Well, sometimes, well, I get up. I got up this morning and I get up, like today I am up. I am up here, cuz I get up in the morning." (he continues…)

It is apparent from the sample that Juan does not have language function. He attempts to provide the rules for what would be called "the time before school" when the students are outside "playing around." And, his explanation is directed to someone else, which means he is aware of the purpose of sharing spoken language. Both of these elements mean that Juan is concrete in his thinking (7–11 years old), which is age appropriate, but he has continued to add structures without the language function for some of the time, quantity, quality concepts. For example, when he talks about the time element of "before school" he begins to retag and retell his ideas. This *redundancy* means that Juan does not have a clear meaning for the time concepts. Likewise, when he uses a quantifier, "first" to talk about the time period, his talking becomes redundant, which suggests he does not have the formal meaning of these quantifiers. This quantifier issue overlaps with Juan's issues of time as well. For example, when he tries to determine what the original topic was, he uses the word "first," a time and quantity marker. He also has some qualifier issues; such as when he tries to ask about the topic of discussion.

Activity: Why is Juan's language so redundant? What does his redundancy have to do with time, quantity, and quality?

Juan's inability to use the time, quantity, and quality words clearly in specific ways suggests that he is *restricted* in his ability to use English, a time-based language. Because Juan has difficulty understanding the language function of time, he also has trouble understanding time-based activities such as when assignments are due, how to plan or organize his activities, how to be on time, and when to do his work so that his homework is not late. More about time and quantity will be found in Chapter 15.

Look at the sample again. Notice that Juan is using grammatical sentences in an attempt to share information in a conversation which is how language functions; but, he is not able to be clear in his meaning. His inability to be specific in meaning results in ***tangential*** utterances. This ***tangentiality*** in the classroom also results in Juan having difficulty following through with directions or tasks. So, intervention with an emphasis on building conceptual meaning will be helpful. As Juan acquires more conceptual meaning, then the external redundancy will decrease. He will be able to be specific in his use of words.

Activity: Why is Juan sometimes tangential in his thinking? What will help him become less redundant?

Language function means that Juan should be able to use specific language for a variety of purposes including academics. Juan needs to be able to use his language as a tool for clarifying his meaning and for learning academic concepts. For example, the cartoon in Figure 10.3 shows Juan coming to school on time. This clarity of visual thinking about how to be at school on time helps provide Juan with the concepts he needs to begin to understand the relationship between time and his actions as an agent.

A single cartoon provides Juan with the meaning of how he relates to one event or one activity. But, Juan has many activities at school and at home so he needs to understand how his actions relate to others to be functioning at the language level. In order for Juan to understand that his activities don't always look the same and that unplanned events do happen, Juan will need to learn how to replace frames in a sequence of activity (like a cartoon), as he develops better language *flexibility*. Figure 10.4 shows the choice that Juan has to make between being at baseball practice on time so he can play or eating a snack and being late to practice and not being able to play because he is late. By drawing Juan in the spaces, he is learning how the space of events takes time. And, by seeing himself in these activities, he is able to begin to understand the meaning of the specific time, quantity, quality, and space words.

Juan gets ready for school...
7:10
Yawn
At 7:10 Juan wakes up, gets dressed, makes his bed and then walks to the kitchen to eat breakfast.
7:25
At 7:25 Juan eats breakfast and then puts his dishes in the sink before walking to the bathroom.
7:40
At 7:40 Juan uses the toilet, washes his hands and face, brushes his teeth and combs his hair before leaving for school.
7:55
Juan
History
Math
SCHOOL
At 7:55 Juan puts his school books, papers and lunch sack in his backpack so he can take them to school.
8:02
Bus STOP
At 8:02 Juan puts on his shoes, coat and backpack and then leaves the house to walk to the bus stop.
8:05
DISTRICT
Bus Stop
At 8:05 Juan walks to the bus stop and then waits for the school bus to pick him up and take him to school.

8:17
Sch
At 8:17 Juan steps off the bus, walks toward the school and then enters the building.
8:20
Room 8
At 8:20 Juan walks down the hall to his classroom, enters his room and then prepares for class.
8:23
At 8:23 Juan takes out his books, papers and pencils from his backpack and sets them on his desk.
8:25
At 8:25 Juan hangs up his backpack and coat and then walks back to his desk.
8:29
Good morning class
At 8:29 Juan sits in his chair and makes a picture of what the teacher is going to say when the bell rings.
8:30
At 8:30 the bell rings with Juan at his desk thinking about being a learner.

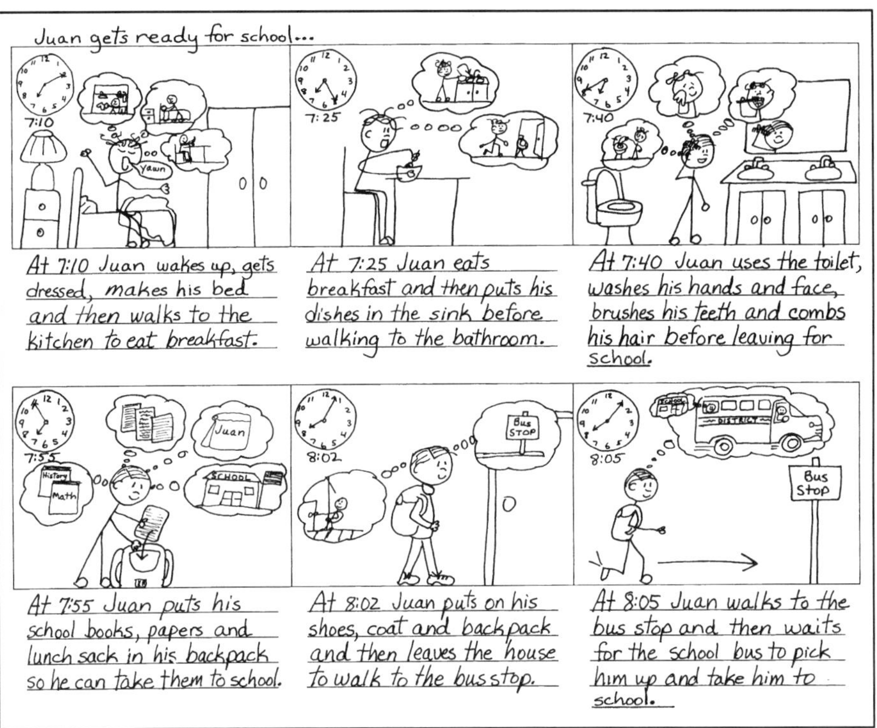

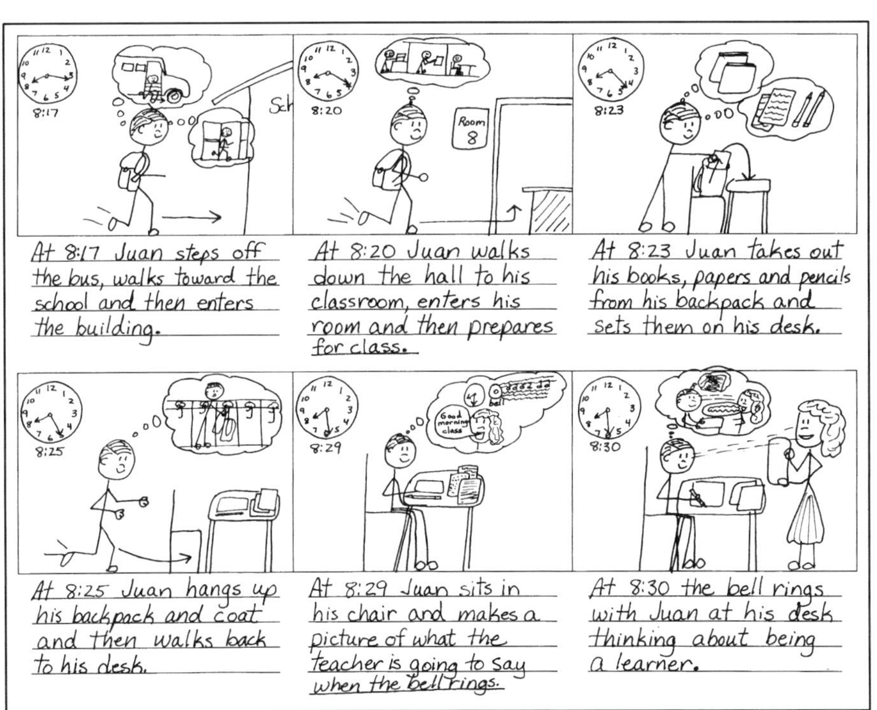

Figure 10.3 Juan is learning about being on time

OOL
When it is 3:00 the school bell rings and Juan leaves school to walk home.
14 15 16
22
APRIL
After Juan arrives home, he puts his backpack away and then checks his calendar.
3:25
15
4:00 baseball game
APRIL
Juan sees that today, April 15, he has a baseball game at 4:00. The clock on the wall says 3:25.
APRIL
Juan thinks about what he needs to do before the game: change clothes, eat snack and bike to the baseball field.
3:30
First Juan goes to his room to change into his baseball uniform. It is now 3:30.
Once Juan is dressed in his uniform, he puts his mitt, cleats, ball and bat in his sports bag. It is now 3:40.

3:50
With his gear in hand, Juan walks to the kitchen to fix a snack so he will have energy to play. While he thinks about his snack choices, time is going by. When Juan looks at the clock he sees that he only has 10 minutes to get to the ball field. He thinks about his choices.
3:50
If Juan jumps on his bike right now, he will arrive at the field by 4:00.
4:00
Hi Juan!
If Juan arrives at the field by 4:00, he will be on time and the coach will allow him to play in the game.
crackers
If Juan stops to eat a snack before riding his bike to the ballgame, he will arrive at the field at 4:10.
You're late
Sit on the bench
If Juan arrives late (4:10) to the game, the coach will not allow him to play in the game because he didn't care enough to arrive on time.

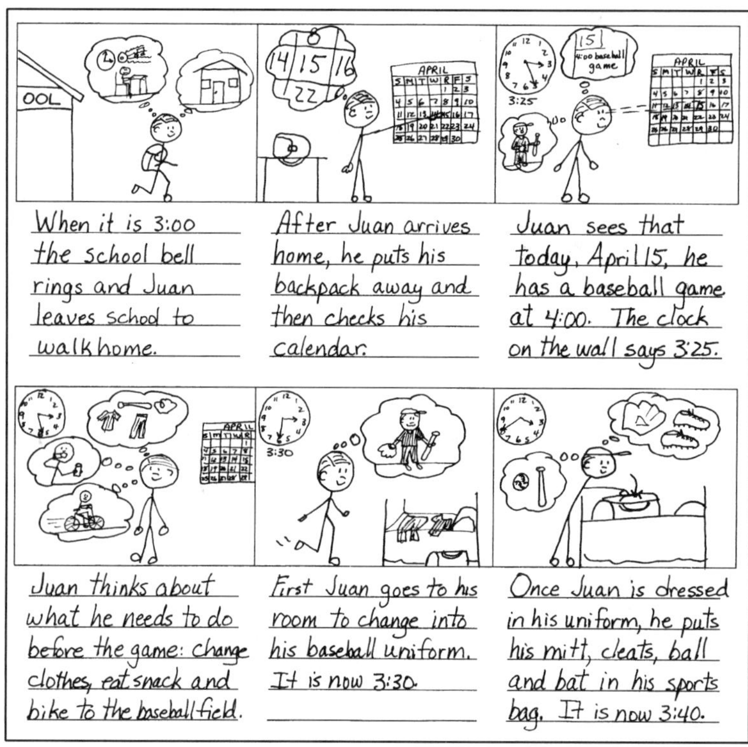

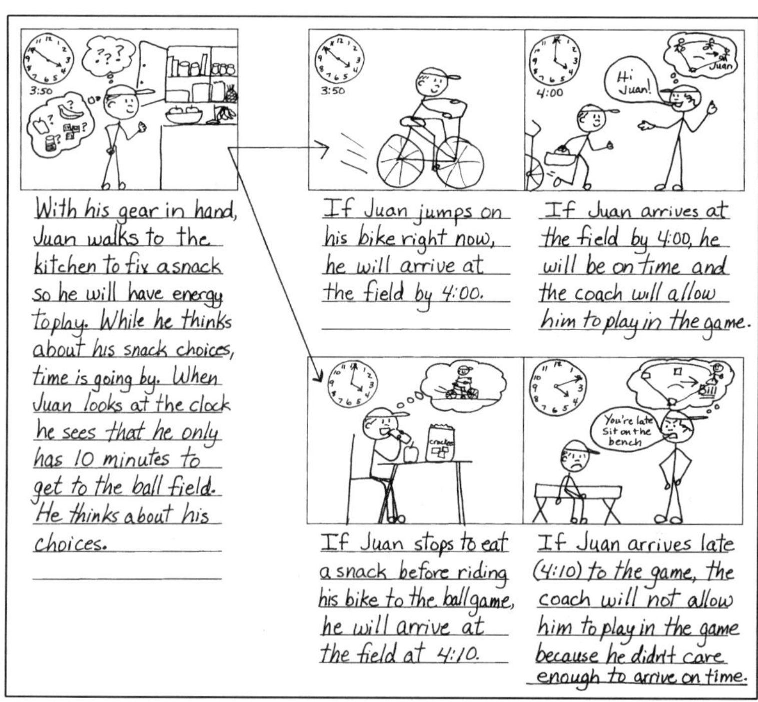

Figure 10.4 Juan learns about being on time and making choices to be on time

Activity: Why does Juan need to see himself in relationship to what he does to begin to understand where he is in space at a given time?

As Juan begins to learn about the thinking-language strategies that he needs to use to be able to relate to others clearly, then he is able to advocate better for himself. Box 10.1 shows an example of Juan's strategies. These strategies are based on the following: Juan is at the concrete level of thinking but struggles with language function specifically related to time, quantity, quality, and space. Since he lacks time-based use of English (an auditory language), then he must be visual in thinking. These strategies emphasize a visual way of thinking by utilizing the Viconic Language Methods™ of imposing characteristics of visual languages onto the use of English.

The strategies are language-based functions that connect the way a person thinks with the use of language as a tool. Language provides the thinker with strategies for learning to be literate; that is, for speaking, listening, thinking, viewing, reading, writing, and calculating. Juan's strategies are designed to help him have a way to think about learning and to learn about thinking.

Activity: What is the purpose of language-based strategies?

Box 10.1 Juan's meta-cognitive language strategies for learning to think and be literate

Juan's strategies:

1. Before I write words, I draw my ideas into a cartoon strip and then write my ideas below each picture.
2. Before I ask a question in class, I make a picture in my head… If my picture is clear, I ask my question. If my picture is not clear, I sketch what I know and then ask.
3. If there is something I want to say but others are talking, I write my idea down so I don't forget my idea.
4. If I am unsure what to do, I look around and see what most of the other students are doing and try to make a mental picture of what I look like doing what they are doing.
5. If I don't know what others are doing, I can ask the teacher (raise my hand first) or I can read the board or I can ask a friend (if it is student talking time).
6. When I read, I read silently so the sound of my voice or others' voices do not make my mental pictures disappear.
7. As I read, I make mental pictures and then make visual notes to go with the pictures. Visual notes are pictures with some words.

8. To get pictures about material I read, I scan the headings, pictures, end notes, chapter questions, anything that is not solid words (text) and try to think with mental pictures what I am going to see when I read.
9. To help with understanding the reading and to help write the words like they are supposed to look (spelling), I will use vocabulary sheets. These sheets will show how to bubble ideas and make the ideas into shapes that have pictures of meaning attached. I can close my eyes and see those shapes I have drawn. When I want to write that idea, I just remember the way the shape looks in my mind. Sometimes, I can use my hand to do some air writing to recall the movement of the shape.
10. For math, I draw the meaning of the numbers and problems so that I can make mental pictures of what the numbers mean. I can also make sheets that connect the numbers to their meanings or concepts like a vocabulary sheet.
11. To plan, like doing my homework and turning it in, I have to cartoon and measure the space something takes and then put it in three places to help me remember when to do something (see Chapter 11).

Activity: Explain why these strategies are needed to help Juan acquire more language function.

The purpose of these strategies is to help Juan understand how to use language as a tool which is what language function is all about. If he cannot use his language to perform the academic tasks, he will function at the preoperational level where the world revolves around him and where he has no one else in his picture which means that he will be dependent on others for life. Only when individuals are able to function at the concrete level of language function are they independent; able to function on their own.

To summarize Juan's language-learning assessment, three questions for language assessment were addressed:

1. How does Juan learn concepts? Juan learns new concepts best when using his visual thinking system. The language sample shows that Juan talks about what he sees and has difficulty with time-based concepts which are auditory in nature and an auditory component of English.
2. What is Juan's learning rate? His learning rate is okay. This is determined by the fact that he has learned a lot of ideas and has lots to say but not all of the auditory concepts are well developed.
3. What can the adults do to help Juan learn better? Provide Juan with semantic therapy that helps develop the way his language functions for learning and for academic tasks. Part of this therapy includes assisting Juan in learning how to develop concepts through his own use of visual-motor language strategies.

Activity: How does Juan learn best? How do you know his learning system uses a visual way of thinking?

Sicily

Sicily is a third grade, nine-year-old female. She has had numerous evaluations to determine why she is not learning to read and write. Prior to collecting the following language sample, Sicily had been administered 17 different batteries of tests. The results were conflicting: Sicily had trouble with visual perception but her strength was in visual memory. The following language sample was collected from Sicily:

> "Sicily, what do you do on a typical day?"
>
> "Well, um…" (long pause)
>
> "What do you do on a school day?"
>
> "I colored this and I paint for the water. We had to color for the water. Teacher gave us craylors."
>
> "Tell me about your whole day."
>
> "The school bus, and the bus go pick up the kids and you. I colored this faster. I forgot to color this. I work some books. I had to go to another class, and the dan, said you'll can. I got to another room. The teacher say, 'Pick up your book and you'll have to go and work.' You can color a book and you can do all that. You can the teacher say. You'll can look. The teacher get us candies. You put a yellow thing paper. You put the happy face and you can. The teacher get us some color books and colors. Our teacher not. Our teacher you'll can do homework or look book. Me, my brothers ride the bus. We ride #9 bus. And we pick up everybody. Everybody not want to go to school. Why they call?"
>
> "I don't know."
>
> "Why everybody go to school. Our teacher said, 'Where everybody?' There miss. They——(unintelligible)."

From the language sample, the three main questions must first be answered: How does Sicily learn best? What is her rate of learning? What can the adults do to help her?

As Sicily is over eight years old, her language structures should be grammatical. Even though she attempts to engage in a conversation with the adult, she does not have grammatical structures for all of her ideas. For example, most of the utterances are restricted. "I work some books" could mean "I did some work in the books" or "I worked some in the books" or "I worked in some books." Without the correct time marker or tense, it is difficult to know exactly what Sicily means. Another example of the lack of grammatical utterances is "Our teacher not." The listener is not sure if Sicily is using this utterance to negate the idea that her teacher does not provide coloring books, paint books, candies, or happy faces. Or, maybe Sicily means her teacher is not at school. Again, without ideas that connect in time and are grammatical, it is difficult to determine a conversational meaning. Furthermore, Sicily does not use the word order in a way that represents the typical English subject-verb-object (SVO) form. For example, when she says, "the dan, said you'll can" there is no referent to "dan." And, there is no person in school by the name of Dan. So, is this an ***auditory misperception***?[1] Did she mean "man?" And, this is an error in syntax. Syntax refers to word order and her word order is not typical for English if "dan" is a noun for a subject.

Like Charley (Chapter 9) who was functioning at the pre-language level, Sicily is struggling with the underlying meaning of the semantics of some of the basic relationships necessary for grammatical structures to develop. The difference between her ability to think about others and her language development is a gap. On one hand, Sicily wants to share her information with the adult in a conversational manner typical of a 7–11-year-old language function (unlike Charley); on the other hand, she is not able to understand all of the relationships surrounding agents, their actions and objects, typical of a 3–7-year-old pre-language thinker. This means that Sicily has the cognitive ability of being concrete but *not* the neuro-semantic development of a child her age.

Activity: What is the semantic level of concept understanding for Sicily? What is the evidence?

There are other, non-typical types of errors in Sicily's sample. For example, she has difficulty staying with the topic. As a result she talks about other topics. For example, the evaluator wants to know what she does at school and she talks about sick children not getting on the bus, and so forth. Such changes in topic without letting the listener share in the switch of topic are considered ***off-topic*** utterances. These types of *off-topic* utterances indicate that the speaker is not socially maintaining the conversational referent of language function. The significance of these *off-topic* utterances is that it affects her ability to be independent socially and her ability to maintain language function with someone else.

Sicily has some auditory processing issues as indicated by the fact that she has not learned the structures of what she hears other speakers utter, but also by the fact that she creates her own words or ***neologisms***. For example, when she is talking about water colors (paints), Sicily creates a new tag, "craylors," something between a crayon (probably) and a color or a paint. *Neologisms* can be a combination of phonological and morphological structures like "craylors" for crayons and crayolas. Or, "copheliter" is a rearrangement of sound sequences for helicopter. Or, *neologisms* can be based on certain meaningful features like shape. One child defined every word on a vocabulary test based on shape. An umbrella is a round circle over the head, pancakes were circles with syrup, tables were squares with legs, people were rectangles with circles, and so forth. *Neologisms* indicate that the person is struggling to perceive the sound features or semantic features (Chapters 1–3) as patterns to form conventional concepts.

Activity: What are some of the problems in Sicily's oral language that indicate she is struggling with learning the auditory components of English?

Sicily also makes ***associations*** between ideas. For example, when she talks about the happy faces as rewards; she associates the happy face with what the other teacher doesn't do. This

1 Sicily may be intending to produce a word that she thinks sounds like "dan" but is really not that sequence of sounds.

type of association is the one of the purposes of rewarding a child. The child connects the reward of a happy face with doing her work. However, she thinks about one classroom (probably mentally sees herself in the first classroom) and then she thinks about seeing herself in another classroom so she talks about the other classroom. It is a random *association.* In fact, in the youth of the US, it is not uncommon for a person to introduce these changes in topic as "Here is something random." Sicily is not able to make such changes in topic or content from the listener's perspective; in other words, she does not let the listener know she has changed topics.

Activity: What are neologisms and associations?

Sicily also has some ***semantic word errors***. She refers to a substitute teacher as the Dan. It is structurally an error but also a semantic error. Sicily does not know that the names of people are not objects but agents. Therefore, she makes a surface error in use because she does not understand that the name of a person represents who the person is, an agent, not an object. Sometimes *semantic word errors* are more obvious. For example, Juan asked what the next discussion was on when he meant "What did we begin talking about?" or "What was the original topic?" Juan's use of the word "discussion" is a semantic word error. He does not have enough meaning of the word to use it correctly.

There are also times that Sicily's oral language becomes unintelligible to the listener. These are not errors in the motor ability to pronounce the words (articulation) but in Sicily's inability to know mentally what the sounds are that go with the motor movements of her mouth. This lack of phonological processing for specific ideas means that she has an *auditory misperception. Auditory misperceptions* occur specifically for a sequence of sound patterns that a speaker does not have the meaning adequately visualized or mentally shaped. For example, when Sicily tried to talk about students missing school, Sicily had to think about what her teacher said in relationship to the students not at school. This is concrete in developmental cognition. But, then Sicily had to add her meaning about why the students were not on the bus. Sicily's interpretation that "the missing students" were sick and would be missed was too semantically difficult for Sicily; so she becomes unintelligible in production. Remember that when the semantic meaning is too complex, the language structures will drop in complexity.

Sicily stays on the topic very well but occasionally strays off into tangent ideas. For example, she talks about what rewards the teacher provides instead of directly talking about what she does at school. This is called *tangentiality.* It is the same problem that Juan exhibited. Both students need more conceptual information to be able to understand the concrete level concepts that they are trying to use in their language when they are maintaining a conversation.

Activity: What are some of the neuro-atypical types of errors that Sicily shows in her language?

Notice that in the process of collecting a sample for Sicily, the evaluator changed the level of the prompt from "typical day," which is an auditory time-based task, to a concrete task, "school day," to help make the conversation easier. Sicily still had trouble with the conversational task. As the conversational task was difficult for Sicily and therefore difficult to understand, the adult asked Sicily to talk about an event-based picture (see Figure 10.5).

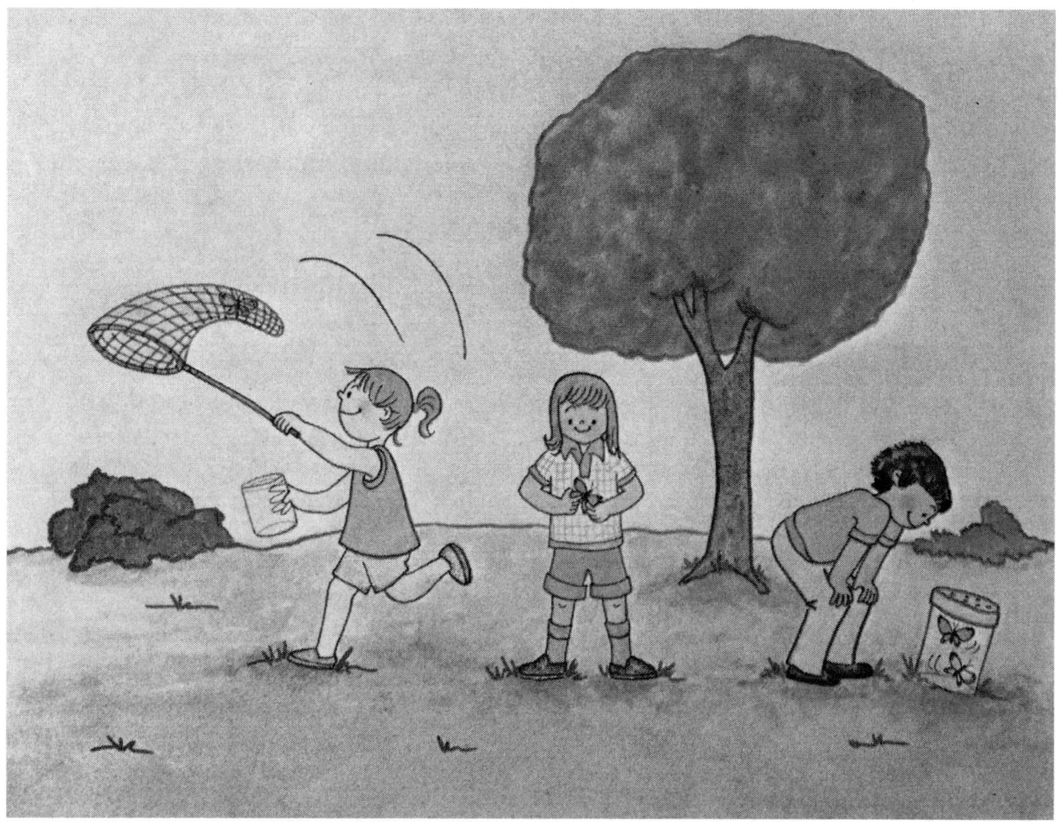

Figure 10.5 Catching the butterflies

As the reader may recall from earlier chapters, a picture like this provides a lot of language for the child (Arwood *et al.*, 2009). Sicily looked at the picture and began to talk about it.

> This girl holdin' the net. This boy catchin' the butterflies. This girl standin'. This jar on the ground. The end.

Remember *language function* uses grammatical adult-like structures. Even though Sicily socially and cognitively tries to maintain a conversation with the adult like a child of her age, the language structures do not show adult-like grammar. For example, some of the function words (functors) like the copula, to be form, "is," is omitted in "This girl holdin' the net." Also, notice that the ideas are not connected. What does "holdin' the net" have to do with "catchin' the butterflies"? The typical expansions, extensions, and modulations of structures are incomplete resulting in restricted language. Sicily is using a pre-language function to express her ideas even though the task has been simplified to talking about an event-based picture. So, does Sicily not know the story-like meaning of what she sees in the picture? Or, does Sicily understand what she sees but does not have the language structures?

Most formalized tests[2] will check for whether or not Sicily has the structures of language. She has passed at grade level a formal vocabulary test and a sentence structure test and an articulation test. Furthermore, even if the reader did not have all of those test results, compare Sicily's ideas in the spontaneous (conversation-like) sample against the sample to the picture. In the spontaneous sample, Sicily actually produced a single complex grammatical sentence: "Pick up your book and you'll have to go and work." This means she can produce the structures. It is possible that this is a direct quotation of what the teacher actually said. In other words, Sicily can borrow others' words. But, her spontaneous ideas indicate that she does not have the underlying meaning of what she sees in the picture or in the classroom. At this point, many professionals will immediately assume that Sicily does not have the physical, real experience of what she sees in the picture which is why she cannot talk about it.

This explanation is naive because one of the functions of language is "displacement," the ability to talk about things that are not in the here-and-now and therefore have never been physically experienced. *Language function is a cognitive experience.* Language function allows a person to talk about "Ancient Egypt" without ever visiting there or to plan an exploration into space without benefit of anyone else's experience. Sicily should be able to talk about what she sees in the picture, if she has language function which most children by eight years of age would have, whether or not she has ever physically experienced what she sees in the picture.

Activity: Why is language function related to thinking about ideas that are not necessarily part of a person's physical experience?

Because Sicily's ideas do not make a story, that is, she does not connect the "who" with the "what" or provide a "where" or "when" for the whole story, the author asked Sicily to listen to the author tell a story. The author told an elaborate story while pointing to the various ideas she was talking about. The story went something like this:

> This is a story about three children, Misty, Sicily, and Billy. Misty told Sicily and Billy that she wanted to catch some butterflies and that she needed Sicily and Billy to help her. Sicily and Billy said they would help Misty catch the butterflies. So, Misty, Sicily, and Billy walked to the park to catch the butterflies. Misty took the net so that she could catch the butterflies in her net while Billy took the jar to put the butterflies in and Sicily said she would help carry the butterflies.

The author then asked Sicily to tell the story about Misty, Sicily, and Billy. Sicily said, "This girl holdin' the net. This boy catchin' the butterflies. This girl standin'. This jar on the ground." The author attempted to connect the ideas for Sicily:

> Right. This girl is holding the net so that she can catch a butterfly in her net. Then she will put the butterfly that is in her net into the jar. While she is catching the butterfly and putting it into the jar, her friend over here is also catching a butterfly with his hands. Sicily, what is the girl doing with her net?

2 Formalized tests are developed across populations in a standard fashion that uses statistical processes to determine what the majority of test takers will respond to specific test items. These tests are widely accepted as the only measures used to determine academic progress or eligibility for services. However, not all formalized tests have acceptable standardized measurement data.

Sicily responded, "She holdin' the net." "And, what will she do with the net?" Sicily responded, "I don't know."

Remember that there are always three questions to answer: How does Sicily learn concepts the best? What is her rate of learning? And what can the adults do to help Sicily? As Sicily is not changing the meaning of what she sees based on the sound of the author's voice pointing out the ideas to Sicily (acoustic with visual) and because she has not developed a full grammar of English, an auditory language while living in an enriched auditory environment, she is not able to use auditory input for learning concepts. Further, Sicily is not seeing how the ideas connect in the picture even when the connections are pointed out several different ways. Therefore, she is not learning concepts by seeing what people talk about. The remaining option is that she learns the shapes of what she sees.

Activity: How is Sicily learning concepts the best?

Shapes develop from the movements of the hands or lips writing and/or saying the words (Arwood & Kaulitz, 2007). So, the author asked Sicily to write about the butterflies to see how movement of her hand helped or didn't help her language function. Figure 10.6 shows her writing.

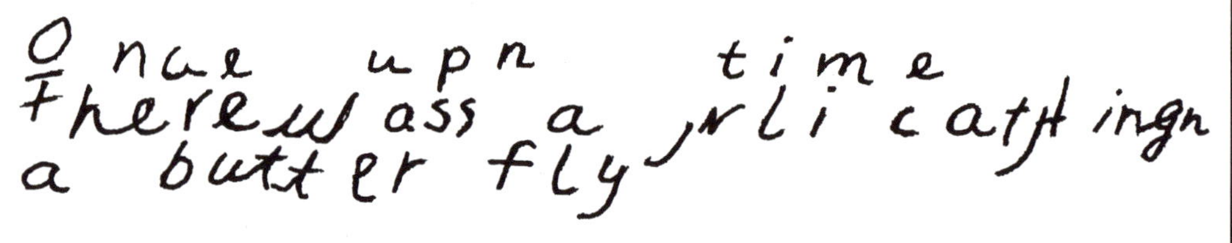

Figure 10.6 Sicily's writing

Note that the writing has huge spaces between ideas or words. These spaces represent where the letters or words are put on the page in relationship to Sicily's body. In other words, she is seeing the ideas as if she were positioned on the page. Figure 10.7 shows where she is on the page.

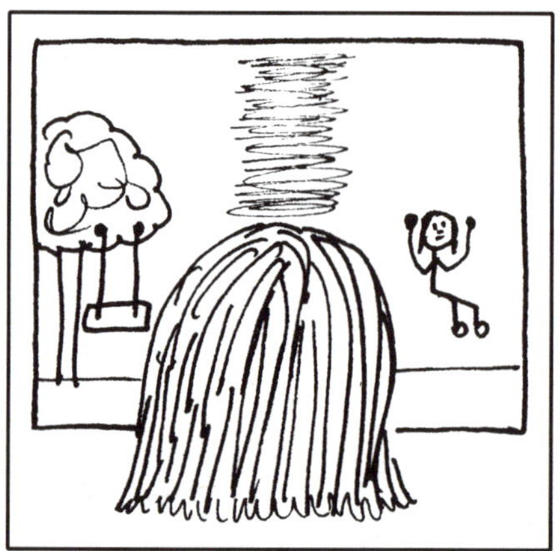

Figure 10.7 Sicily positioned over the middle of the paper

Because the human body is divided into quadrants and because Sicily said she could see what to write with the paper on her upper right-hand quadrant, the *author put the picture directly in front of Sicily* so that her body was across all four quadrants. The author then asked her, "How many pictures do you see?" Sicily said, "Four." This means that Sicily may have adequate acuity of vision but she sees her world as separate quadrants. Figure 10.8 shows how the human brain processes a "b" written in the upper right-hand quadrant of the body by a right-handed person is seen as four different letters. The eyes are positioned at "eye level" of the body. The right hand writes the "b" and the brain sees all the other letters. The learner is able to assign meaning to the letter as a sound, "bee," and therefore recognizes the one pattern, "b," as a concept and the other patterns are ignored.

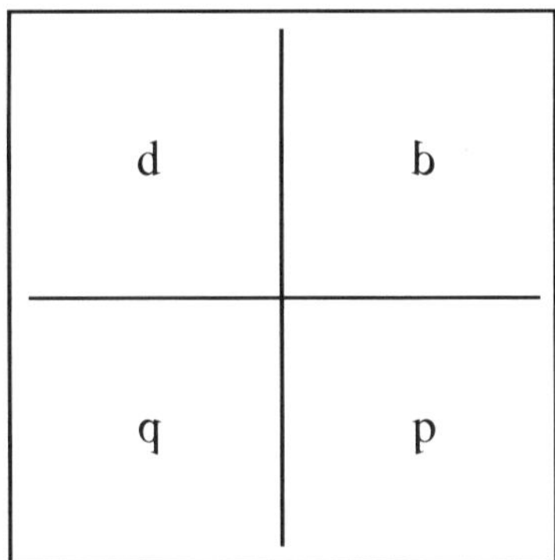

Figure 10.8 The four quadrants of a person's body as seen by the eyes

Sicily is not able to use sound to make concepts so she is not able to sort out the visual patterns of the letters as sounds. Therefore, she sees all the various patterns in relationship to her body, instead of in relationship to her mind. Knowing that the motor task of writing with the picture and paper positioned correctly helped Sicily produce the patterns that matched her thinking, the author asked Sicily to draw a picture about what she does at home. The author wanted to see what happens when the picture is a drawing, not letters. Again, the author put the paper for the drawing directly in front of Sicily. In this way, she was seeing the drawing in all four quadrants in relationship to her body. Remember Sicily had trouble with seeing the people in the butterfly picture as an event. She saw the separate people and their actions as separate relationships. Sicily was asked to draw her story. Figure 10.9 shows what Sicily drew.

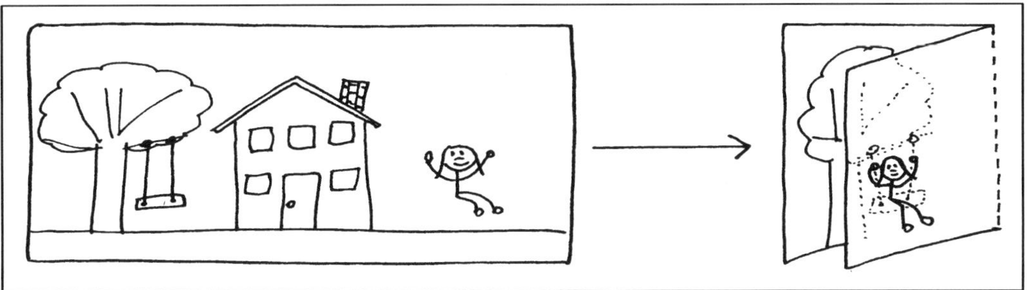

Figure 10.9 Sicily draws a girl swinging

The author asked Sicily to tell about her picture. Sicily said, "I am swinging." The author asked her to point to the part of the picture that shows Sicily swinging. She pointed to the swing. The author said, "Sicily, there is no one on the swing." So Sicily pointed with her other hand to the girl in the picture. Then the author said, "Sicily, the girl is not on the swing." Sicily looked at the picture. The author moved the whole picture over to Sicily's right upper quadrant and Sicily immediately drew herself onto the swing and said, "Oh! That's me there on the swing." Look at Sicily's picture. Notice, that if you fold the picture the girl is on the swing. Sicily is literally seeing the girl on the swing because she does not have the language to see the space in the middle. By moving the paper into one quadrant she is able to see the space.

Activity: Why did Sicily draw the picture of her swinging as two separate ideas, but on one paper?

The author moved Sicily's paper over to her right side since she writes with her right hand and positioned the paper above eye level. The author then wrote with Sicily hand-over-hand. See Figure 10.10.

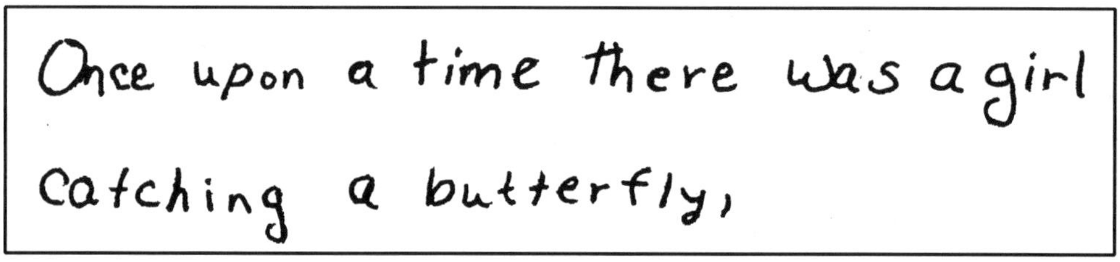

Once upon a time there was a girl
catching a butterfly,

Figure 10.10 Sicily writes with the author

Sicily said she could write. So, the author released her hand. Figure 10.11 shows her writing with the paper moved.

were
There was some
Oncee upon a time chern
catching butterflys. Misty was
catching a brutterfly, Billy
was woching the other
brutteflys in a jar.

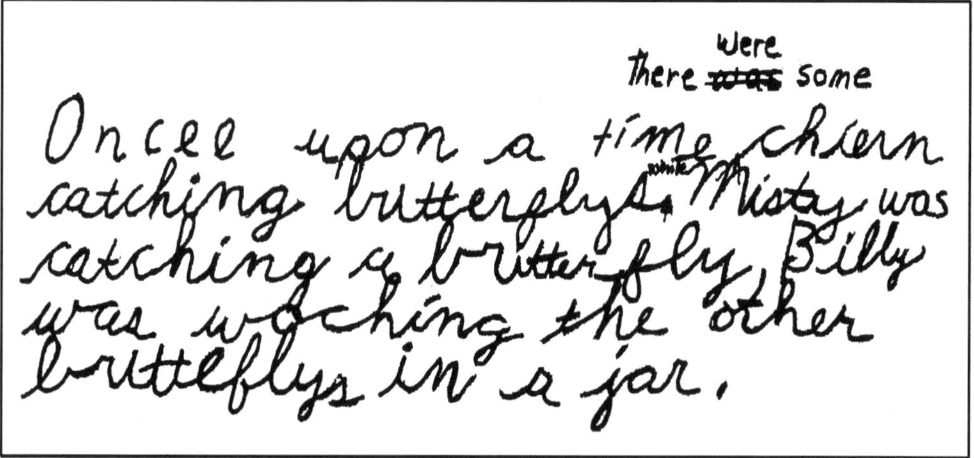

Figure 10.11 Sicily writing with the paper moved

The difference between Figures 10.6 and 10.11 is amazing. Her writing switched to cursive and she wrote the story. When she read back what she wrote, she orally completed the grammar and the author put in the corrections that Sicily said. The motor use of shapes on her right side made a huge difference in her processing of grammar as well as the story.

Sicily is able to know what she sees when the information is limited to the right side (she uses her right hand to write) and above eye level. The writing improved because, first, the author gave her the language with a picture, with an oral explanation, and with the writing of the mouth shapes, second, the paper was in the upper right-hand quadrant so she could see what her hand produced, and third, the author had used pointing and visually cuing of her mouth movements so Sicily could see the overlapping shapes. Because the motor shapes with drawings worked, this was the approach used in therapy with Sicily to help her language function for better literacy. Figure 10.12 shows the format of what was used in therapy. Sicily would write the story from her picture dictionary entries and the adult would help her put the dictionary entries into a conventional form with meaningful pictographs for the concepts to develop the language (print) that goes with the pictures.

Some children, Sicily, Billy and Misty, wanted to catch some butterflies as part of their insect collection.
Picture Dictionary
Sicily
butterflies
insect
catch
wings
holding
watching
children
collection

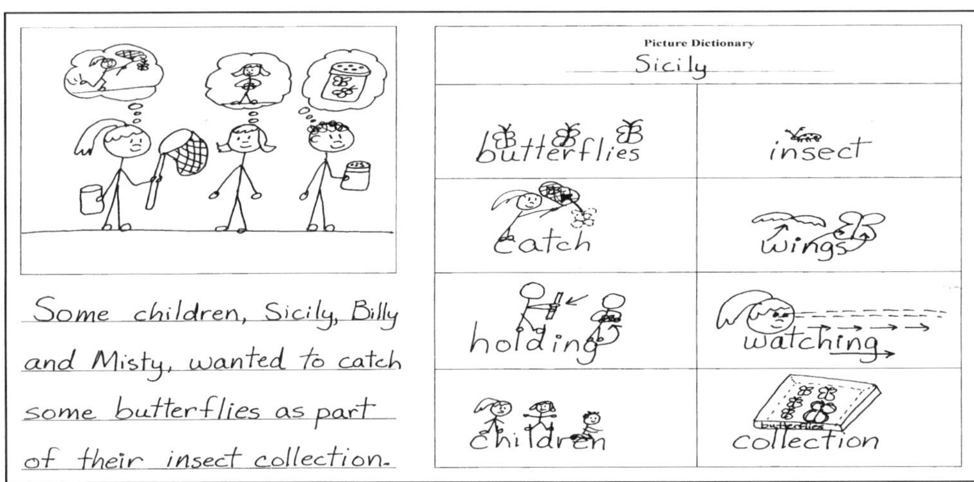

Figure 10.12 Sicily writes and draws about her concepts

Once Sicily was able to use writing as a sequence of shaped patterns that matched with pictured concepts that she drew about in her upper right-hand quadrant, she began to be successful in school. Please note that Sicily, like the other students discussed in this book, does not use the sound of concepts to learn new meanings, but is able to think in the visual concepts of the meaning of spoken words. In this way, the students learn to translate the auditory culture into meaning that allows them to have the strategies to be successful at school and in society. To be independent in society, a person must be able to function at the language level.

Activity: What are some of the reasons that the language level of thinking is so important to functioning in society?

Summary

A person with language function is able to maintain conversation with another person. Conversation requires shared conventional meaning. Therefore, conversation in an auditory language like English requires the speaker to be able to use grammatical utterances that are clear in meaning and connect with time-based words or markers like appropriate use of tense.

Neuro-typical learners develop a language function around seven to eight years of age, and therefore demonstrate adult grammatical structures at this age. Language function allows an individual to displace ideas from the here-and-now into examples and rules that have concrete meaning. In other words, language function allows a person to talk about ideas they have never physically experienced and are carried out by people who are not in the thinker's own experience.

Not everyone develops a language function that matches cognitive function or ability. For example, a person who thinks concretely may not develop language function. By intervening with methods that match the thinker's way of forming concepts, strategies can help a learner develop concepts so that language becomes more displaced, flexible, productive, semantically complex, and less redundant. In this way, the person develops a concrete language function that allows him to participate independently in society.

Applications

- Try to find some classroom materials designed for teaching time, space, quantity, and quality as part of language...if this is difficult, it is because these semantic components of language are often ignored.
- Develop a list of skills that an independent adult must have to be a citizen. How many of these skills depend on a language function that tools literacy?

Chapter 11

LINGUISTIC THINKERS

Learner objectives: Chapter 11

Upon completion of this chapter, the reader should be able to:

1. Explain what characteristics a linguistic thinker has.
2. Explain how time, quantity, space, and quality function at the linguistic level.
3. Provide some examples of strategies to help a person function more at a linguistic level.
4. Explain how to help flowchart the meaning of ideas so as to increase the learning of formal concepts.
5. Explain how the lack of linguistic function affects literacy.
6. Explain how improving the function of language as a tool improves literacy processes, especially reading and writing.

I know multiple ways of seeing the same movie.
I can watch multiple screens at the same time.
I can rewind the movie or the teacher's spoken words.
I even have my own copying system.

Linguistic function is the pinnacle of language development. Grammatical sentences express complex ways to *displace* ideas beyond what is seen, touched, or felt. *Conversations* about government, politics, economics, historical accuracy, philosophy, religion, for example, go beyond personal opinion and facts and into theory and policy, mores of ethics, and application of principles. In an auditory culture that uses an auditory language like English, ideas connect with *time-based* arguments to form formal ***propositions*** or messages at the linguistic level of function. This chapter will discuss the characteristics of linguistic thinkers and then discuss the expectations of an auditory society with regards to linguistic function.

Neuro-typical linguistic function

Grammatical language structures that function with the most complexity are linguistic in nature. This means that, at this level, the linguistic function of language provides maximum cognitive *displacement*, *semanticity*, *productivity*, and *flexibility,* while minimizing the external *redundancy* of structures. These maximum functions are a result of the speaker learning concepts as layers of meaning over time. Maximum displacement means that the speaker is able to talk about ideas that cannot be seen, touched, or felt such as concepts of "justice," "government," "respect," "responsibility," "liberty," "consideration," "collaboration," "ancient," "love," "power," "accountability," "thoughtfulness," and "kindness." These ideas are the most "abstract" in that each concept represents a multiplicity of applications. For example, the concept "respect" could be applied to respect for one's self, respect for others' needs, respect for personal property, respect for others' actions, respect for authority, respect for one's feelings and others' feelings, respect for community, respect for values, respect for learning, and so forth (Arwood & Young, 2000). These many applications of a single concept will result in a formal way of thinking. Formal thinking is the ability to use the concepts in a variety of socially acceptable ways for maximum development of meaning.

Activity: What is formal thinking like? What are some language examples of linguistic function?

All concepts at the linguistic level of function are relative to the development of other formal concepts. And, formal applications develop from the multiplicity of concrete, rule governed concepts that relate to each other. This layering and overlapping of conceptual meaning or *semanticity* develops into the linguistic function, the maximum function of language.

Activity: What is maximum displacement? What is formal semanticity?

With the ability to represent ideas with a maximum level of *displacemen*t and *semanticity*, a learner is able to create concepts about the mind, of the mind, through the mind, and separate from the two-dimensional, neuro-physical brain. This unique human capacity to create knowledge of discovery such as "thinking" about "thinking" is what neuroscientists and educators attempt to understand when their images show that the brain is synergistic and the "whole is greater than the parts" (Arwood, 1983, 1991a; Basor, 2006; Compagni & Manderscheid, 2006; Peirce, 2000). The neural networks that develop to provide the overarching development of learning capacity known as the formal mind require the most cerebral feedback and therefore the highest level of linguistic function. Linguistic function stems from the interactive cognitive and social applications of language, across multiple uses of concepts in a variety of settings. The social application is from society determining the most productive and flexible applications of the cognitive displacement and semanticity of formal thinking.

Activity: Why is linguistic function an expression of both social and cognitive thinking?

Formal thinking or linguistic function provides for maximum *productivity* in the application of learning to be literate. Maximum productivity is the ability to use language as a cognitive tool to generate ideas without physical experience. For example, with maximum productivity, a thinker is able to create concepts about working in outer space or at the bottom of the ocean without ever being in space or swimming at the bottom of the ocean. This type of productivity places no limits on language function. Likewise, the person who has maximum linguistic productivity is also able to use language in a variety of places—work, academia, travel, home, community, and so forth. For example, a person with maximum flexibility might be asked to travel to Egypt tomorrow. Even though the person has never been to Egypt, he is able to know what he needs to take for clothes, paperwork, money, and can be ready to go by morning. The flexible producer of maximum language is able to "think" through this formal process and "take care" of loose ends within multi-tasking. Of course, this hypothetical example assumes that the traveler has the resources for taking care of family and work related issues and that the organization and planning is specific to how the brain functions.

Activity: What is maximum flexibility and maximum productivity? How do these two linguistic functions interact with maximum displacement and semanticity?

The formal thinker is able to problem solve, resource, critically plan, and organize ideas independent of others. Thinking and doing are abstractly intertwined. This means that the formal linguistic thinker is able to create new ideas from what is not known and problem solve from taking the perspectives of others. Being able to conceptualize about the "unknown" is purely a cognitive function. For example, a formal thinker is able to take all of the past knowledge about airplanes and build an airbus that flies on its first outing because this thinker can interconnect all the conceptual pieces into a bigger picture, something no one has ever seen, touched, or felt. This type of conceptual interconnectedness is true ***symbolization***, the act of creating the meaning of more complex concepts from symbols, not from physical experience. For example, sometimes adults will say, "I am a hands-on learner." If that is really true, then this learner cannot function above the preoperational level of pre-language function: The hands-on learner functions in the here-and-now where ideas are as one sees, touches, and feels. This restricted function limits the amount of *displacement*, *semanticity*, *flexibility*, and *productivity*. This adult who thinks she or he is a hands-on learner is probably not aware of how language can function as a tool for cognitive development.

Activity: What is the difference between a physical experience and a cognitive experience?

Higher order thinking and problem solving require maximum linguistic function to be able to analyze and evaluate all possible options from others' perspectives. For example, to learn about the physics of a sound wave can occur with words. That does not mean that an experiment with musical strings would not enhance one's knowledge about pitch, loudness, and time of a sound wave, but this "hands-on" experiment has no meaning without language. For example, recall a time when a science teacher demonstrated an experiment and then asked students to write up what they learned. Without language that explained what the students saw in the demonstration, the students did not know the conceptual meaning of the experiment. Students can describe the experiment but not necessarily be able to talk about the higher order conceptual relationships of the experiment.

With linguistic function, a learner is able to watch the experiment and then use mental language to think about how to resource, such as how to read the science book to learn about the meaning of the teacher's science experiment or how to draw or write out the ideas to "see" the meaning of the experiment through avenues of literacy. Linguistic function allows the learner to develop a formal way of problem solving and critical thinking. *Linguistic function gives the learner the mental social and cognitive processes to think about how to learn and how to use language for learning.*

Activity: What does linguistic function do to help a learner think?

As thinking or cognitive development is represented by language function, linguistic function represents formal cognition, the process by which thinking is layered over and over into more and more complex concepts. At the earliest level, newborn babies are acquiring sensory input but by the time they are 18–24 months, they are able to respond with motor acts that represent what they know about the *pre-language semantic relationships of agents, their actions, and the context's objects.* These semantic relationships overlap in meaning to begin to create layers of concepts representing limited or restricted ideas about the child being the center of others' acts and objects, *preoperational development of pre-language function.* At the next level, the preoperational ideas and relationships overlap creating layers of meaning that create a concrete or rule-governed level of meaning. The same scaffolding process of overlapping layers of meaning into more complex concepts occurs across the developmental stages to eventually form linguistic function. At the *linguistic level of function or thinking* the layers of meaning are symbolized abstractions of concepts that include social processes of ethics and integrity.

Table 11.1 shows the levels of cognitive function as language develops for the concept "table" (Arwood & McInroy, 1995).

Table 11.1 Stages of thinking and language functions

Neuro-typical development	Pre-language function	Language function	Linguistic function
Sensori-motor thinking (0–2 years)	Pre-production limited structures The concept "table" is seen as a place for the bottle.	NA	NA
Preoperational thinking (3–7 years)	Restricted structures The concept "table" is talked about in relationship to the child's actions.	NA	NA
Concrete thinking (7–11 years)	NA	Shared conversation and grammatical structures The concept "table" is talked about as a type of furniture like the one in the dining room, the bedroom, the family room, next door, at school, etc.	NA

Formal thinking (11+ years)	NA	NA	Maximum: displacement semanticity productivity flexibility limited: redundancy The concept "table" is uniquely abstract: "Please table that motion until we have served notice to the public."

Activity: What are the levels of meaningful acquisition for concepts?

Social-cognitive linguistic development

Concepts are social and cognitive in nature. In this way, learning is a socio-cognitive process. Because language represents these social and cognitive concepts, language is intertwined in the development of social and cognitive layering of concepts. As language developmentally increases so does cognition. And, as the child thinks about his or her own "self," the child's thinking *displaces* and the child begins to think about others. In this way, the child is learning the social concepts as well as the cognitive concepts.

Similarly, the social development means that children with more development about social concepts are able to think about others. At the formal level, this ability to be socially cognizant of others allows the linguistic thinker to experience empathy, walk in the shoes of others, problem solve from others' perspectives, and so forth.

Activity: Explain how concepts represent both social and cognitive development.

As social and cognitive development increases, the mind also develops into being able to understand more formal, abstract and symbolized forms of language. However, this linguistic function of social and cognitive development tends to increase through the processes of literacy. Literacy includes thinking, viewing, listening, speaking, reading, writing, and calculating. Each of these literacy processes use language as a tool. Language at a concrete level of function scaffolds the meaning of concepts for the learner into more formal, abstract concepts. Therefore, the more literate a person becomes the better developed is the cognitive and social development. Being literate helps develop cognitive development at the formal level of linguistic function.

Children, who are able to develop literacy at a concrete level of thinking or higher and have grammatical use of language structures, are able to function at the linguistic level provided that they have the opportunity to use their language as a tool. Society expects individuals to function at the concrete level of language function or to function at a higher level. This means that for individuals to function socially and cognitively within the mainstream of society, they must be at the concrete level of language function or higher, at the linguistic level of function.

Activity: Why is a concrete language function needed to develop an abstract, linguistic function?

Those with restricted language function (pre-language level) will be marginalized as they do not have access to the language of society's rules for how to think and function cognitively and socially. Even though individuals with pre-language function do not operate in the mainstream of society's expectations, they may develop a formal level of concept development in a specific area. For example, maybe a person spends most days studying insects. This person may show restricted social development and therefore function as a pre-language thinker. But, the same individual may be able to tell about insects. This telling about insects may be very rote or quite animated from the individual's own interest in the subject. However, thinking about another person's perspective about insects may not be understood. So, this thinker tells about insects again and again and again, not thinking that the other person may not be interested in insects. Deep understanding of a particular ***semantic field*** of concepts such as insects only provides formal conceptualization, not linguistic function. Linguistic function must cross social and cognitive areas of symbolized development for maximum *displacement*, *semanticity*, *productivity*, *flexibility*, and *limited redundancy*.

Individuals can be very talented in a particular conceptual area but still struggle with social or cognitive developmental functions in other areas of their lives. This latter issue has possible widespread effects on society. More about these effects will be provided later in this chapter.

Activity: What is the relationship between linguistic function and conceptual development? Why does linguistic function require both a cognitive and social component?

Not all learners are able to think at the formal level of linguistic function. In fact, it is estimated that around 30 percent of the regular population thinks at a restricted level of function: using blaming language such as "It's your fault," victim language such as "You made me angry," and single person language such as "my classroom," "my students," or "my ideas." These thinkers are in the preoperational level of cognitive thought and often function at the social level of the world revolving around them. At this level, these thinkers do not imagine other people in their mental pictures and they are not higher order thinkers or problem solvers. Most of the time, they do not have access of linguistic social and cognitive function.

Society expects a concrete, rule-governed level of function so that thinking is about how people work together, function in a classroom together, live in a family or community together, and share experiences together. Language is about "our story" such as "We got a new pet at school today." Individuals at this level think about themselves in a mental picture or with head language that is about "others" such as families, classrooms, and employment situations. These individuals may show an occasional use of linguistic function and sometimes, under stress, may function as a pre-language thinker.

At the formal, linguistic level of function, decisions are made as a process of analyzing what is best for the greater good. Ethics, rather than rules, dictate what is socially acceptable. Principles, rather than simple right and wrong, provide the rationale for action. Thinking is a symbolic linguistic function.

Activity: What are the three conceptual levels of thinking as they relate to language development and function?

Symbolic thinking

Since English is a time-based, alphabetic language that is inflectional and global in nature, a linguistic thinker must be able to use the properties of English for symbolic thinking. In other words, a linguistic thinker of English uses the language with maximum time-based concepts in a variety of literacy forms. English conveys time in a multiplicity of ways: time words, time endings, time phrases, time concepts. Therefore, a linguistic thinker is able to use English in a time-based way.

A speaker with linguistic function refers to shared ideas with symbolic forms of complex sentence structure. The ideas, which are also called arguments, are then interconnected through time elements to form an auditory proposition or message that is greater than the sum of the arguments. For example: "Yesterday I went to the store to buy some flowers, but I forgot to take my wallet. So, I had to come back home and get it." The first idea is about something that already happened: "Yesterday" and "went." The speaker tells the listener "what he did" and then connects that idea with a temporal element, "but" to indicate that something related to the first idea happened: "He forgot his wallet." With these words, the listener is to infer that the speaker could not "buy" the flowers because he forgot his wallet. The little word "so" connects both the idea that the speaker wanted to buy some flowers but forgot his wallet with what happened next: The speaker went home to get his wallet. The inferred meaning of what the speaker did with his wallet, which is to go back and buy the flowers, is a greater meaning than the separate sentences. *The three ideas interconnected in time to form a proposition, a message that is greater than its parts.*

Activity: What is a proposition?

If three sentences are produced without such temporal (time-based) connections, then the parts will not create a proposition. For example: "I like to ride my horse. My horse is spirited. Other people don't want to ride her." These three ideas do not interconnect with temporal meaning and therefore the listener is not sure why other people do not ride the speaker's horse. Now watch what happens when the ideas are temporally interconnected. "I like to ride my horse but she is so spirited that others don't want to ride her." The meaning of the three sentences combined by temporal words is greater than the parts: The listener knows that people are probably afraid to ride the horse because it is so spirited; that is, the horse might "buck off" its riders who could be hurt.

At the formal linguistic level of function, language creates auditory propositions that are time based. This ability to produce these propositions assists in the development of literacy skills (reading, writing, thinking, viewing, listening, speaking, and calculating) that are pro-social in nature. Pro-social thinking includes the learner's ability to interconnect ideas of others with present or future ideas. For example, "I want to have friends. Friends are important to me. Sally is my friend." These separate ideas are not interconnected with time-based elements. Interconnect the ideas: "Sally is a very important person to me because she is my friend and I value good friends." This ability to interconnect social and cognitive ideas allows a person to think about others in a linguistic manner. In this way, the linguistic thinker is able to think about others and how they think. By being able to view from other people's perspectives, the linguistic thinker is able to develop higher order thinking about social development. People who live in an auditory culture, and who possess linguistic function of English, experience a match between their thinking and their culture. Their development of literacy is at a formal, linguistic level of function.

Activity: How do time-based elements create propositions? How does the social and cognitive development of ideas help develop linguistic function?

Neuro-atypical linguistic function

When people develop a lot of language structures and are older than about 11 years of age, most professionals do not recognize that there is a language problem. In other words, a speaker who produces a lot of language structures is viewed as exhibiting adequate language. But, "possessing" language structures is not language function. The function of language is about thinking. And, at the linguistic level, thinking is formal in nature. This section describes the development of language structures without the linguistic function and the formal ability to think about a cognitive area of development such as dinosaurs, but not having linguistic function for social or other cognitive areas of development.

The brain of most learners is ready for the abstract, formal linguistic thinking at around 11 years of age. Common ideas have developed concrete meanings that layer to form the most *displaced* meanings for *productive* and *flexible* language function. This means that formal, linguistic function does not happen until age 11. Therefore, people who are over 11 years of age are expected (by society) to understand formal concepts such as "steal." However, remember that not all neuro-typical people function at the formal level and society expects only a concrete, rule-governed level of understanding. Therefore, society expects a person to understand a formal concept like "steal" only at the rule-governed or concrete level: "Don't take things." However, when formal concepts are used and individuals do not understand the rules (concrete) or the formal function of the words, there are social or cognitive effects. For example, a 15-year-old has a television set in his hand, the same television that was in the backseat of a car that a person is loading. "You stole my TV." The 15-year-old responds, "No, I didn't. I didn't steal anything." The person loading his car says, "I saw you take that TV out of my car." The 15-year-old says, "I didn't take your TV." The adult says, "I saw that hand (points to his hand) take that TV from that (points to the backseat of the car) car." The 15-year-old says, "Yeah."

This example of the 15-year-old is based on several true stories where the person who has stolen an item or items rebukes the concepts of "steal" which is formal and "take" which is concrete, but admits to the author the preoperational task of possessing hands that do something. This is a neuro-atypical function of language development. These individuals are functioning at a preoperational level of thinking about themselves. Others and others' things are not in their pictures. Furthermore, they "know" that "steal" is "bad" and they do not see themselves as bad; therefore, they cannot steal. As this individual and other individuals who have stolen items have told the author, the TV (or any other item) was not in anybody else's possession or hand, therefore the TV does not belong to anybody. Again, having the object as part of the agent is preoperational in nature. At the concrete level, the person understands the rule about taking something that a person does not buy is wrong.

Only at the formal level does a person really understand the concept "steal." Steal is formal in that it performs an action (see Chapter 3 about performatives) that the mind creates when the concept functions with language assigned. The formal rules for the concept of "steal" are semantic in nature and include: Knowing that when one sees an object that one did not buy then someone else bought the object; and whoever bought the object owns the object. Furthermore, the rules of society include: Taking an object that does not belong to one is wrong and a person should be punished for wrong doing. Both socially and cognitively, linguistic functioning is important to society. If 70 percent or more of the general population do not function at the formal level, then 70 percent or more of the general population do not understand concepts like "steal," "lie," "marry," "government," "justice," "liberty," at a formal level. Of these 70 percent, about 40 percent are able to understand these concepts as rules: "It is wrong to steal or lie." "Government is big business." "Everyone should have justice." These sentences are borrowed "sayings" that are like rules to live by. However, that leaves 30 percent or more who do not live by the rules. These individuals understand formal concepts at a preoperational level. They depend on society to control their lack of understanding through social services, unhealthy or dependent family relationships, and/or by forms of incarceration.

Activity: What happens when a person does not understand a formal concept like "steal" at a formal level? What is the difference between concrete and preoperational thinking about formal concepts like "steal?"

A person may develop enough language structures to appear to maintain a language conversation (see Chapter 10 about language function) but not have the understanding of formal concepts like "steal" or "justice." Keep in mind that this person with all of the language structures is able to "imitate" the acoustic pattern of the formal concept and therefore the person can "say" the word but still not understand the meaning of the produced word at a formal level. For example, many individuals who are diagnosed with various learning affected labels such as ADHD (attention deficit hyperactivity disorders), ASD (autism spectrum disorders including Asperger syndrome), FAS (fetal alcohol syndrome or effects), or SLD (specific learning disabilities such as dyslexia, dysgraphia, dyscalculia) are able to develop significant adult-like vocabularies, especially in an interest area, but still not have linguistic function for formal social and cognitive development. For example, a person with an autism spectrum disorder may be able to show a variety of literacy processes for numbers related to accounting; but, this same person may not be able to fit into a social cocktail hour. Most diagnostic labels, such as ASD or SLD, are determined, in part, by cognitive and/or social differences which in turn have a language component.

Activity: Explain how a person might demonstrate a lot of language development but still not understand very abstract concepts like "respect" or "steal" at a formal, linguistic level of function.

Being able to function at the language or linguistic level requires that a person is able to function socially and cognitively in the way that society expects (rule governed) as well as across the multiple settings. Therefore, educators need to understand that a child who is a "genius" with numbers but who is not reading and writing will be restricted both socially and cognitively in language function. Therefore, schools must consider how to increase thinking for critical analysis, problem solving, and planning as part of their curriculum if schools want students to be able to function socially and cognitively at their best. Imitating others' patterns for correct facts, right answers, and repetition of skills or language structures does not provide students with language or linguistic function. Remember that linguistic function is ideal but society only expects the rule-governed language function level.

Activity: Why should schools provide students with language opportunities for critical thinking if schools want students to function in the mainstream of society?

How a person's language functions is always a mirror of how a person learns concepts. If the educator knows how a person learns concepts, intervention may be planned to match the person's strength in learning concepts. Remember intervention emphasis is not on teaching language structures; the emphasis is on language function or thinking that affects social and cognitive development.

The following sample is taken from an adolescent in an attempt to assess him for his language function which will provide the basis to appropriate intervention:

He struggled with the prompt "What do you do on a typical day?" When the student said that the town was building a new Home Depot store, the evaluator asked, "What will you do when you go to the new store?"

> Well, I don't know. I haven't looked over there. Um, not directly, you know. I haven't looked all over. Um, um, the reason I have 20 some dollars is because see um, I see, I don't, of course, I don't get paid anything if, I, um don't work for anything, you know. Um, which I think I would be kind of spoiled to get something just without work. And, so I, so I um, um, so I well, um what happens is, you would normally think at first that a route was fun. It isn't fun when you get used to it, you know for a little while. Um, so, so, what I did, I get, I help Arnold on, on the certain part of the route, only do certain ones like now I do 7, used to do 13, used to do 6, sometimes I did 1, not 2, but sometimes, 14, and 3, and 8, but used to do 9, but now I do 7, but it's just like a hill because a big hill would be a mountain, used to do 13, but now I do 7. Um, well, there's this hill, it's long, but it isn't, it isn't big, you know. Used to do 13, used to do 6, not 9, sometimes 2, not a long route but a big route, will, it's like long but it, it isn't. I would get the route, well I think it was fun but it isn't. We first started out on the paper route, didn't we? Well, I help Arnold, on some routes, not the long part, well it is like a hill and I help him on the hill…

The adult finally cut Cliff's conversation off.

This young teen, Cliff, is in general education and he should have a linguistic way of thinking or functioning. This means that his oral language should show maximum understanding of displaced ideas (*maximum displacement*), formal concepts (*maximum semanticity*), the ability to talk productively about ideas in the past with someone in the present (*maximum productivity*), and with efficiency (*maximum flexibility* along with limited external *redundancy*). Even though Cliff uses a lot of sentence structures he does not have linguistic function.

The usual assessment questions are asked and addressed:

1. How does he learn concepts the best? Because he does not use time to connect his ideas into a chronological story, he is not using time-based English. English is a time-based, auditory language; so, he does not learn concepts with an auditory system but a visual system.
2. What is his rate of learning? Cliff has learned lots of structures. Anytime a speaker has lots of language structures, then his learning rate is average or above.
3. What can educators do to help Cliff? Cliff has a visual way of thinking; so the educators may want to use some VLMs (Viconic Language Methods™) to help him learn about time and how to organize his thinking so that he speaks, reads, and writes with a linguistic function.

Educators thought Cliff had developed a lot of language structures but from assessing his language function, it was evident that he had not developed linguistic thinking. Therefore, his reading and writing problems were a result of learning that affects his thinking, but he did not really have a problem with the development of language structures. By helping Cliff develop better language function, at more of a linguistic level, then his academic as well as social skills improved. The following sample of intervention shows how VLMs provided Cliff with context, spatial use of ideas (instead of time-based ideas), and a visual-motor way of organizing his thinking. Once his thinking was organized, he showed solid writing.

The first step of the process was to help Cliff modify his use of reading and writing strategies into better thinking based on how he learned. So, he was asked to read a grade level passage,[1] and then use his oral language to tell about what he read.

> Mark Twain's name is famous throughout the world for his tales of Tom Sawyer and Huck Finn.
>
> Twain tried many kinds of work, though, before he became an author. He worked as a printer, river pilot, soldier, and newspaper reporter and editor.
>
> In 1865, he and a friend, Jim Gillis, were in the California mountains of Calaveras County prospecting for gold. The two young men spent the rainy times in the tavern of the mining camp.
>
> One rainy day at the tavern they met an old prospector, Ben Coon. Coon spent hours telling endless tales, all in a flat, monotonous tone of voice and with a deadpan face. Twain and Gillis thought that the old prospector's stories were excruciatingly funny because of the way he told his stories with absolutely no expression or suggestion of humor.
>
> A few afternoons later, Coon told them a ridiculous anecdote about a jumping frog. Twain thought the story was so amusing that he decided to write the story of the jumping frog, He sent it east to a friend, who had it published. The story caught the fancy of the public and was given the name "The Celebrated Jumping Frog of Calaveras County."

1 This passage is from the Sucher-Allread Oral Reading Test which is no longer in print.

Reading out loud was difficult because the sound of Cliff's own voice makes the pictures of what he is seeing on the page disappear. But, he tried to tell what he could remember:

> It's about Mark Twain…first became a writer, and…how him and his friend were in California in Calaveras Country and they met this old guy that…uh, kept… telling tales with absolutely no expression, and with really like low and deep voice, and how he sent a few, sent it back to a writer, and got it published and the name was the uh, The Something jumping frog.

Cliff's oral language does not show the type of functions that stand alone for conversation to be understood without inferring or interpreting the meaning for Cliff.

Cliff was then given a choice to write about the story or draw the story. Most students his age have been told in a variety of ways that writing must come before drawing, so he opted to write even though drawing would have been easier. As he began to write, he squirmed, perspiration poured down his face, and so he asked to re-read the passage silently. This is really a good strategy for Cliff, as he is a visual-motor thinker. So, he was given the passage to read silently. All children with visual systems should be taught to silently scan for the ideas on the page rather than practice over and over the sounds of the words for oral fluency. Scanning is accomplished by putting the material flat on the table, with the reader's eyes looking out over the paper that is positioned in the upper quadrant of the side the child writes with. Then the educator shows the reader how to use his or her hand to scan the words lightly as the reader sees the print so as to create a visual-motor scan of what the reader sees. He then attempted to write, still struggling all the way through the 15-minute process. Figure 1.1 shows his writing.

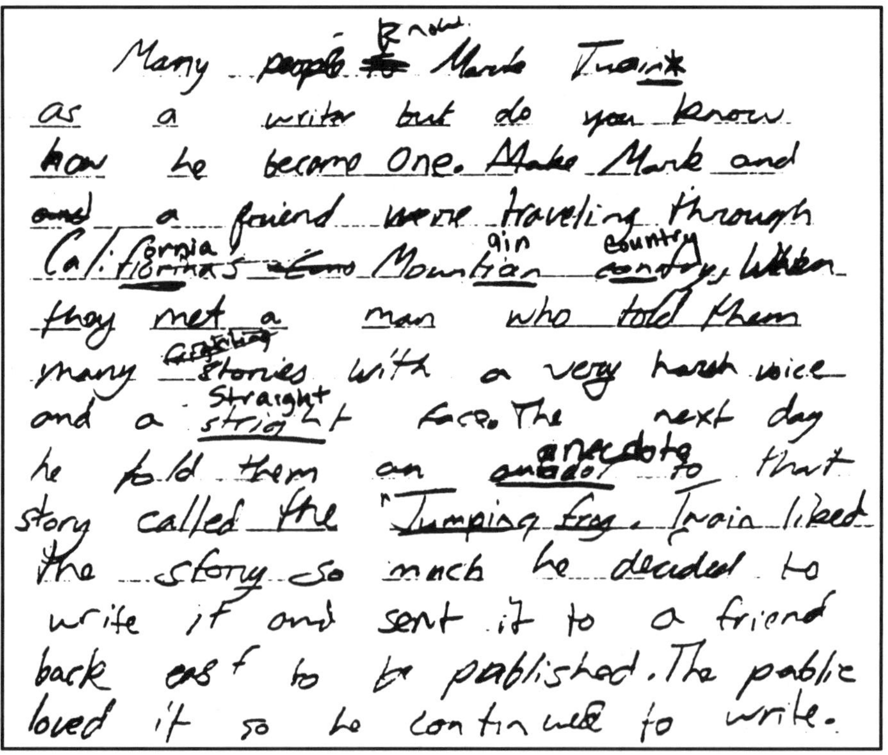

Figure 11.1 Cliff's writing

Cliff was then asked to cartoon what he remembered of the story. Figure 11.2 is his cartoon. Note that he mentally understood what "cartoon" meant and he needed no additional instructions.

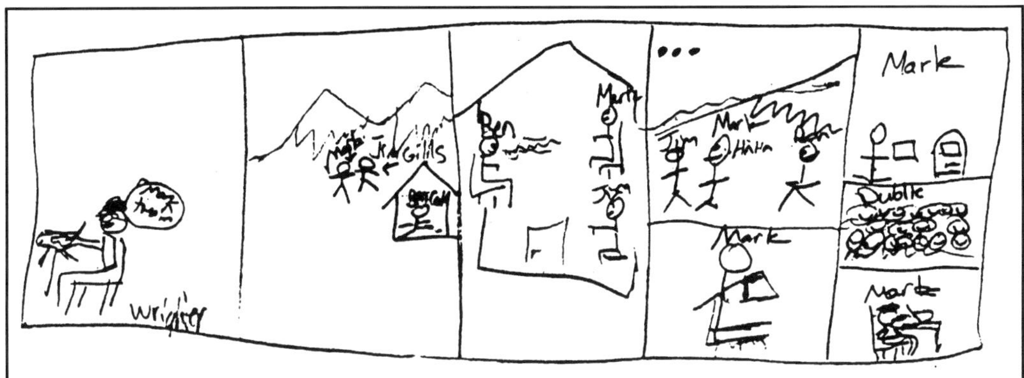

Figure 11.2 Cliff's cartoon

If the drawing helped Cliff organize his thinking, then drawing should help him with his oral language as well as his writing. So, he was asked to tell the story to the cartoon; that is, while he looked at the pictures of the cartoon. The following is Cliff's oral language as he talked about the pictures and literally pointed to the picture.

> Many people know Mark Twain as a writer, and he's writing a book (he points to the picture). And this (points) is before when he was in the mountains with his friends and then there (points) he had many jobs. He was a publisher, an editor, un, a something pilot, and a printer. And, uh, one day he was hiking through the mountains with his friends, one's name Jim, and they went into a tavern, and Ben Cook, an old associate or something, and he told them long tedious, not tedious, what's the word, end-less tales, and he had a very serious face, and then the next day, after he tells him the stories, Ben tells him an anecdote to that story called the "Jumping Frog" and Mark Twain likes it a lot and decides to write about it and then he sends it off to get it published by a friend back East, and the public loves it so he becomes a writer.

Cliff was able to tell a lot more details, but, who, what, where, when, why, and how of the story are still not connected. English connects these ideas with time-based elements. By scanning silently and by drawing a cartoon he was able to retrieve a lot of what he saw as print on the page, but he still needs more visual-motor layers to create the language function that will stand alone for conversation and linguistically will represent the functions of English.

Because Cliff is thinking in a visual-motor way, he is given another visual-motor layer by asking him to put words to his pictures. He literally wrote words to one picture about Mark Twain (see Figure 11.3).

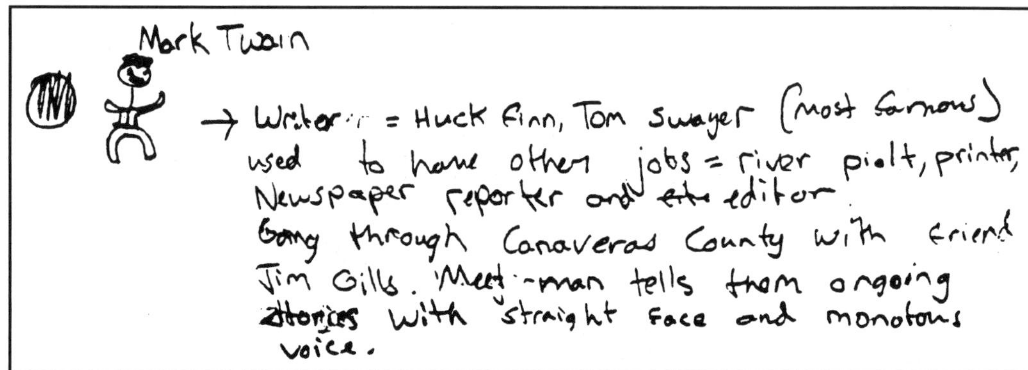

Figure 11.3 Cliff's words in isolation to the one picture

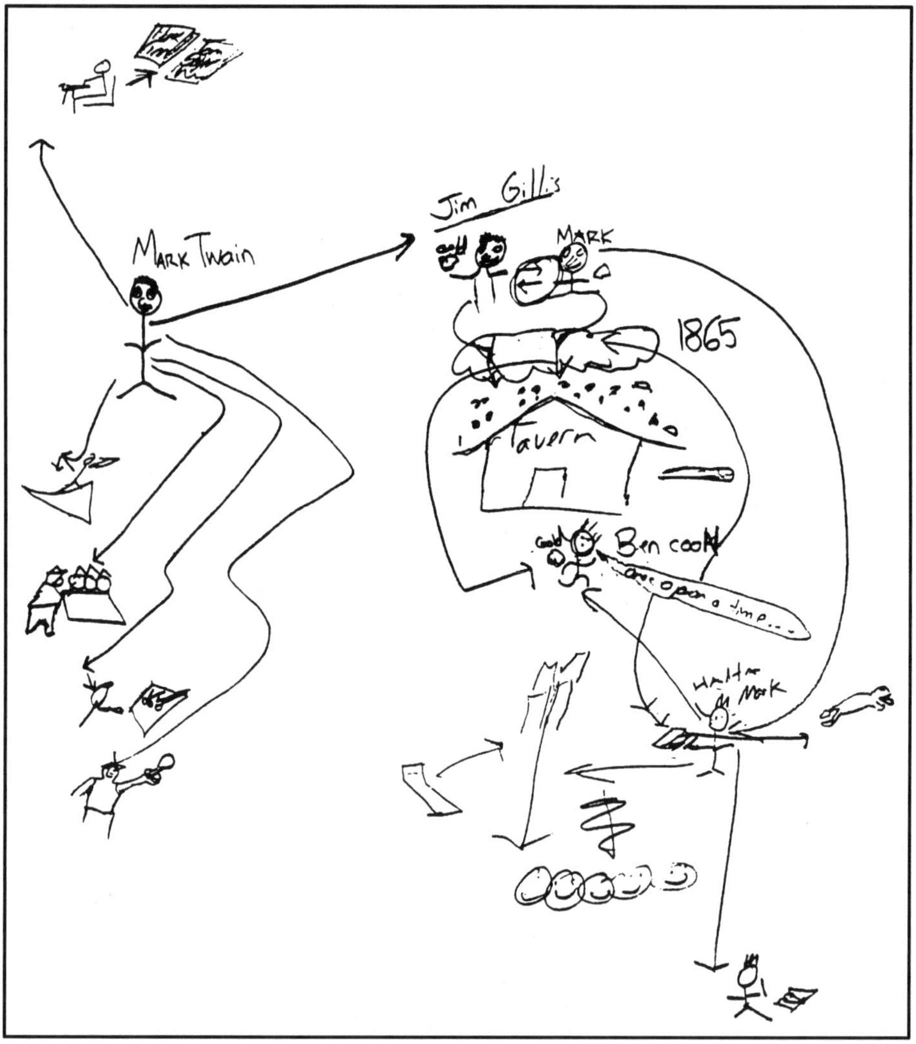

Figure 11.4 Cliff's flowchart to translate thinking to writing

The educator told Cliff that she wanted a set of pictures in place of the words but not as a cartoon to show how the ideas were connected in a "flowchart." Cliff immediately drew a flowchart (see Figure 11.4).

This drawing had more details: why they went into a tavern, who was there, what they did, when they did it, and even some about how and what they did.

Since all of the expanded functions (who, what, where, why, how, and when) were included, Cliff was asked to use his flowchart to write his ideas about what he read. He quickly began to write (see Figure 11.5).

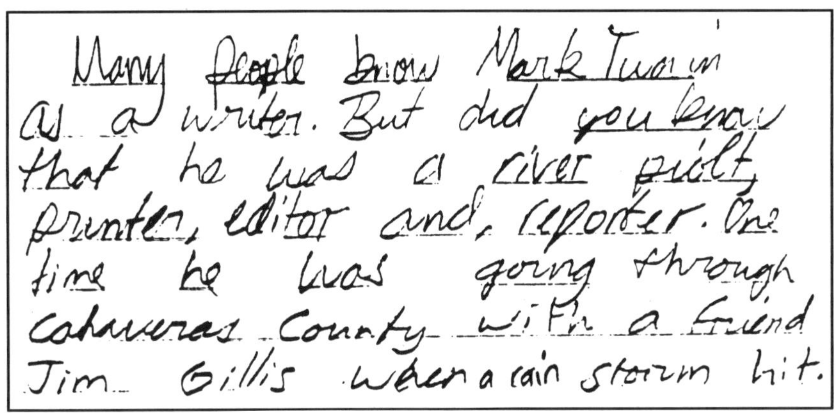

Many people know Mark Twain as a writer. But did you know that he was a river pilot, printer, editor and reporter. One time he was going through Calaveras County with a friend Jim Gillis when a rain storm hit.

Figure 11.5 Cliff's writing after gaining language for thinking

Even though he wanted to continue, he was stopped as the 45 minutes from beginning to end of this session had run out. It literally took him seconds to write this paragraph.

Drawing what Cliff read helped him put visual ideas that he gained from the print on the page into a static form. Then he could refine the drawings with words and the words with drawings until his thinking emerged into more linguistic function. At that point, he was able to organize the language of the drawing, match the print of the passage to his thinking, and write what he was able to understand.

Activity: What were the intervention steps for Cliff?

All students with visual systems should be encouraged to draw before they write. The drawings can be complete pictures of stick figure stories like used in primary grades (see Chapter 13), or cartooned stories like used in intermediate grades (see Chapter 14), or pictographed symbols for middle school, teens, and adults (see Chapter 15). By drawing the ideas onto a piece of paper, the visual thinker is able to refer back to what he drew while writing or speaking.

Writing the words to the exact pictures did not help Cliff understand the concepts so he was asked to make the visual connections of the ideas (pictures with arrows connecting pictures) as a visual flowchart. This provides Cliff with the ability to see how the ideas interconnect. This type of formal thinking on paper allows individuals with the formal ability to see how formal concepts interconnect. Remember that formal concepts have multiple relationships which is why drawing the ideas and then the connections with arrows provide the learner with a visual way of seeing the interconnections among ideas.

Notice that Cliff was asked to write about the passage after his drawing helped him organize his thinking. The result of the help with his thinking was better writing, not only in terms of legibility but also conceptually. One of the most important principles of language function is as follows: *When the meaning of the task becomes more difficult, the production level goes down.* This means, when Cliff had to explain the formal relationships among the characters of the passage and "how Mark Twain became a writer" his oral language, read language, and written language productions were not good. However, when his thinking about what he saw in print was organized, then he was able to draw what he knew, refine the meaning of the connections among the concepts (flowchart), and write at a formal, time-based linguistic level.

Cliff's ability to write his ideas fluently did not come from working on language structures such as grammar, punctuation, vocabulary, or writing skills, but Cliff's ability came from helping him refine his thinking so that his ideas were organized and his concepts more complete. *In other words, if an educator increases a thinker's conceptualization, then the thinker's literacy products improve. But, working on products does not help thinking.*

Activity: What are the two principles about production and comprehension that were described in the previous section?

Cliff's inability to read and write at grade level was the result of the lack of teaching him how to think with his learning system. By providing Cliff with language strategies to translate his visual thinking into auditory English, he was able to begin to use his language as a tool for improved reading and writing. The amount of time that it took to work Cliff through the various visual-motor translations about Mark Twain took only 45 minutes. He then went home and pulled out a magazine about one of his hobbies, skate boarding, and proceeded to do the same process. His parents were amazed that with the translation process in effect, that Cliff could read and write. Cliff was described as a non-reader and a non-writer at the time he came in to be assessed, which meant that Cliff was not learning to use his language as a tool to become literate. When he was given the language tools, he could read and write at a linguistic level because he could think about what he was reading and writing in the way that he learns concepts. The result of Cliff being able to use his visual system to access higher level thinking is symbolic language for better thinking and problem solving.

Activity: How does learning concepts affect reading and writing for linguistic function?

Specific language errors

For individuals who are able to think at a formal level in a specific area of conceptual development, but who do not have linguistic function, there are some other language issues in addition to organization by time-based properties of English. Specific errors in language function are often noticed: (1) Lack of ***referential clarity***, (2) misperceptions that result in ***misconceptions***, (3) problems with focus ***on-topic***, and (4) a lack of ***natural language***.

1. Lack of *referential clarity* results in vague or non-specific language. For example, notice that in Cliff's sample, the reader is not sure how Mark Twain and his friend were traveling through the mountains, who they met, when they met, where they

met, how they met, and why they told stories. Cliff's inability to articulate these specifics stems from his own inability to organize his mental pictures. When he was talking about earning money from his paper route to use at the store, he never really connected the job to the referent of what he was going to do at the store. Cliff has visual mental thoughts, but Cliff does not know that his spoken or written words do not match his mental thoughts. And, Cliff is not aware that others do not have the same mental pictures that he does and that others are not able to see his mental pictures. At the formal level of linguistic function, his language should reflect his clarity of thought.

Activity: What is referential clarity?

2. Because people who think in a visual meta-cognition live in an auditory culture, then they often do not receive information in a visual way. Therefore, they attempt to use the spoken word in the way that they perceive it. For example, Cliff struggles with the concept of long as in the length of a route and a hill that is steep but not high like a mountain. These concepts are all part of linguistic qualifiers that relate to space and size. So, his perception of a route (area) is not long or tall and he cannot conceptualize how to tell the listener about these differences in a paper route. As a result of his lack of clear understanding of these auditory, linguistic terms which he has heard but probably has never seen drawn out or compared visually, his oral language becomes very redundant as he tries to explain what he means. With linguistic function, a person should be able to be succinct in talking, speaking, or writing. And, at the linguistic level, the space, time, quantity, and quality words are specific in meaning.

Activity: How is a misperception a cultural aspect? How does a misperception result in a misconception?

3. Problems with staying *on-topic* (for off-topic errors in thinking, see Chapter 10) at the linguistic level come from not being able to use the auditory concepts in formal ways. For example, because Cliff is so redundant in his speech, then he gets off-topic and begins to talk about tangential or related ideas. This means that he is not able to stay with the topic that he started talking about. Eventually he asks about "what they were discussing" but continues to talk since he knows that he did not complete his own thinking. This type of tangential thinking results in a lack of focus and ability to stay on topic.

Activity: Why might a person who has a lot of language structures but lacks linguistic function become tangential and lose focus in a conversation?

4. The lack of *natural language* results from borrowing others' ideas and then attempting to share those ideas. For example, plagiarism is quite widespread in the colleges because so many students have learned to regurgitate what they read or to write down exactly what they hear (phonographic ability is not auditory) and to receive praise and rewards for the imitation of patterns. But, such copying is

not conceptual in nature and lacks linguistic function. So, when the person with lots of language structures does not understand certain concepts, then he or she may borrow ideas—patterns that others produced. When these patterns are written down as one's own ideas, then the person plagiarizes, whether intentional or not. When others' ideas are spoken, they sound unnatural because the speaker has not processed the meaning of the concepts so the speech is mechanical, robot-like, and/or lacks natural prosody. Cliff had a little problem with natural language when he talked about the different numbers to the different routes. His speech became monotone and robot-like as if he was just going through the numbers of the routes as mental images that he listed. Sometimes, the monotony is so dramatic that the speaker's speech lacks almost all natural ideas.

Activity: What helped Cliff develop more natural language function?

Language structures alone will not create the flow of natural, shared language prosody that cognitively functions to create meaning that is greater than the parts. The following sample (Figure 11.6) was written by a student who copied his ideas from a book, but he could not answer any questions about what he wrote. This means that he borrowed the language and did not understand the meaning. The result was that he did not use his own, natural language to put the ideas of the author into his own thinking.

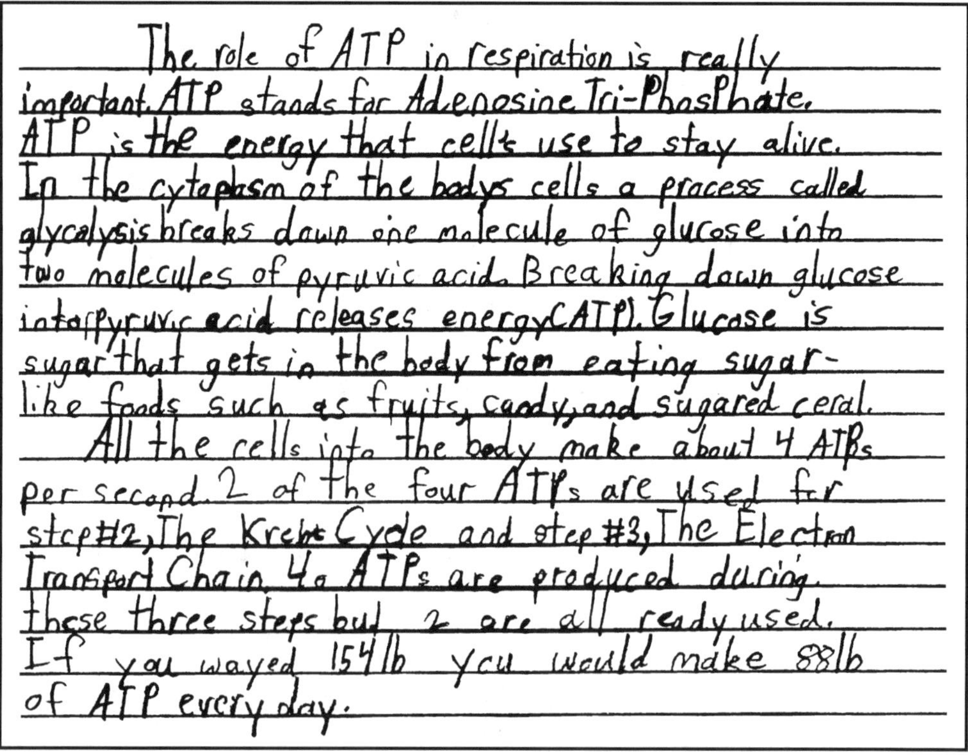

The role of ATP in respiration is really important. ATP stands for Adenosine Tri-PhosPhate. ATP is the energy that cell's use to stay alive. In the cytaphsm of the bodys cells a process called glycolysis breaks down one molecule of glucose into two molecules of pyruvic acid. Breaking down glucose into(pyruvic acid releases energy(ATP). Glucose is sugar that gets in the body from eating sugar-like foods such as fruits, candy, and sugared ceral.

All the cells into the body make about 4 ATPs per second. 2 of the four ATPs are used for step#2, The Krebs Cycle and step #3, The Electron Transport Chain. 4o ATPs are produced during these three steps but 2 are all ready used. If you wayed 154lb you would make 88lb of ATP every day.

Figure 11.6 Copying to "sound good"

The educator helped him draw out his ideas starting with putting him on the page and then connecting the ideas to him. Cognitively, when the learner is on the page, the drawing is preoperational in nature. All new concepts are learned best at the preoperational level. As the ideas are connected to the learner, then the concepts are raised to a concrete level. Finally the concepts are retagged with formal ideas such as "adenosine tri-phosphate." Figure 11.7 shows the flowchart of visual thoughts that this young man drew with the help of an educator.

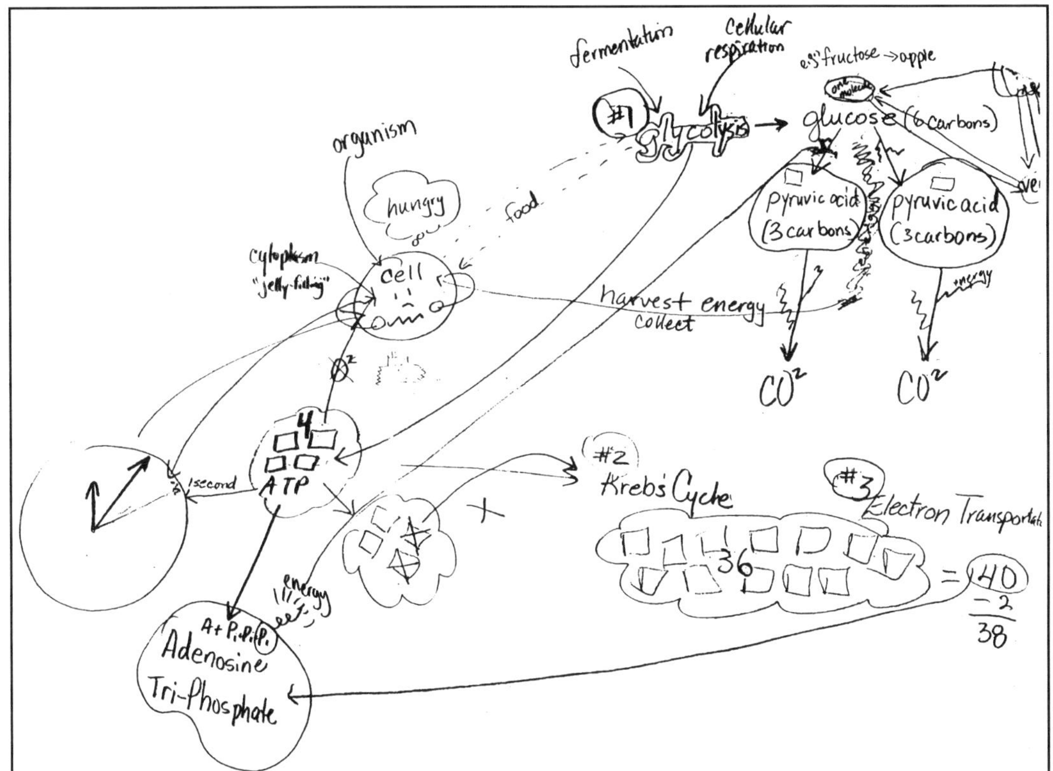

Figure 11.7 Visual picture of the formal concepts

Without the use of natural language, the learner could not comprehend the meaning of his copied words. By helping him "see" the concepts of the print, he had a much better understanding of the meaning of the words. Once he had ample thinking, he was able to write his own ideas with his natural language. Remember that when a person thinks with natural language, the person has attached meaning to the ideas which puts the ideas into semantic memory, a long term memory function.

Without natural language, spoken or written, a learner is left to copy, imitate, or regurgitate others' ideas. As students grow up, copying others' ideas in order to get the only correct answer, they lose the function of their language. Likewise, they do not learn to comprehend ideas from others' meanings. Many college students, who grow up copying what others say (or write) to get the right answer, often do not learn to use their own language to understand spoken or written ideas. This copying of patterns results in many college students struggling to understand new text material, so, many college students choose to not read their textbooks.

They do not understand the words on the page. The words are patterns and the students do not have sufficient language about the topic to be able to put the written patterns into their own natural language for understanding. And, they do not have the strategies to translate the auditory language on the page of the textbook into visual thinking strategies for learning.

Summary

Linguistic function is based on the maximum development of displacement, semanticity, flexibility, and productivity with efficient use of language structures (limited redundancy). If a person is older than about 11 years of age, this person should demonstrate linguistic function. Without linguistic function, the person may exhibit the use of a lot of language structures without the time-based connections for succinct English. If a person learns a lot of language structures but cannot use the linguistic function, the person borrows or copies the language about linguistic concepts, concepts that cannot be seen, touched, or felt. The result is the use of unnatural language and lower socio-cognitive functioning. Chapter 12 describes the social and behavioral effects of language that lacks linguistic function.

Applications

- Determine how much knowledge students have about a content area by asking them some why and how questions about their area of study.
- Ask some students over the age of 11 about some linguistic concepts; for example: What is a country? What is a continent? What is an eclipse? What is a government? What is respect? What is geography? Record the answers to see if the students have linguistic function.

Chapter 12

LANGUAGE FUNCTION AFFECTS BEHAVIOR

Learner objectives: Chapter 12

Upon completion of this chapter, the reader should be able to:

1. Define how language function affects behavior.
2. Explain the relationship between learning and social development.
3. Describe the relationship between language and social development.
4. Explain the continuum of anti-social development.
5. Explain the continuum of pro-social development.
6. Define social competence and how social competence develops.

Learning to behave is
neither right or wrong.
The right and wrong of language
is social behavior.

Up to this point, the author has emphasized the relationship between learning, language, and thinking. But with cognitive development, a learner also acquires social concepts which represent social skills. These skills or patterns represent a thinker's underlying cognition. Therefore, learning language is both a social and a cognitive process. "Learning to think" is how language functions. *"Learning to behave" is the social function of language*. For example, an infant moves her body in response to the input of sensory stimuli to develop the brain and its cognitive component. Years later, this infant, who is now a teen, makes choices about how she will respond to her parents' rules. The teen's actions or behaviors reflect what she has cognitively learned about her choices. The teen's cognition or language function determines the options for choice, and the teen's behavior reflects her social development. Both social and cognitive functions are developmental products of the Neuro-Semantic Language Learning System. *People learn to think and be social. Likewise, "thinking to learn" is both social and cognitive.* Language becomes the tool for higher order ***pro-social*** development as well as advanced problem solving or ***critical thinking***. This chapter will describe the way that learning to behave is a language function.

Neuro-typical behavior

Learning to behave is both a cognitive and a social process. As the learning system activates the development of cognition, the learner also becomes social. Language development reflects the interdependence between social and cognitive development. Therefore, linguistic cognitive function is the product of learning to think at a formal level, and social competence is the ability to initiate and maintain healthy relationships or social competence at this same formal, linguistic level. Table 12.1 shows the relationship between language development and social function.

Table 12.1 The relationship between social learning and cognitive learning according to developmental products

	Social learning Adult assigns meaning	**Social development Behavior**	**Cognitive function Language**	**Cognitive development Conceptualization**
0–2	Adult maintains with baby. Baby does something, caregiver does something (child is dependent on caregiver)	Reflexes→ Motor Develops into gazes, points, reaches, etc… dependent on others for safety (extension of world)	Pre-production or silent emerging to telegraphic production such as "mama juice" (pre-language function)	Agent-action-object (non-verbal) becomes verbal basic semantic relationships (sensori-motor thinking)
2–7	Caregivers maintain with child. Relationships are based on one person or "I based" (dependent on others)	Child acts toward others according to child's own needs… dependent on others to interpret what is okay behavior (child's behavior is about self…agent)	Shows restricted and limited function…my toys, my school, my rules (pre-language function)	Child is center to the world. Child shows agent-action-object; egocentric. Child is in his own picture. Thinking is in the "here-and-now" (preoperational thinking)
7–11	Child shares in relationships according to societal rules. Child can initiate and maintain relationships. Relationships are mutually based or "we based" (independent)	Child is independent in actions…is able to follow others' rules and maintains socially expected behaviors; rules are followed (shared expectations of behavior; agent to agent)	Shows grammatically complete ideas in conversation with all literacy processes being conventional. Person can read, write, think, view, listen, speak, calculate about what others read, write, talk, and so forth (language function)	Child is able to think about others (agents) in relationships. Thinking is about others (agents) in relationship to society's rules (concrete thinking)
11+	Learner acts on behalf of the greater society…social learning is about the "greater good" where "the whole is greater than the parts" (ethical and principle dependent)	Thinker is capable of initiating and maintaining healthy relationships (social competence; take other people's perspectives)	Language is time based and functions as a tool for learning; efficient use of language (linguistic function)	Learner is able to think with maximum displacement, semanticity, flexibility, and productivity (formal thinking)

Table 12.1 shows several socially important issues related to behavior and thinking:

1. The neuro-typical learner is able to be independent in thinking and behavior at the concrete, language function of a 7–11-year-old. This means that individuals who reach the concrete level of thinking and who possess language function at a concrete level can function according to society's expectations based on rules.
2. In contrast to the first point, a person who does not develop language function beyond the "here-and-now" of thinking of themselves at the preoperational level will not fit into dominant culture of society and therefore will be dependent on other forms of agency: incarceration, schools, families, social welfare systems, and so forth.
3. Concrete thinking with conventional language function of a 7–11-year-old is rule governed and parallel to today's rule-governed society. Today's society is a rule-governed, legalistic type of culture.
4. In contrast to point number 3, a person who is not capable of following rules in society will also not show conventional language function. The person may have lots of language structures, but the structures will not show the function of being able to maintain a conventional, shared conversation. Maintaining a conversation is a two-way process that exemplifies the conversationalist's ability to think, view, listen, and speak from another person's perspective. Parents and educators who think they are having a conversation with a child or student by using "20 questions" or following the child's or student's flow of thinking and speaking are *not* really having a conversation. To function independently, a person must be able to use enough language function to carry a conversation.
5. In Table 12.1, it is apparent that thinking in the "here-and-now" is not only a cognitive function but also a social function. The individual is central to all behavior and therefore others must maintain with the "self-centered" individual. This egocentric behavior is *only* neuro-typical for the 3–7-year-old child, not the adult who thinks only of self needs. (Table 12.2 will show the anti-social behavior at the various learning and development levels.)
6. In Table 12.1, notice that social competence is also a cognitive function of language. Language provides the learner with the development of concepts related to "self," a cognitive function. Social competence occurs at the formal level. Since only about 30 percent of society functions at that formal level, then only about 30 percent of the members of the dominant culture become socially competent.
7. Thinking about behavior and learning to behave are not the same. A person learns to think and learns to behave through the Neuro-Semantic Learning Language System. Others assign social and cognitive meaning in a way that scaffolds the concepts through the learning language process. This process is synergistic. For example, increase the cognitive function of a given set of ideas such as "bomb building" and the social development may not increase. However, increase the language function about the social outcomes of bomb building and the person's social development such as responsibility and accountability also increase.
8. Development is a product of the learning system. Tap into the learning system and the social, cognitive, and language developmental products all increase. But, working on the individual developmental products will not increase a person's overall cognitive and social function. For example, teaching a child the social

skills of how to say hello does not help the child function at a higher cognitive level of social learning. However, when a child learns how to use language to talk to others in a variety of situations, then the child begins to develop cognitive functions related to how to talk to others. Adding developmental products as a curricular strategy does not affect the way a person thinks or acts based on learning.

9. Language function reflects both cognitive and social function. As a person learns to use language, the learner's thinking (cognition) and socialization (social development) also increase. A child who learns sufficient layers of cognition about how to relate to others with various forms of literacy is learning to be socially competent. But, learning only about facts, rules, and specific content areas will not provide a thinker with social competence, the ability to initiate and maintain healthy relationships. More about healthy relationships follows.

Activity: Summarize the relationship between social and cognitive development as it relates to learning how to function with language (concepts in Table 12.1).

Social competence

From looking at the data in Table 12.1, it is apparent that the ultimate level of learning to behave falls into the development of ***social competence***. Social competence is found at the linguistic level of social learning and development. A person who is socially competent is able to initiate and maintain healthy relationships. There are three important aspects of this definition:

1. To initiate a relationship means to start up a conversation, to ask someone to engage in an activity, or to develop a "dating" sort of relationship where time is spent with another person.
2. To maintain a relationship is much more than just "doing" activities with another person. Maintaining a relationship implies a give-and-take relationship where participants exchange the lead in initiating the shared activities.
3. To have a healthy relationship means that initiating and maintaining the relationship is mutually beneficial to the health and well-being of all people involved. There is a mutually pro-social benefit in engaging in a healthy, interdependent relationship.

Activity: What is social competence?

In healthy relationships, all parties share in the conventions of the relationship with mutual regard and respect for each other's desires, interests, passions, and concerns. Each person's identity is independent in the relationship and the relationship benefits each person's well-being. Although many people are able to initiate with others, they may not be able to maintain a relationship, let alone a healthy relationship. Unhealthy relationships create a situation where individual independence is not respected and the value of the relationship is anti-social in nature. The balance between developing pro-social behavior that leads to social competence when a thinker is able to use a linguistic function about relationships is important to understand in the learning processes. The following section discusses social development as a continuum from behavioral disorders that emerge as a result of anti-social behavior to social competence that emerges from pro-social behavior.

Activity: What does a healthy relationship promote?

Social development of relationships

People who are socially competent are able to initiate and maintain healthy relationships in part because they have linguistic function about their social development. Social competence comes from years of pro-social experiences. Pro-social experiences encourage social learning of concepts that promote positive assignment of meaning to behavior. For example, people in pro-social relationships receive nurturance, support, safety or healthy protection, credit, recognition, and appreciation for "who" they are as well as "what" they do. Over time, pro-social experiences develop healthy friendships and spousal relationships for all parties.

Language is a social tool for the cognitive function of the development of pro-social development. For example, people show gratitude for actions, a shared pride in accomplishments, and give credit as well as recognition for others' ideas and activities. Language sounds like this:

> Thank you for your help with setting the table. I appreciate the many kind things you do to help around the house. Your contributions are beneficial to making the household a comfortable place for us to live.

Or:

> I really enjoyed watching you play soccer today. I recognized your willingness to share the ball with the other players and to take constructive criticism from the coach. I am so proud at how you are learning to contribute to the work of others. I appreciate the many ways you show your enthusiasm for being a team player.

Pro-social development occurs from the assigning of support, nurturance, and safety with language that results in formal social competence. The language example shows support for the child's interest in soccer, nurturance for developing him as a person who does acts that others pride, and who believe in the child's own welfare or safety.

Activity: What is pro-social language like?

In contrast to pro-social behavior is *anti-social* behavior. Anti-social behavior is a lack of cognitive function that does not support, nurture, and provide safety. Language that creates anti-social development of concepts sounds like this:

> You are pathetic. I don't know why I bother with you. You should have taken control and kicked the ball when you had it. You know that is the only way to win a soccer game. What is wrong with you? What were you thinking?

This language shows that the speaker does not support the child's decision making nor does the language nurture the child's own development of becoming an independent thinker who feels safe in his actions or choices of behavior.

Activity: What does anti-social language sound like?

Social learning of concepts

Learning the concepts of how to be social and therefore how to behave conventionally is based on how others assign meaning to a thinker's behavior or actions as well as how well a person is able to use language to assign meaning to his or her actions and behavior. This process of social learning occurs through the Neuro-Semantic Language Learning System. All concepts scaffold, including those that represent social development. Likewise, both pro-social and anti-social behaviors are cyclic in nature; an increase in pro-social learning increases pro-social development and an increase in anti-social learning increases anti-social development. This cyclic nature mirrors the process of learning concepts described as part of the Neuro-Semantic Language Learning Theory.

When caregivers assign meaning to children's behaviors, then the children's perceptions of their behavior result in the layering of concepts (Chapter 3). In the case of social concepts, the layers are pro-social or anti-social in nature. *Either the layers become more pro-social eventually resulting in social competence or the layers become more anti-social where behavior becomes more aggressive eventually resulting in more violent behavior.* Many scholars, in addressing anti-social behavior, report that large numbers of general education students engage in anti-social behavior (e.g., Walker, Kavanagh, Stiller, Golly, Severson, & Feil, 1998). Anti-social behavior socially spreads like a disease. One child assigns the negative meaning to another child based on the first child's negative experiences at home and so the second child assigns negative meaning to someone else and so forth. The cycle of anti-social behavior increases.

Activity: How does anti-social behavior spread?

Pro-social development has positive outcomes but, typically, does not spread the same way. In this dominant culture, the individual is valued in terms of *wha*t the individual is able to achieve. Therefore, a person's accomplishments in terms of "whats" is valued, not a person's "who." Pro-social learning values the "who" of a person, not the "whats." Therefore, it is easier in the dominant culture to perpetuate the anti-social development because the "whats" are more important in this culture. This propensity for encouraging the development of "whats" such as a "win" in soccer rather than the development of team play or a "who" is further supported by the use of material or extrinsic rewards and punishers. Many behavior specialists report that anti-social behavior that is punished through a system of rewards and punishers becomes more aggressive and eventually leads to violence. In other words, the actual use of rewards to improve behavior has a negative factor by assigning meaning to the anti-social development of aggression which can lead to violence (e.g., Leonard, 1988).

Activity: Is pro-social development like anti-social development? Why or why not?

These findings are not surprising when put into the context of the Neuro-Semantic Language Learning Theory. For every reward given to a child, there is a second message: Without the reward the child's acts or thinking are not adequate. For every child who receives a reward, there is some child who feels punished because he did not receive the reward. All rewards are punishers and all punishers are rewards; they assign the value of a "what" to behaviors; they do not support, nurture, or protect because they are not conceptually based in language function (Arwood & Young, 2000).

Within the learning system, concepts develop from the sensory input that forms perceptual patterns. Therefore, experiences determine the type of sensory input as well as the types of patterns that are offered. Likewise, caregivers provide an assignment of meaning to the child's behavior that in turn provides more sensory input and more patterns. If the adult's input assigns pro-social meaning to the child's actions or behaviors, the child learns pro-social concepts. Pro-social assignment of meaning scaffolds the development of concepts about supporting, nurturing, and protecting the child. If the adult's input assigns anti-social meaning to the child's actions or behaviors, then the child learns anti-social meaning.

The same actions or behaviors provide opposite assignment of meaning:

Pro-social assignment of meaning

I really enjoyed watching you play soccer today. I recognized your willingness to share the ball with the other players and to take constructive criticism from the coach. I am so proud at how you are learning to contribute to the work of others. I appreciate the many ways you show your enthusiasm for playing soccer with others.

Anti-social assignment of meaning

Don't you know better? You should have kicked the ball. Don't give the ball to someone else. That gives them the glory. You are so stupid. You don't get it, do you? You really need to take some lessons on how to win. Winning is everything. If you don't win then why play? Get smart or get out.

On one hand, the adult assigns pro-social meaning to the child's actions and the child learns concepts about how to be an agent separate from the playing of soccer, a what. On the other hand, the child with an anti-social assignment of meaning learns that he is not smart unless he wins. His self-concept is wrapped up in whether or not he wins the soccer game. His social development is about "what" he does, not "who" he is. And, winning soccer is about him playing soccer, not about how he plays on a team of soccer players. The anti-social assignment of meaning results in the child growing older but socially remaining at a preoperational, pre-language level of function. This type of thinking results in low self-esteem which sets up the cycle of devaluing others. Low self-esteem is related to how well a person thinks he can achieve. Part of this thinking about achievement is based on what others say. Developing a person's "who" or self is about an interdependence between others assigning meaning and acquiring the language to assign meaning to one's own acts or to others' actions.

Activity: How does different language promote a person's thinking about who he or she is?

How a person thinks about self-achievement or self-esteem or how a person conceptualizes the cognitive function of being an agent (self-concept) is dependent on learning the concepts about social expectations from others assigning meaning to behavior or actions. Learning to behave in the way that society expects is both social and cognitive in nature. Social and cognitive development is a function of the Neuro-Semantic Language Learning System where learning to behave is a conceptual development that stems from neuronal circuits of concepts learned from the environment's input that forms concepts for language function.

Activity: Explain how the Neuro-Semantic Language Learning Theory affects social development.

Cognitive function of social development

Learning to be social is a neuro-typical, pro-social learning process that occurs across developmental stages. However, when anti-social development results from the learner not being able to understand the cultural input or the input being anti-social, then the learner develops an anti-social, neuro-atypical system. In other words, even though the people in the child's environment assign pro-social meaning, the child has to have the Neuro-Semantic Language Learning System that will allow the child to understand the input. Table 12.2 shows the anti-social behavior for the various levels of learning and development.

Table 12.2 The relationship between social learning and cognitive learning for anti-social behavior

	Social learning Adult assigns meaning	**Social development Behavior**	**Cognitive function Language**	**Cognitive development Conceptualization**	**Anti-social behavior**
0–2	Adult maintains with baby. Baby does something, caregiver does something (baby is dependent)	Reflexes→Motor output; gaze, points, reaches, etc...dependent on others for safety (baby is extension of world)	Pre-production or silent emerges to telegraphic utterances such as "mama juice" (pre-language function)	Agent-action-object (non-verbal) becomes verbal... (sensori-motor thinking)	Crying, hitting, biting, scratching, self-stimulating, enraged, acts on sensory smells, licks
2–7	Caregivers maintain with child. Relationships are based on one person or "I based" (dependent on others)	Child acts toward others according to child's own needs...dependent on others to interpret what is okay behavior (child's behavior is about self... agent)	Shows restricted and limited function...my toys, my school, my rules (pre-language function)	Child is center to the world. Child shows agent-action-object; egocentric. Child is in his own picture. Thinking is in the "here-and-now" (preoperational thinking)	Blaming behavior, name calling, my needs, my wants, sorrow or hurt is about me; e.g., hitting someone doesn't hurt unless it hurts my hand

7–11	Child shares the relationship according to rules. Child can initiate and maintain relationships. Relationships are mutually based or "we based" (independent)	Child is independent in actions…is able to follow others' rules and maintains socially expected behaviors (shared expectations for behavior; agent to agent)	Shows grammatically complete ideas in conversation with all literacy processes being conventional. Person can read, write, think, view, listen, speak, calculate about what others read, write, talk, and so forth (language function)	Child is able to think about others (agents) in relationships. Thinking is about others (agents) in relationship to society's rules (concrete thinking)	Do unto others as they do unto you…rules can be manipulated; rules used to determine what is right or wrong; e.g., "I didn't break the law" even though everyone lost their money because of my actions
11+	Learner acts on behalf of the greater society… social learning is about the "greater good" where "the whole is greater than the parts" (ethical and principle dependent)	Actions are ethical and principled and thinker is capable of initiating and maintaining healthy relationships. (social competence; take other people's perspectives)	Language is time based and functions as a tool for learning; language is efficient (linguistic function)	Learner is able to think with maximum displacement, semanticity, flexibility, and productivity (formal thinking)	Not applicable

Activity: What are examples of anti-social behavior?

In Table 12.2, different behavior shows different levels of social and cognitive learning. Cognitive development parallels the person's thinking about being social. People are capable of becoming psycho-socially "stuck" at one of the levels. For example, a 12-year-old non-verbal male, who rocks, kicks, hits, bites, is displaying the anti-social behavior of a two-year old. Or an adult who yells, screams, throws items, or can't remember a situation after it occurs, is also functioning at the sensori-motor level of development. It should be noted that Table 12.2 not only shows the level of development and social learning but also offers a visual display of intervention options. For example, a 12-year-old who is non-verbal and kicking and biting needs to learn some of the cognitive, pro-social concepts about agency to function differently. This male's behavior reflects his social and cognitive learning. Extinguishing the negative behaviors will not work because such a methodology does not provide him with any pro-social conceptual learning to take the place of the anti-social behavior.

Activity: What does sensori-motor atypical social learning look like in terms of cognitive development?

Understanding how social development occurs also relates to adult behavior. An adult who is experiencing "adult tantrums" or meltdowns needs therapy to help develop his thinking of himself. Adult tantrums often result in violent acts such as throwing objects, hitting, killing, etc. Because the adult is at a first or sensory level of functioning, the adult is not "thinking" conceptually. Sometimes the adult does not even remember tantrum types of acts. Memory for these acts would involve the use of concepts or thinking that would be at the preoperational or higher levels. For some of these people who have these types of tantrums, using VLMs such as drawing the person into a picture where he can actually see himself behave raises his thinking to a preoperational level where he can now begin to "think" and receive help. This does not mean this adult does not have some chemical or medical problem as well, but he needs help with seeing how he is an agent with or without medical intervention in order to begin to think differently.

Activity: What is the sensori-motor behavior level of social development like?

At the second level of the social and cognitive development (preoperational thinking and pre-language function), the learner's behavior centers on his own actions. The person who thinks in a preoperational way of social and cognitive learning is learning about himself. So, anti-social behavior at this level shows the learner's own needs and wants such as demanding one's own way and blaming others for actions. Language at this anti-social level is *not* nurturing, supporting, and protecting. Instead, it is "abusive" psychologically as the teen or adult caught at this level must blame others using name calling and words of devaluation. For example, "You are unprofessional" (without any evidence or rationale). "This work is pathetic" (personal judgment, not a statement of fact). "You are the bane of my existence" (blames others for feelings and beliefs). "You are mean" (no evidence for statement). "You are ugly" (personal attack based on judgment). "Those people are those types" (overgeneralization).

These types of statements show that the speaker's language function is anti-social in nature because the speaker is at a preoperational social level of cognitive development. In other words, this type of language reflects the speaker's social learning. The speaker is thinking at a level of social development that reflects preoperational cognition, where the person lashes out from his or her own experience. When a speaker uses this type of anti-social language, the assignment of meaning to the listener is also anti-social. The listener is receiving the anti-social messages. This results in "bullying;" bullying is a type of personal attack that abuses or attempts to control others. The bully negatively impacts the listener whether or not the listener is trying to ignore the input. The input exists and the listener receives the input. Bio-physical studies (e.g., McEwen, 2008) show that this type of input negatively affects body functions such as raising flight or fight hormones, increasing cardiovascular output and the subsequent bodily effects.

A listener's attempt to use language to compensate for the effects of "bullying" such as "self-talk" helps but does not completely compensate for the physiological effects of abusive language. For example, the boss calls a worker's proposal "pathetic." The worker thinks, "Everyone at work thinks this work is great so it can't be pathetic." Intellectually, the worker knows that the work, not the worker, is viewed as "pathetic." Others like the work, so the worker knows that not everyone believes the work is pathetic. This type of language function helps maintain the worker's own social well-being. But, the effects of the bullying are still bio-physically present. And, this worker has sufficient language to mitigate the effects. This is why bullying is so dangerous in the schools; for those students who are vulnerable because their own social and cognitive learning is at the concrete or preoperational level, they become what they hear at a deep cognitive level whether or not they start out at the level. For example, if they receive messages about "stupid," "idiot," "dumb idea," "should know better," "try harder," "student of your low caliber," and so forth, they will begin to believe that they are not as smart as others. Even if they brag about "being smart," their actions (bragging) show that they don't believe they are smart but need others to assign that meaning. Bullying that occurs for those people who are socially and/or cognitively functioning at the preoperational level creates the "meaning" of "who" the person is at that level. These individuals do not have enough language to try to compensate. Bullying of those who are at a concrete or formal social and cognitive level still has detrimental effects on individuals' self-beliefs and physical well-being.

Activity: Why is bullying of individuals who are at a preoperational level so dangerous?

The second, preoperational, pre-language level of cognitive learning is the social level at which most individuals with behavior disorders or individuals who have long histories of incarceration function. Individuals who are not able to move beyond being a victim and must recreate settings always to be a victim are also functioning at this level. Blaming and being blamed is a vicious preoperational, anti-social cycle of cognitive development.

At this pre-language level of functioning, the individual is able to think about what he or she sees or hears. For example, a visual thinker at this cognitive level is able to see his hands and feet and part of his body. Therefore, his feet kick and his hands pick up the bat or TV, but he does not see his face or himself. When a person functioning at this social level is asked about behavior, the person denies such accusations. For example, "Did you steal that TV?" was said to a teen who was observed taking a TV from an unlocked car. While holding the TV, the teen said, "No, I don't steal." Remember the concept "steal" is formal in cognitive development. So, the adult asked, "Did you take that TV?" Again, the teen denied the action, "No, I didn't take this TV." So, the adult asked, "Did that hand (pointing to his hand) pick up that TV (pointing to TV)?" to which the teen said, "Yes." This teen's choice of behavior is limited to the here-and-now, to behaviors that can be literally seen, touched, and felt. His cognitive functioning for behavioral choices is as good as his language functions. And, his social learning is as good as he is able to understand others' language function. Others' language function works for him only when he can "see" what others say. He has not learned the auditory language of what "steal" or "take" mean in relationship to other people's belongings.

Activity: How does thinking affect behavior? How does language affect understanding of behavior?

The author has worked with many, many children and adults who, literally, do not understand the very words that they can utter or respond to. Words are auditory in nature (Chapters 4–6) and are not visual in nature. Therefore, words can be uttered or repeated as acoustic patterns without understanding the underlying meaning. The aforementioned teen who stole the TV not only could use the word "steal" but also could tell you that "stealing" is bad and he was not bad. *Speaking is also a process of literacy which requires an understanding of what the person is saying.* As that teen functioned at a "pre-language" level of meaning for "steal" it is also not surprising that his lack of language function could also be seen in other areas of literacy, specifically with reading and writing. His lack of literacy skills is not surprising, as literacy is culturally viewed as a set of auditory skills and abilities that are taught in auditory ways. Because he functions in the here-and-now, he does not understand the meaning of language that is inferred and logically deduced from spoken ideas, such as for concepts like "steal" or even "take." In this teen's mind, "steal" refers to something that a person takes from someone else but there were no people in the car that had the TV. Therefore, he did not take the TV, and, that means, he also did not steal the TV. His mental picture of "steal" did not match his thinking about what he did. Furthermore, "stealing is bad" and he does not see himself as bad. Therefore, he would not steal and he could not steal. "Take" refers to reaching out the arm to grasp something like a child's hand or a piece of food. He could not literally "take" the TV; he had to "pick up" the TV. His language function is limited and restricted. As a result his behavior is also socially and cognitively restricted to what he can see said or written. He sees part of his body pick up the TV so that he knows. For all of the other meaning, he does not know he is a part of "stealing" or "taking."

Activity: How does the way a person learns concepts affect a person's thinking?

In order for the teen who stole the TV to function at a higher level of literacy, he would need educators to teach him with more visual thinking types of methods. Reading and writing with VLMs would help him see himself and his behavior as part of the concepts of steal and take. Drawing out the concept of steal actually allowed him to see what he had done because then "steal" had more meaning. He realized that steal has to do with ownership and property that belongs to others whether or not the owners are there with their belongings. Because the teen did not pay for the TV at a store, he did not have ownership; and because the person who left the TV in the car bought the TV, the person who left the TV in the car had ownership. Matching educational methods to the way a person acquires the concepts represented in language helps provide more social and cognitive learning for higher order thinking. Behavior is a social and cognitive representation of thinking.

Activity: Why do some people struggle with behavior even when they appear to understand societal rules such as "not stealing?"

Society's social expectations

Society is a large, symbolic agent that represents the concrete actions of the individuals that make up society. Therefore, society's social expectations are formal in nature because these expectations cannot be seen, touched, or felt. However, the concrete actions of individuals can be seen. For example, "respect" is a formal concept that requires a lot of actions that represent many concrete concepts such as acts that show respect for self, respect for others, respect for property, respect for ideas, and so forth. In order to develop a formal, linguistic understanding of "respect," a thinker would have to experience a lot of language meaning assigned to acts such as:

> I am glad you hung up your clothes. By hanging up your clothes, it is apparent that you have respect for your things, the money that your parents work hard to earn to buy the clothes, for your self and your belongings and for your health as hanging up your clothes keeps your room cleaner.

This type of positive assignment of meaning helps a person learn what respect really means. Respect is a formal concept with many, many concrete meanings.

Activity: Explain why formal concepts have to have lots of concrete meanings.

These formal societal concepts are learned through many different applications of meaning. This same child who hangs up his clothes at home also hears the teacher at school say:

> Bart, I am so glad that you helped Mary pick up her desk to move it. Your actions show that you respect Mary's desire to move her desk; and, it also shows that you don't want her to hurt her back or scrape the floor which shows that you also respect the janitor's time. If Mary had to move her desk by herself then she might have scraped the floor and the janitor would have spent a lot of her time cleaning the marks. Thank you for being so respectful of others.

Bart has home messages and school messages about the concept "respect." He is learning that the formal, linguistic concept of respect has many, many meanings. In order for Bart to learn the formal meaning of respect, then many individuals within society must assign the social value of the meaning of respect in many ways. In this way, Bart is learning the socio-cognitive linguistic function of "respect."

Activity: How do formal social concepts like "respect" become learned?

Individuals who do not understand the formal concepts have a greater chance of becoming more anti-social. For example, Charlotte, who thinks with a visual meta-cognition, may not understand the inferred meaning from a parent who casually says, "Thanks for hanging up your clothes." Without Charlotte's mother using more words to paint a mental picture, Charlotte does not know why the parent says "thanks." As a young child, Charlotte wants to please the adult so she does whatever the parent thanks her for, even though she does not really understand why she is being thanked. Charlotte begins to make "friends" and begins to visit their homes. In many of the homes, the friends do not hang up their clothes. They walk across the clothes, toss the clothes, shove them under the bed, and so forth. When these friends visit Charlotte's room they make comments: "Your room is so clean. Your mother must be a clean freak." Charlotte is trying to "fit-in" (fitting-in is a social function of children around 7–11 years of age) with her friends so she now sees her mom as a "clean freak." Without the rationale for why Charlotte's mom likes the clothes hung up, Charlotte must choose between her mom's thanks and her friends' approval of what Charlotte does. *Note that approval is about "what" a person does, not acceptance of who the person is.*

Activity: How can the lack of understanding result in anti-social behavior such as name calling?

Developmentally, without the language for understanding respect at a formal level, Charlotte takes an anti-social stand: "I am not going to be a 'clean freak' like my mom." Charlotte may not even know what "clean freak" means but she realizes that if it is a "name" it must be bad and she doesn't want her "friends" to see her in that way.

In order for Charlotte and many, many other learners to become socially competent, to learn the social concepts that society expects, and to be a positive influence as a citizen, they must have the language for the social concepts that are valued by society. These concepts might include: accountability, citizenship, responsibility, respect, nurturance, acceptance, credit, recognition, values, integrity, trustworthiness, loyalty, friendship, and many others. Figure 12.1 shows the work of a student learning the meanings of many words that he needs to turn his anti-social behavior into more pro-social behavior. The more language function he acquired, the better his behavior became.

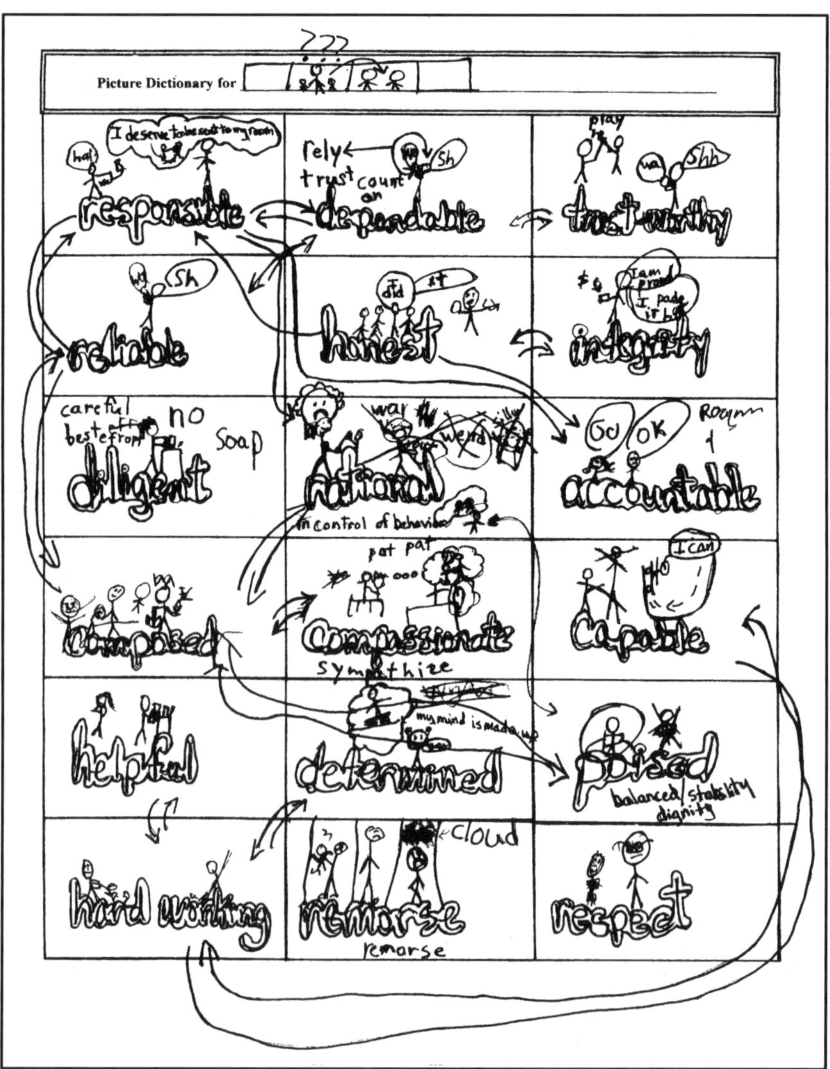

Figure 12.1 A vocabulary dictionary of social words needed for linguistic function of formal concepts

Table 12.3 shows the development of the formal concept "respect."

Table 12.3 How concepts like respect develop socially over time

0–2 years	3–7 years	7–11 years	11+ years
Caregivers meet the baby's individual physical needs. They show a physical respect for the baby's being.	The child is becoming an agent and the caregivers use the word respect when talking with the child about his actions, his needs, his wants, his behavior.	The child knows that respect refers to many different behaviors such as respect for parents, respect for teachers, respect for belongings, respect for siblings, and so forth.	The early adolescent knows that respect refers to how people value others; their interests, desires, passions, and needs in relationship to acts of respect. The adolescent is developing relationships based on mutual regard and respect.

Activity: Explain how formal social concepts like respect are acquired.

The meaning of concepts comes from the experiences of a learner. These experiences are culturally and linguistic specific to a group or groups. In many schools today, there are rules about what is valued. Some of these rules are written as part of a "positive behavior support (PSB) system" (Horner, 2000). But, the author has found that most of the students who need the greatest understanding of these rules do not have enough language function to understand rules like "be kind," "be responsible," "be respectful," "be caring," and so forth. It would make more sense to develop a rich language approach to behavior so that teachers would draw, write, talk, show students many, many acts of what pro-social behavior looks like when it is called "responsible" or "accountable." *Learners can acquire the meaning of concepts about social behavior only if they have the learning system to support how these concepts are being taught.*

Activity: How does language determine the meaning of social concepts like responsibility?

Language and social development

By now, the reader probably recognizes that the way others use language to assign meaning to behavior impacts a learner's social being. The assignment of meaning might be pro-social or anti-social in nature. The greater the pro-social assignment of meaning the more likely the person understands more of society's social expectations. Likewise, the more anti-social the assignment of meaning is to behavior, the more likely the learner's behavior goes against society's rules or expectations. Of course, genetics (genotype) makes a difference, but research shows that generational effects (phenotypes) may become genetic in nature as well (e.g., Franke, Leboyer, Gänsicke, Weiftenbach, Biancalana, Cornillet-Lefebre, Croquette, *et al.*, 1998; Holmes, Murphy, & Crawley, 2003). So, *learning to be social is both a cognitive or conceptual development of meaning as well as a language function.*

Table 12.4 shows the continuum of expectations across pro-social and anti-social development.

Table 12.4 Pro-social and anti-social continuum

	0–2 years	**3–7 years**	**7–11 years**	**11+ years**
Pro-social behavior	Acts receive positive support from others so that child feels comfort as an extension of others who are agents.	Acts to others and by others are mutually regarded as positive but based on what a person does, not who a person is.	Acts are intended to help and support others so multiple supportive relationships are developed for groups or teams.	Social competence; support, nurtures, and protects the initiation and maintenance of healthy relationships.
Anti-social behavior	Acts receive little or any support from others; neglect, abuse, or inconsistent acts may be received.	Acts to and by others are viewed as fault, blame, victim-based; bullying may begin.	Bullying is mutual; aggressive acts are admired or credited by others; relationships are based on what is gained.	Societal protection is warranted to provide others with safety from the acts of this person; and/or relationships are based on abusive premises.

In Table 12.4 it is apparent that the concepts about becoming a social being are based on the language others use to assign meaning to behavior and on how the thinker applies his knowledge to his own acts. A thinker's knowledge is rooted in his conceptual development of language function. Therefore, learning to behave according to societal expectations is both a social and a cognitive function of language; language that others use to assign meaning as well as a product of the development of language function of the learner. For example, friendship should be a valuable tool that society deems important, as social competence is defined in terms of initiating and maintaining healthy social relationships.

From the definition of social competence, friendship refers to those friends who mutually initiate and maintain healthy social relationships. But, the development of the concept of friendship is most interesting. Because "friends" are about others, preoperational thinkers can use the word "friend" but not really have friends because their thinking restricts agency to being about themselves. For example, a college student once told the author that her concept of friendship is about what is in the relationship for her. If a drug dealer was positive toward her, then she would have a drug dealer as a friend. This is often what is referred to as "fickle friendship." In pro-social development, six-year-olds who are still preoperational in thinking often express a fickle friendship mentality. Fickle friendship sounds like this: "Sally is my friend. She played ball with me." But the next day: "I don't like Sally. She played on the swings." Likewise, the drug dealer would be the college student's friend as long as the drug dealer's actions weren't toward her. The drug dealer could sell drugs to others and could steal from others and could get others addicted to drugs or put in jail but the drug dealer would still be a friend according to this college student. Friendship for this college student is about what is in the relationship for the student. There is no mutual regard. This college student had a long history of being involved in unhealthy and abusive relationships. People who are older than the typical six-year-old and who function at this level of social development are as pro-social as their language about social relationships determines. If they think they are central or preoperational to all activities, relationships act upon them but are not mutually developed. Their language will reflect such social, here-and-now thinking.

Activity: How does language reflect a person's thinking about being a friend?

Social concepts like respect, responsibility, or friendship are also part of society's beliefs and values. For example, technology has provided the opportunity to create computer linkages that connect people. People create their own page about themselves and then others who also have an account to the same website are able to connect via computer. Sometimes, there is an invitation to the page to "be a friend;" so, with the stroke of a few keys, a person is added as a friend. Some people participate in the process like a game of how many people they can sign up as "friends." But who are these people? What are their relationships to one another? Society has deemed friendship a process of communicating rather than a process of mutual regard with shared conversations toward pro-social development. The language of friendship has new twenty-first-century electronic meaning. Society values "friends" as knowledge of communication.

On the other hand, society has also begun to realize that the meaning for how to get along with others is a necessary part of socialization so programs in schools designed to teach social skills to general education students as well as those with special needs have developed. Whenever a society values a social concept, then the meaning of that concept is passed along and does not have to be taught. But, when a value changes so that it has to be taught, then the general public does not intrinsically value the concept which is why it has to be taught. *Society helps determine whether a behavior, an act, a belief, a social concept is valued.*

Activity: How does society represent the value of social behaviors?

Summary

Language function represents both the social and cognitive function of learning through the Neuro-Semantic Language Learning System. As a child acquires more meaning about social concepts, the child changes his or her behavior to reflect the cognitive understanding of social learning. This social learning is on a continuum where pro-social behavior and conceptual understanding increases the language function toward social competence and anti-social behavior or understanding results in more negative or abusive behavior as deemed by society.

Because social concepts are learned, a thinker will learn these concepts as well as he or she is able to acquire the meaning of the environmental input. If the learner is a visual thinker, then higher order social thinking requires the use of visual inputs such as VLMs in order for the learner to understand the social meaning of concepts that cannot be seen, touched, or felt like "respect" or "friendship." Learning to behave is a social and cognitive process of development.

Applications

- Look at a newspaper and determine what articles are pro-social and what articles are anti-social in nature.
- Write down ten rules about people that you have developed. Are your rules mostly anti-social or pro-social in nature?

PART IV

EDUCATIONAL APPLICATIONS OF LANGUAGE FUNCTION

How Do We Apply This Knowledge about Language to the Classroom?

The purpose of Part IV is to apply the knowledge about assessment, diagnosis, and intervention based on language function to the educational setting. Three different chapters represent three different levels of development: Primary or pre-language function (pre-kindergarten to third grade for Chapter 13), intermediate or language function (fourth grade to sixth grade for Chapter 14), and advanced or linguistic function (older than sixth grade for Chapter 15). The final chapter, Chapter 16, addresses the overall research basis for the applications.

Each chapter provides examples of how to use Viconic Language Methods™ in the classroom. Chapter 13 highlights Bonnie Robb's first grade, primary class. Robb is a Milken Teaching Award recipient for outstanding teaching. Her application of the Neuro-Semantic Language Learning Theory to the classroom through VLMs is described. Applications in this chapter are for children who are groupable, preoperational thinkers. For neuro-typical learners, the age that corresponds with these thinkers is from three to seven years.

Chapter 14 highlights Alyse Rostamizadeh, who typically teaches between fourth and sixth grades and is a leader among her peers as an outstanding teacher. This chapter provides VLMs for children who think concretely. Many of her examples showcase the relationships among literacy processes, language, and content. Her classroom examples provide the reader with how to make content the focus of better literacy.

Chapter 15 addresses those individuals and groups who are able to think with formal cognition, but who struggle with linguistic functions such as time-based organization or multi-tasking of events and ideas. This chapter highlights two professionals, Norman Stremming, who works with middle school and high school age students, and Dr. Joanna Kaakinen, who works with college students.

Chapter 16 describes the research evidence of VLMs based on the Neuro-Semantic Language Learning Theory. This chapter provides the umbrella for understanding the process of data collection of methods that emphasize learning, not teaching, so that a paradigm shift is valid. This chapter offers the history of evidence-based data that provides the need to shift from language structure to language function, from teacher to student driven data, from products to processes, from patterns to concepts, and from imitating skills to socio-cognitive thinking for higher order problem solving.

Chapter 13

THE LANGUAGE-BASED PRIMARY CLASSROOM

Learner objectives: Chapter 13

Upon completion of this chapter, the reader should be able to:

1. Develop language-based literacy lessons for children in primary grades.
2. Explain why sound-based programs may not develop thinking and viewing as part of literacy in primary grades.
3. Explain the purpose of Viconic Language Methods™ for primary grade children.
4. Describe why the emphasis on language function in the primary grades may still produce success on the testing of basic skills (phonics, phonemic awareness, and so forth).
5. Explain at least three different VLMs for use with primary grade children.

See the smiling children, so happy to learn!
Give them ideas...don't test them.
Assign meaning...don't test them.
Nurture them...don't punish them.

The goal of the primary education classroom is to provide the young child with the fundamental foundations for becoming literate. Culturally, the medium for teaching literacy is the English language. Primary teachers use English to give directions, to teach skills, to assign meaning to behavior, and so forth. English is the basis for the child's ***literacy***. *Literacy includes the semantic processes of speaking, reading, writing, thinking, viewing, listening, and calculating* (Cooper, 2006).

In order to develop effective programs for teaching a child to speak, read, write, think, view, listen, and calculate, a decision about what constitutes English must occur. Early in this book, the author provided the reader with two basic ways of viewing language: as a set of structures, or, as a process of learning functions. If primary teachers view English as a set of additive structures such as sounds, words, sentences, parts of speech, and vocabulary, then the programs for teaching English teach sounds to form words, words to form sentences, parts of speech to improve grammar, and vocabulary to improve meaning. These additive structures are the bases for most literacy programs since the late 1950s and, for the most part, continue to be. However, in the previous chapters, the reader learned that a child acquires language functions through the Neuro-Semantic Language Learning System and that becoming literate (speaking, reading, writing, thinking, viewing, listening, and calculating) is *greater than adding language structures* (Chapters 1–3).

The child learns the language structures from those speakers around the child; the child learns to think in the meaning the child acquires from what the child perceives. A neuro-typical child acquires and uses English as a natural, representative *function* of the child's *thinking*. Therefore, it is only logical that primary educational programs should be based on the underlying semantic or thinking properties of language-learning. Structures or products of the learning system develop from the way that language functions for learning concepts. Utilizing the Neuro-Semantic Language Learning Theory provides educators with knowledge about how products that represent literacy come from the underlying learning of language. This chapter explores effective practices based on language functions, not structures, for learning English as the foundational tool to becoming literate.

Literacy

Literacy results from a person *learning* to read, write, speak, think, view, listen, and calculate. Each of these psychological processes requires the learner to be able to think in the meaning of the process. For example, for a child to be able to understand the print on a page, the child must be able to recognize the patterns of print and assign a concept or meaning to those patterns. In other words, the process of reading utilizes the same language acquisition system found in the development of speaking or oral language: First, the child sees the print (sensory input), second, the child's neurological system recognizes the sensory input as patterns (sight of a pattern, or sound of a pattern, or sight and sound of a pattern), and third, the child uses his or her knowledge to assign meaning (concepts) to the patterns. In order to share those concepts with someone else, the child must use learned language structures to represent the child's thinking. Remember that a child's thinking is language function.

Activity: If literacy is seen as a set of structures, what is the focus for programs designed to develop literacy? If literacy is seen as the process of acquiring language functions, what is the focus for programs designed to develop literacy?

The neuro-semantic learning system utilizes the same set of processes for any literacy function: reading, writing, speaking, thinking, viewing, listening, and calculating. The learner must be able to receive the input, neurologically recognize the patterns of the input, and the child's neuro-biological system must be able to attach meaning to those patterns which is conceptualization, and then, if desired, share the process with others through language. As previously discussed, the child will learn concepts only in the way the child's learning system is able to convert patterns into concepts. So, visual thinkers who think in visual concepts learn new concepts with a visual overlap of visual or motor (shape-based) patterns. Since 85 percent or greater of the general education population think in a visual way, it is logical that the patterns for becoming literate should be provided in the way that the majority of children form concepts or think in order to maximize inclusive effectiveness.

Activity: As learning concepts is integral to being able to understand the meaning of literacy processes such as reading, writing, and calculating, how would the majority of thinkers need material presented to be able to learn to be literate?

This knowledge that most learners think in a visual meta-cognition coupled with knowledge about the learning system challenges the logic of utilizing literacy practices that are auditory in nature. Auditory literacy practices utilize sound-based programs where children must learn the sounds of parts of words, like letter and sound combinations, in order to read, because English is an auditory language. Then, utilizing the same auditory practices, children are taught to use spelling to learn to write. Writing is taught as an auditory practice of putting letters with sounds to write words. Decoding and encoding sounds and letters to read and write are auditory literacy practices that assume the learners acquire conceptual knowledge in an auditory way. However, only 15 percent of the population thinks in an auditory way. The patterns used to teach reading and writing are auditory, but the patterns could be visual-motor. If the patterns for teaching children were visual-motor in nature, then more students would be able to learn the concepts of literacy easier and in a more natural way.

Activity: Why would the majority of learners benefit from a literacy program designed to promote a visual way to decode?

This means that children would learn to be literate based on concepts or thinking; they would be learning more than just the decoding and encoding of additive language patterns or structures. Remember literacy includes the processes of thinking, speaking, viewing, and listening—not just the trained or memorized imitation of patterns of sounds and letters that replicate the sound-calling for practices related to reading and writing. Thinking is a process of literacy. Literacy involves functional language! *Learning to be literate requires educators to align methods with the child's thinking system, if functional language is an expected outcome.*

Activity: What is literacy? Explain why most people teach early literacy as an auditory task.

Literacy develops from language function

Literacy is defined as seven processes, not seven products. Processes are functions of the learning system while products or structures are taught patterns—the copying, imitating, memorizing of patterns. Patterns can be taught as skills or products, but becoming literate requires more than just the imitation and testing of products. Literacy requires cognitive functioning of language. Literacy is *thinking*. Literacy is functional language. Through functional language, the learner turns patterns into concepts that are language-based for the purpose of taking meaning off the page known as *reading*; *writing* one's ideas to someone else to understand; sharing conversations of ideas or *speaking*; turning what others say into mental pictures or *listening*, understanding what others think or *viewing*, and being able to manipulate numbers for *calculating* or problem solving. These seven functions of the language learning system develop as a child's language develops a level of functioning or thinking that allows the child to use language as a literacy tool.

Activity: What are the seven processes of language function that develop literacy?

State-of-the-art literacy practices

Numerous sound-based auditory programs have been developed as curriculum packages for teaching literacy skills as products. Within these programs, much time is spent on the use of "practicing" the sounds of patterns to be able to "read" and to write those "sounds as letters." However, with 40 years in the field of education, this author has worked with thousands of children and adults (Arwood, 1983, 1991a; Arwood & Brown, 2002; Lucas, 1978, 1980) who are frustrated with the primary sound-based practices or who feel they have been failed by these auditory practices (Chapter 6). Teachers are frustrated because so many children struggle to make sense out of the sound exercises. Some parents or adults feel that the system failed them when they realize that they cannot read with comprehension; because, they were not taught to read the way they learn concepts. Much emotion is vested in the "right way" to teach a child to read or become literate (e.g., Smith, 1992, 2004).

As a professor in education, this author has also worked with hundreds of in-service teachers and hundreds of pre-service teachers who teach the sound-based practices of programs only to turn around and try to help make meaning out of the sounds with other types of classroom activities. As one veteran second grade teacher said, "In the morning we do the reading and writing programs to satisfy the principal and the district adoption committee. In the afternoon, I teach them to read and write." As an observer in this teacher's classroom, the morning time was stressful for everyone with lots of externally needed rewards to keep students doing the worksheets and the scripts. In the afternoon, the teacher told a story and then the students would talk about the story, draw the pictures, tell their ideas to the teacher. The teacher would write down their ideas for them. The students would then research their ideas to refine their drawings, make their own stories to write, and so forth.

The room was calm in the afternoon and there were no rewards or punishers. It was quite apparent to the author that the afternoon session closely matched the way the students meaningfully learned language. On the other hand, the morning emphasis on practicing the parts of words as sounds and letters did not have enough meaning and therefore did not match the children's way of acquiring concepts. Like most children today, these students thought in visual concepts or pictures. It should be noted that this was a metro classroom of second graders that represent the general population. No one in the classroom was on an individualized education program (IEP) or diagnosed with a learning-language problem.

Activity: What are some of the natural language functions that are not part of the teaching of language products?

Learning to be literate is most effective when the teaching practices match the way children *learn* concepts. Therefore, for most children, providing them with visual patterns of concepts will match their visual thinking systems and should provide the most effective way to teach them to be literate with language function. Remember that "visual" refers to the way the learner creates concepts, not a style or preference or a modality. Therefore, what is known about "visual language functions" must be applied to English. Earlier in this book, the application of visual language functions to English was introduced as Viconics. Methods based on Viconics are called Viconic Language Methods. The remainder of this chapter provides the reader with how a primary classroom teacher supports her children to be literate while matching their learning systems with appropriate visual practices for translating English, an auditory language, into a visual language function.

Primary literacy practices

Primary literacy practices are designed to teach three to eight-year-old children. Previous chapters described these children as preoperational thinkers, where their world revolves around them. From their egocentric position in the world, they quickly learn language structures that represent their rapid acquisition of concepts or language functions. By eight years of age, they have already acquired adult-like grammatical structures, are able to tell expanded stories related to themselves, engage in early conversational practices, and begin to think about how they socially fit into groups. During this time, children depend on caregivers to use lots of language to provide a scaffold of meaning that builds their conceptual knowledge into the rich, concrete language function of an eight-year-old. And, for many students at this age, the majority of their waking hours is spent with educators, teachers, nannies, sitters, and caregivers. So, the burden of language development rests with the educational system. *Developing concrete language function should be the primary purpose of school. And, the foundation of literacy skills should emerge as a product of the language processes.*

Activity: What should be the purpose of language for the primary age student?

Model language-based first grade classroom

Bonnie Robb, M.Ed., is a first grade teacher in a Portland, Oregon classroom. As a veteran teacher of 15 years, she has learned to make her classroom a place where language functions as the purpose, rather than the product, of the classroom (Arwood *et al*., 2005; Arwood & Robb, 2008). Her classroom is described as an inner city classroom where 80 percent of the students currently receive free or reduced lunches, where the mobility of students is around 52 percent a year, where there are more than 30 different languages within a K–8 school, where she has students with seven or eight different languages per year in her room, where her average class size is about 22 (17–26) per year, and where there are few resources from parents to support the students. The majority of students come into her class with little English or a lack of English development.

Activity: What is the demographic like for Robb's classroom?

When Robb first started teaching first grade, she had already been licensed as a reading specialist, had a master's degree in education, and soon became licensed in the teaching of children with English as a second language. She had state-of-the-art coursework in these areas, but she also realized that too many of her students were not able to engage in the sound-based literacy methods.

Robb realized that her students needed language development; so she collected samples of language to determine how her students learned language the best and to see at what language level each student functioned. Over a five-year period, language samples were collected the first day of school from all of her students. These samples showed at least one-third of her students were at a pre-production level of pre-language function. The other two-thirds of the students had language structures, but their language was also still restricted in function. Out of the 125 students over the five-year period, 124 were visual in thinking. Because the majority of students in Robb's classroom typically have lots of ideas and many language structures, most teachers would assume that they had the language function to add literacy processes. These processes would then be typically tested for how many patterns that the students had learned.[1] Because Robb had the background in language and collected samples, she realized that her students did not have adequate language to support the literacy programs.

Activity: How do most of Robb's students think?

After her first year of data, Robb collaborated with the author, a university professor, over a four-year period to shift her teaching from an auditory approach to a classroom that emphasized the learning of English language functions (Arwood & Robb, 2008) by utilizing Viconic Language Methods. During this time, she collected data each year on the children's language and again later in the year to determine language progress.

Robb also tested her students on the mandatory district sound-based tests to see if her students were able to show the products even though the emphasis in her classroom was on language function, not language structures. In other words, Robb did not and does not teach the splinter skills of sounds, letters, spelling of words, and so forth. All learning about the products comes from the process of engaging in language-based activities. In 2009, she received a Milken Teaching Award for her outstanding teaching. Table 13.1 shows some examples of Robb's students' language in September and then four months later. The first three are English language learners (ELLs), the second two are not ELLs, and the last one is a child with an IEP who is being served in Robb's classroom.[2]

1 The students learn a lot of patterns toward passing the testing of the same patterns. But, later in academia when language is needed to understand content, which is around the fifth grade, students show a decline in their ability to read, write, and calculate. In order to reverse this decline in the US, language functions need to be emphasized in literacy, not the imitation and memorization of language structures or patterns.

2 The child receives all of his services through the classroom teacher, Robb.

Table 13.1 Language learning as part of the primary classroom curriculum

September samples	January samples
Out there pickin' corn, and, and, der planting, (cue) corn (cue) pickin'	The family is picking apples cuz maybe they want to take them home so they can take them home; so, they can eat em, they are picking apples cuz they make you healthy. Apples make you stronger. Apples can make you healthy. They like apples.
There's a kitty, and then, it got out (cue) (cue) was em.	They are picking apples and putting them in the basket. This little boy, this grandma is getting apples and putting them in the basket and he is holding the basket (points) and the dog is biting his shoe.
The cat, um, came out da garbage (cue) because he wanted to get out	When the kids were putting oranges and apples inside the bag, some accidentally fell out and the dad slipped on em and fell on the ground
Um, there was a cat came out the garbage (cue) two boys got scared	He went to the hospital cuz he has chicken pox and he had to have this thing (points) under his tongue. I guess he is going to get a shot. His mom is right here. And the man, a doctor, is going to give him a shot.
You can use it to write or to unlock the house… there were some people who were pulling corn out of there (content doesn't match picture)	The grandma is trying to get apples and so is the uncle. The girl and boy are helping by putting them (points to apples) in the basket to wash them so they can eat them. And the dog is pulling his leg. Maybe they will wash them for apple pie or other recipes like apple sauce or fruit cobbler
Build pants (plants) corn (cue) um, um, um, um going to pull green stuff off (cue) draw da way (cue) shovelin, holdin bucket [this child has known brain injury from craniostenosis]	Dad is picking the apples to give to the kids and things. The parents pick the apples and the dog bites it (points to pants leg). The woman looks at the dog, then the dog bites the woman. The dog made a hole in his pants and then he went back to his house the pickin and putin in the basket. The Dad is picking the apples, walking to home. She (points) put 6 more in, dog walk home, And the dog got, the dog got down. They walked safely (content still not complete)

Data collected in this classroom provides evidence of best practices. Robb graphed her data over eight years to show her students' performances. During her first year of teaching, before she changed to emphasizing language function, using best practices for sound-based reading (remember she was a reading specialist), 71 percent of her English language learners did not meet the requirements of the district test, which means only 29 percent of the English language learners did meet the requirements. When Robb began using language function as the basis for teaching literacy, the numbers turned around: 75 percent of the students met the standards and only 25 percent did not meet the standards during the second year. By the fourth year (also 100% for years 5, 6, 7), she had 100 percent passing. The eighth year Robb had 92 percent passing; one ELL student had only one-word utterances in September in her L1 which means she had a language disability, not a language difference. She was the 8 percent who did not meet the standards. She did show remarkable gains. The district aggregates the children with special needs into the class data. For Robb's other students, including some children with severe learning or language disabilities, she showed only 59 percent met her first year teaching when Robb used literacy practices based on sound-based methods. When she began to emphasize language on the second year, the number passing jumped to 83 percent, with 95 percent passing by the third year. The fourth year, she had two students with severe disabilities related to brain trauma and injury. For the last four years she has had over 90 percent passing. Her passing scores are significantly higher than the typical first grade classroom in the district. It should also be noted that she did not teach to the test. In fact, the excellent test performance by the students was a result of her emphasis on helping the students become literate through language functions of literacy, not through teaching the parts emphasized on the tests.

Figures 13.1 and 13.2 show the data in graph form.

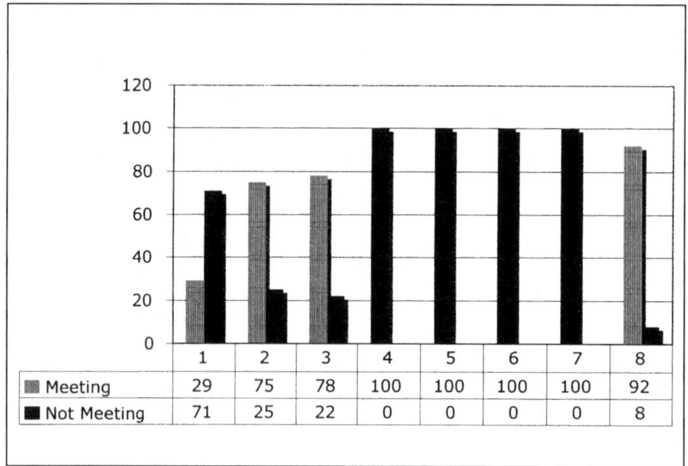

	1	2	3	4	5	6	7	8
Meeting	29	75	78	100	100	100	100	92
Not Meeting	71	25	22	0	0	0	0	8

Figure 13.1 Percentage of English language learners meeting/not meeting reading standards

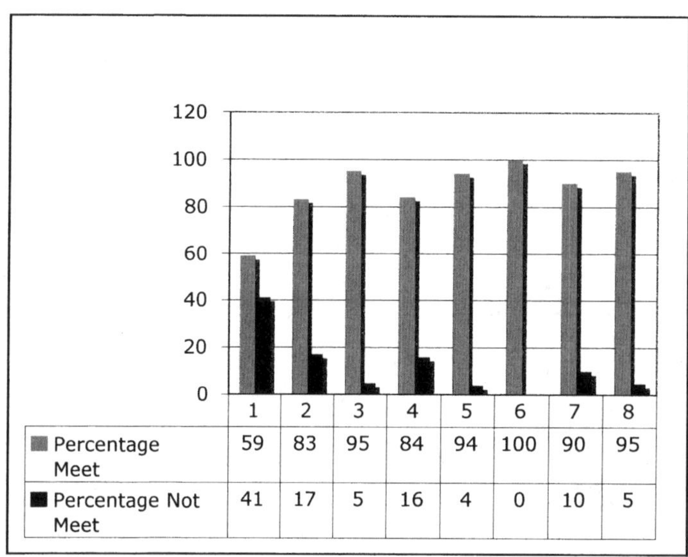

	1	2	3	4	5	6	7	8
Percentage Meet	59	83	95	84	94	100	90	95
Percentage Not Meet	41	17	5	16	4	0	10	5

Figures 13.2 Percentage of students meeting/not meeting reading standards

From this data, it is apparent that not only do children learn language better when they are able to make meaning by using their own learning systems, but also students learn the language structures when the emphasis is on functional language. Furthermore, in Robb's classroom, the English language learners consistently perform as well as those whose first language is English. Students who come from low-income or poverty settings also function at grade level or above in Robb's classroom.

There have been only a few children in Robb's classroom, since she shifted to language function emphases, who have not met benchmarks; these students have special needs. Even these students showed tremendous growth, acted like they socially fit in with the group and often barely missed the target number for reading, writing, and math skills. It should also be noted that between one-third and one-half of Robb's students tested out *exceeding* the expected level by two or more years. Remember, after her first year of collecting data, Robb placed an emphasis on literacy as a function of language, not on language structures.

Activity: Is it possible to test children on state skills of sound-based practices and have them pass the tests when they are not taught the splinter skills?

Language strategies for the primary grades

Because English is an auditory language, researchers and educators assume (Chapter 6) that English literacy can only be taught using auditory techniques; more sounds, more ways to learn sounds, more ways to blend sounds, more ways to make meaning from sounds, and so forth. After all, how can a child learn English except with a sound-based approach? This assumption is based on the properties of auditory English and the assumption that learning English is the result of adding language structures together. However, this book has made the case that English is a set of language functions that represent the social and cognitive development of how a person thinks and acts. Therefore, English is more than just a series of additive sound parts. Because English has language function properties such as displacement and flexibility, there are other ways to consider the development of English.

Activity: Why do most people assume that the auditory properties of English must be taught through the addition of sound-based properties?

English is a highly *flexible* language (see linguistic functions in Chapters 3, 4, 5, 6, and 12) which means that English can be *produced* (Chapter 6) in a variety of ways: spoken, written, or signed for example. Because English is so flexible, it does not have to be taught as a series of additive structures. Instead, English as an oral language can be taught in other ways as long as the natural part of language flexibility remains intact. For example, the speaking of oral English may be *seen* as a series of mouth movements that make shapes. English as a written language can be seen as a series of shapes on a page. Each mental shape has a meaning that is like seeing a picture. English can be seen, not just heard. Children with visual thinking systems are able to "see" ideas better than they can hear ideas.

Activity: Is it possible to see English, rather than hear it?

For children who do not hear the sound of English for comprehension, the spoken or orally read sound is background noise. Some of the 85 percent of the school population who think with what they see, are able to attach sound to mental visuals. But for the majority of the 85 percent, seeing an idea is easier than hearing an idea. In other words, many of the 85 percent of the visual thinking children do hear sound but do not have meaning for the sound they hear. In order to develop higher order thinking skills, these children, who do not make sense out of the sound of English, need to learn the concepts of their culture in a visual way as shapes and pictures that will create well-written English. Writing can be a visual-motor task of putting shapes of ideas on paper. In this way, English becomes a shared written language. When the children learn concepts this way, they have a higher language function to be able to think critically, problem solve, and function linguistically. Without the visual way to think, they may not be able to develop the higher order concepts and so they will remain restricted in language functioning.

Activity: Why do visual thinkers need methods of literacy to match the way their language functions in order to develop higher order concepts?

Robb used this information about how visual shapes of mouth or written patterns can be connected with pictures of concepts to create a classroom environment that is safe for all of today's diverse learners. There are five, "anyone can learn," strategies that Robb (2010) has found effective.

First, use Viconic oral language. Robb uses her spoken language as a way to paint pictures for the students so that they can see themselves do academic or behavioral acts as expected. As Robb says, "This is a strategy I can take wherever I go. When the speaker can paint a picture of expectations in the heads of visual learners, their behavior improves. This is quite effective in the general education classroom." For example:

> Boys and girls, it is time for us to walk to the cafeteria to eat our lunches. Before we stand up to walk to the door, I want you to think by making a picture in your head of what you look like when you stand up, push your chair in so no one gets hurt by tripping over a chair and walk slowly to the door so that you don't bump into anyone. So, who wants to show us how to stand up, push the chair in, and walk to the door?

Robb calls on a student at the beginning of school to model these types of behavior rules. She also cartoons them out. See Figure 13.3 for an example of the product. Remember that she cartoons these pictures in real time with the students so they can watch her hand make the shapes of the patterns.

Mrs. Robb says, "It is time to think about walking to the carpet, sitting on the carpet and making pictures in your head of what you see me say."
"First, we each stand up while we think about pushing in our chairs so we do not trip or fall over chairs and we can walk safely to the carpet."
"Then we walk to the carpet thinking about where we will sit on the carpet so we can see the teacher's face and the teacher's paper."
"When we sit on the carpet, we sit where we can see the teacher's mouth move so we can make pictures in our heads about what Mrs. Robb says."

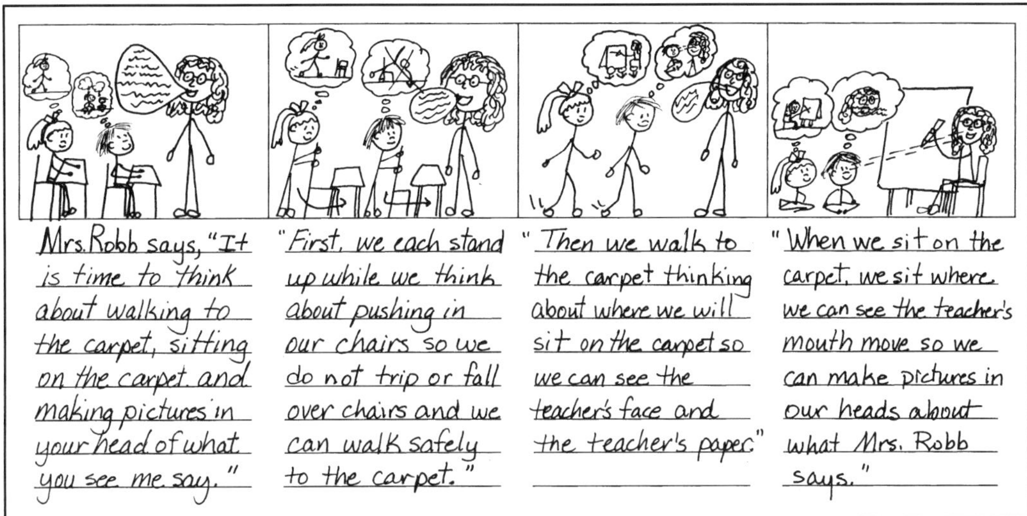

Figure 13.3 Teacher draws a cartoon of a rule

Robb uses Viconic oral language to set up the classroom, to establish limits on behavior, and to help develop academic expectations. Here is another example of making English into more of a visual, relational language (see Chapter 4 for an explanation of a relational language):

> I want us to be safe when we are walking to the cafeteria so we need to put our hands down by our sides so we don't touch anyone else or the walls or the doors along the way. With our hands down by our sides and our mouths closed, then the Kindergarten children won't hear our voices and they will be able to make head pictures so the Kindergarteners can do their work. With our hands by our sides and our lips closed, then we are creating a safe place for the Kindergarten students to work. Also, when we walk to the cafeteria we will want to keep our eyes on the boy or girl in front of us so that if they stopped suddenly we will be able to stop. I don't want any of you to get bumped and get hurt by someone not watching you stop. Also, if we walk in a line where our eyes are on the back of the person in front of us, then we can walk on the side of the hallway where no one else is walking. This is safe because sometimes we are in the hall at the same time the big eighth graders are and we want to be sure to be in our own space.

The lower the language function is for the students, the more details the educator must put into the oral language so that the thinker is able to create visual mental meaning. This type of oral cartooning (Arwood, 1991a) uses relational language and is often very complex (Arwood & Kaulitz, 2007; Arwood *et al.*, 2009) which the author calls "Mabel Mini-Lectures." The following extract shows an example of a Mabel Mini-Lecture used at a store with a child who had little language:

> Wait…stop…I have been hearing the sound of shoes slapping against the hard floor for several minutes. Now I see that it is your feet and shoes running around the store that is making so much noise.

Running feet and noisy feet are okay for outside play, but you are inside, not outside. SO, it is your job to walk your feet through the store.

When you run your feet through the store, you make a lot of noise for the other people in the store. The noise you are making with your feet causes the people who are shopping to think about you and your feet. When they think about you and your feet they forget what they came to the store to buy. When the people forget what to buy, because they are thinking about your feet, they have to stop shopping and try to rethink about what to buy. When the people stop, stand still, and think, they are not getting their shopping done. Because they have to spend time thinking about what to buy, their shopping will take a lot longer to get done. Because you interrupted their shopping with your noisy feet, they will be late getting home, late to make dinner, and late to eat. The people who are at home, waiting for the people who are shopping to bring dinner home, will have to wait longer for the shoppers to get home…the waiting people will be hungry. These hungry people at home will be upset that dinner is not ready because your feet made so much noise that the people shopping could not remember what to buy.

You, running your feet through the store, make a lot of danger for both you and the other people in the store. When you are running your feet through the store, the people can hear your feet, but they cannot see you running because the shelves are so tall. You cannot see where the people are standing in the aisles because the shelves are so tall. Sometime you will run around a shelf at the same time that a person shopping is coming around the other side of the same shelf. The other person who is walking will be able to stop and you will not be able to stop because you are running your feet through the store. You and your running feet will crash into the other person. When your running feet crash your body into the person who is shopping, you will bruise yourself and the other person. The person you hit will be very angry with you and will scold you for running your feet inside the store.

There are other things that can happen if you are running your feet in the store. For example, if you run into someone who is pushing a shopping cart you will hurt yourself badly. You will bruise your tummy when you run into the cart. You may fall on the hard floor and hit your head. If you hit your head hard enough on the floor, you will crack your head open and your head will bleed and you will have a bad headache. If you fall backwards and hit the shelf, all of the food will fall off the shelf and land on your stomach and squish your belly. On this shelf there are a lot of glass jars. If you hit this shelf, the jars of pickles and bottles of steak sauce will fall on you and the floor. When the glass jars and bottles hit the floor the glass will break and fly all over you and the floor. You and the other people will get hit with flying glass and you will get cut and bleed and it will hurt a lot. The broken glass jars and bottles will make a big smelly mess on the floor.

Who is going to clean up the mess? The store people are all busy. The store people have important jobs…some of the store people are working at the cash registers, some of the store people are cutting meat and fish, some of the store people are

> baking bread, some of the store people are cutting deli meat and cheese…none of the store people have time to come and take care of a mess of broken glass jars and bottles…the glass jars and bottles that you caused to fall on the floor because you chose to run through the store.
>
> When you are outside, it is okay to run around, make noise, and have fun. But, when you are in the store your job is to act like a shopper. You are to help push the cart safely down the aisles so that nothing on the shelves gets knocked off and broken, you are to walk close to the adult who brought you to the store so the adult can see you and know you are safe, you are to walk at all times through the store so that you can keep your body under control and make it safe for yourself and for other shoppers.

Although the example provides numerous situations which in turn appears to be a lot of language, it is relational language where the ideas function together to get a mental set of pictures for the listener. Relational language answers the event-based who, what, where, when, why, and how of functional language. Relational language is easy for visual thinkers to make mental pictures because it creates more meaning than the English, "Be quiet; don't run." This succinct English creates very little visual meaning for a visual thinker who is trying to learn to think.

Activity: Why is visual thinking easier with more relational language?

If the teacher or parents use a lot of relational language like the Mabel Mini-Lecture, then the students develop visual concepts or mental pictures. This type of oral language is like putting words to mental pictures about an event, similar to drawing expectations for behavior with oral Viconic Language. The child develops the visual mental pictures to go with the spoken language because the spoken language functions relationally like a visual language would.

Activity: What is relational language? How does a Mabel Mini-Lecture or Oral Cartooning work? Why do these VLMs work for children who are visual thinkers?

The second idea that Robb shares with the reader is she suggests that students and the teacher should draw concepts to increase academic language. Drawing out the expected behaviors, the stories of content about classroom events such as learning about insects provides a visual context for children. Visual thinkers need more context than auditory thinkers. Context is event based and the more information about who, what, where, when, how, and why, the more the children learn about the context or event. For example, for the topic of insects: Who studies insects? Where do they study insects or where do we study insects? When do we study insects? How do we study insects? Why do we study insects? Each of these constituent questions allows for the teacher to scaffold information about insects so that the learner or student who is the one studying about insects is thinking about how, as a learner, the child learns about insects. "Insects" is not the academic unit. The unit is about how children in first grade learn about insects. The context revolves around the students. To put the students into their own pictures, the teacher can begin with an "I story" such as:

> Last night, I was sitting on a chair in my backyard enjoying the fresh air when my dog started to scratch his ear with his paw. He just kept scratching and scratching. Why do you think he was scratching his ear?

The teacher then collects some answers. The students tell their ideas. Someone will probably say the dog might have fleas. So, then the teacher can say, "I wonder what a flea looks like?" (While the teacher is talking she can draw stick figures of her story about being in the backyard, about the dog and an insect with a question mark for the flea.) The teacher then guides the students into researching fleas by looking at books on insects. From their work, the students draw out pictures of stories they have had with insects, they draw out similarities and differences of the insects they saw in the book and from this research decide what makes a bug an insect, and so forth.

Activity: What are two ways that drawing helps students?

Basically, the teacher guides the learning of the content through a scaffolding of drawing, writing, and talking that includes listening, viewing, thinking, and calculating with rich oral language. As Robb says, "Use 'I stories' to increase language development; to introduce all major concepts; and to begin the process of the 'tornado' of layering concepts for learning."

Activity: Why do "I stories" work to establish context? Why does the story of the teacher along with the stories of the students produce context? Why is creating context a VLM for visual thinkers?

Robb's third suggestion is that picture dictionaries should be part of the curriculum: Use picture dictionaries to increase concept/language development, spelling, writing, and reading fluency. Picture dictionaries are part of the reading, writing, and speaking context of children learning the shape of how the written pattern goes with the drawn concept or picture in a way to make visual language. Figure 13.4 shows an example of a picture dictionary that Robb and her students created after telling a story that she drew out with the students.

Activity: What is a picture dictionary? Why do patterns and concepts put together form language?

Fourth, Robb uses writing for everything. Writing is the common ground between oral English and the print of English. Because most students think with visual language, teaching children to understand the meaning of the print on the page is a visual-motor task that matches their thinking. Writing helps the students learn what concepts mean, and developing writing increases their understanding of print on a page for better reading. To learn to write, first they draw ideas based on a common story related to an event. Then, they tell about what they draw and the teacher adds the printed words to the drawn story. See Figures 13.5 and 13.6 for an example. Figure 13.5 shows what the child's writing looked like in September when the child was trying to write with letters and sounds after drawing.

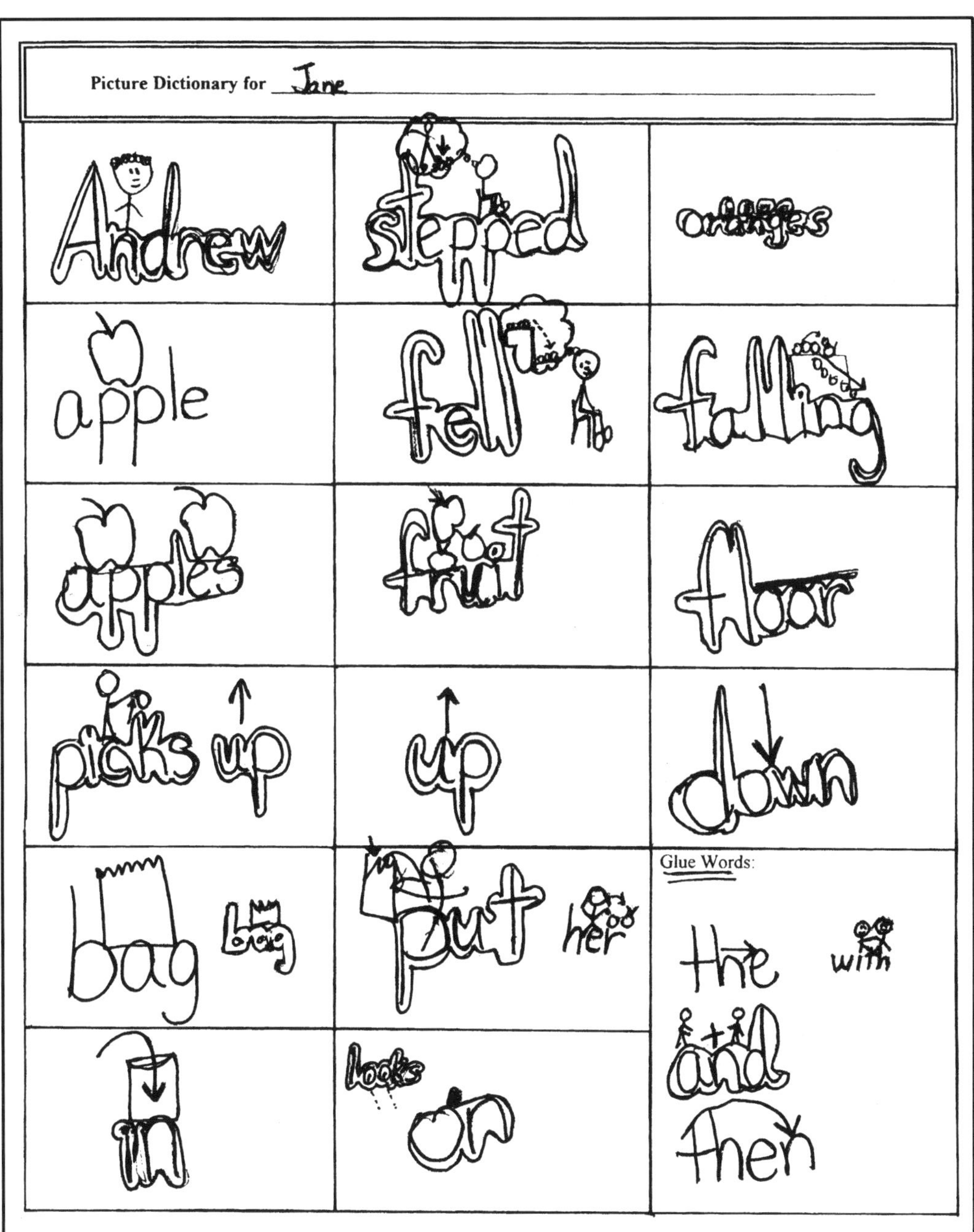

Figure 13.4 Picture dictionary in the primary grades

I loike too glexe
on the cnpYoors.

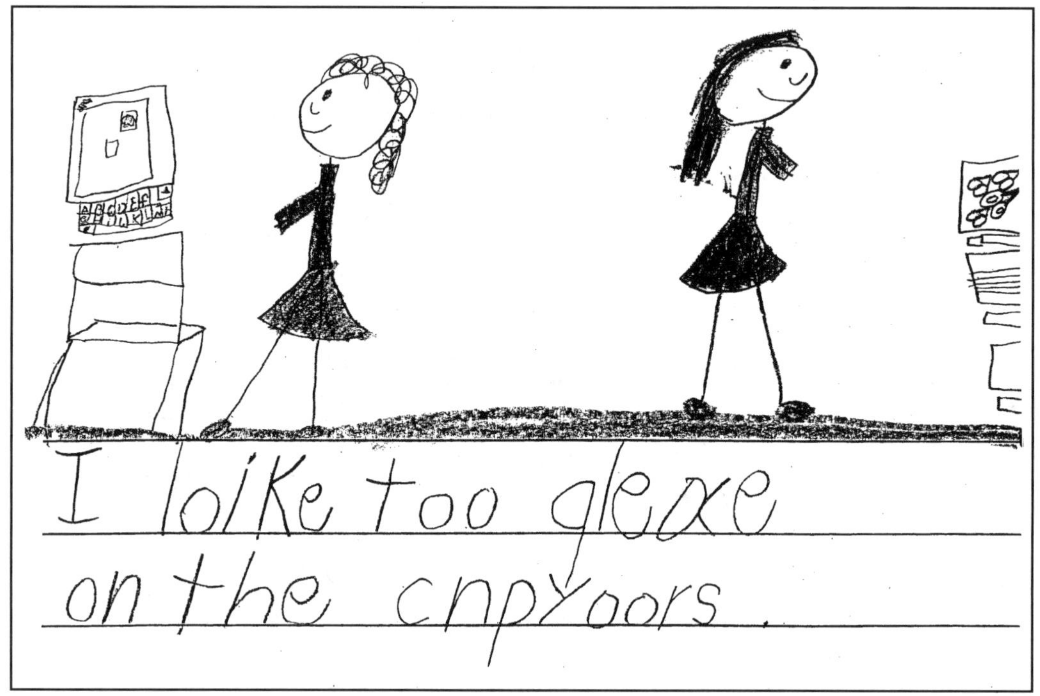

Figure 13.5 A child's writing product in September

Figure 13.6 shows the same child's writing with a prompt but no picture in January of the same academic year after three months of learning to write using a more visual-motor way of seeing the ideas through drawing of concepts with picture dictionaries.

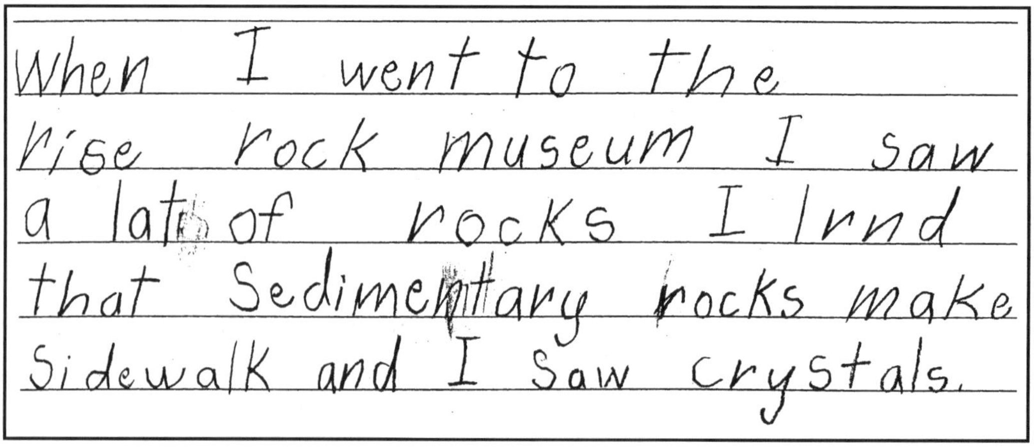

When I went to the
Rise rock museum I saw
a lat of rocks I lrnd
that Sedimentary rocks make
Sidewalk and I Saw crystals.

Figure 13.6 A child's writing product in January

To develop good writers, the writing must be about a shared event such as an "I" story that the teacher draws while telling the story with the whole class. To this story and picture, the students draw their stories. Then the whole class develops a picture dictionary to help write about their own stories. Students are taught to ask for the patterns of words they do not know so they can put those new words in their own picture dictionaries. In this way, students are learning that the words are supposed to be correct or they mean something else. As they draw and write, the teacher monitors by walking around and helping students with ideas about "who, what, where, when, why, and how" as well as with correct patterns and ***learning strategies*** (see Chapters 14 and 15).

While monitoring the class, students tell their stories that go with their drawings. After students tell their stories to their drawings, the teacher labels each child's drawing based on the student's story unless they can label their own drawings. This helps match the picture dictionary entries with the students' language. The students are encouraged to draw a picture onto the word so that the word is a visual-motor pattern and the picture is a concept; and the pattern and concept are attached to each other. The students use their dictionaries for more writing. Basically, learning throughout the day consists of drawing and writing, writing and drawing. Drawing provides the concepts. Writing provides the visual-motor shape of what speaking looks like and therefore the conventions of English for higher order thinking and problem solving.

Activity: What are some steps that can be used to develop writing that is conventional and grammatically meets English standards in the primary grades?

Word walls are made from these relational, contextual events of stories. Spelling is always correct because it is a shaped pattern that is visual, and not a series of sounds. The children tell back what they write, which is how reading improves. Students share stories out loud so there is also a speaking component and a listening component as students are encouraged to watch others' mouths, make mental pictures of what they are saying, and then ask questions about what they saw the other person say. Viewing from others' perspectives and thinking from their own language systems are encouraged to develop as literacy. The same process is also used for developing math concepts.

Becoming literate is based on how the children gain knowledge about their ideas from the way the teacher assigns meaning, just like the way children acquire language concepts for oral functional language. Remember that the teacher can help students produce correctly written patterns by using a hand-over-hand method,[3] where the teacher takes the child's hand and helps the child write.

> It is important for the reader to understand the writing for a visual thinker is like oral language for an auditory thinker: With auditory language we talk to children about all sorts of ideas long before the infant is able to talk. We do this so that the child has the sound-based patterns to begin to form auditory concepts that will underlie the development of language to represent those concepts.

3 Hand-over-hand is the process by which the teacher guides the child through correct written patterns.

For many of the visual thinkers who come to school without a strong language basis, they need to see the written patterns as movements of the hand shapes to form visual-motor patterns that will become written and drawn concepts. We do not need to wait for children to write to have children learn to write just like we do not wait until children speak before we speak to them.

Overlapping visual-motor patterns (hand-over-hand writing or copying with picture dictionary entries, labeling of pictures, group dictionaries where they watch the teacher's hand and mouth move, group drawings where they watch the teacher's hand and mouth move, writing with picture dictionaries about content events, and so forth) create their visual-motor thinking or concepts for better English literacy.

Activity: Why use so much writing? Why not use writing after learning to read? Why does writing ideas rather than letters and sounds fit with the way most children learn concepts?

Finally, Robb says to teach Viconic Language Methods™ as strategies of learning with all students. In the auditory culture, students are given auditory methods for learning: "Listen to the teacher's words." "Use your words." "Don't interrupt when someone else is talking." "Raise your hand when you want to talk." "It's quiet time." "When the bell rings, you need to be in your seat or you will be late." Table 13.2 shows a comparison of what these same auditory phrases sound like when they are adjusted to meet visual thinkers' needs.

Table 13.2 Oral Viconic Language

Listen to the teacher's words.	Watch the teacher's mouth move so you can see what she says.
Use self-talk.	Make a mental picture.
Don't interrupt when someone else is talking.	Keep your lips closed when another person moves their lips and make a head picture of what you see them say. When they stop moving their lips, then it is your turn to tell what your mental picture is about.
Raise your hand when you want to talk.	When you see someone else stop moving their lips, then it is time for you to talk about what you want to say. While you wait to talk about your ideas, draw your mental pictures on a piece of paper so that the sound of their voice does not make your mental pictures go away.
"It's quiet time" (it is inferred that the student realizes that he or she is not to be talking during this time).	When your mouth moves, words fall out onto the floor. The words that fall onto the floor fill up my space and make my pictures go away. When my pictures go away, I cannot think and when I cannot think, I cannot work. When I cannot work, then I do not get my work finished. So, for me to do my work, I need to have you stop moving your lips so your words do not fall out of your mouth and fill up my space and make my pictures go away.
When the bell rings, you need to be in your seat or you will be late.	When you see others sitting down in their seats, it is time for you to sit down too. After you sit down, the bell will ring.

Activity: Why does an auditory culture have to teach most students visual learning strategies for how to use their visual thinking systems?

Language effectiveness

When Robb (2010) was interviewed about the reason for her success in her classroom, she responded this way:

INTERVIEWER: Why is language function important in your classroom?

ROBB: When I use a lot of language, there is a change in the behaviors I can see in the classroom. Language sets up expectations, gives reason for behavior, and children function in the environment because they understand their environment. Language creates enough head language so children can see the "we" and can be rule governed.

INTERVIEWER: The children in your room are very self-controlled but you use no verbal or tangible rewards. How do you account for the way your children socially act?

ROBB: Language develops "self managers" by increasing social language. Rich language allows them to move from the "I" to the "we" which amounts to better social skills, choice making, and better understanding of consequences of actions.

INTERVIEWER: You have had 100 percent success with ELL students in your classroom in the past few years. Why? [Robb is endorsed as a specialist in English Speakers of Other Languages (ESOL) as well as reading in addition to her classroom teaching credential.]

ROBB: Language functions to increase cognitive development. So, when we use drawing that the ELL students are able to see, then they can use their L1 conceptually to understand the English concepts or if they do not have a strong L1, they can learn the concepts. My students understand concepts beyond the yes/no fill in the blank level. They can answer the why question, give because answers, and think globally! I emphasize how language functions to increase language skills in the classroom, which leads to an increase in skills and standardized testing scores. Emphasis on thinking with language mitigates the effects of poverty and ELL on achievement... Language is powerful! Adjusting what I do to meet their conceptual learning needs through Viconic Language Methods is awesome.

INTERVIEWER: Why do you do so much writing? And, I noticed that your major writing block is in the afternoon and the students are calm and leave your classroom calm. Why?

ROBB: Language functions to increase and refine writing. This allows writing to be used as a tool for learning and language acquisition, not just an outcome. Because so many of my students are able to think visually and use their drawings when they write, then writing becomes a visual-motor process, not a sound-based process. We do a lot of writing all day long but the more they write their ideas in a visual-motor way, the more they are matching the writing to the way they are learning. This means they can leave the classroom calm, after they have spent time thinking and learning in their visual way.

INTERVIEWER: Speaking of being calm, I noticed that their bodies become really still when you start to draw out the concepts of your stories. Why?

ROBB: They are watching my hand move. The movement of my hand creates the shape of ideas. Since they think in a visual way, then the shapes are like puzzle pieces that create a picture. When I draw or write, they are thinking about the movement of the shape of my hand, not the sounds or letters of what I am writing.

INTERVIEWER: How can they pass tests that are checking for oral fluency, writing letters and sounds, and numbers when you emphasize language?

ROBB: Those tests measure how well the students can perform acts that involve saying, reading, writing patterns. Patterns are only meaningful when they will form concepts. By giving the students visual patterns [sight and movement] that go with the visual concepts or pictures, they are learning more than patterns for decoding, they are learning the concepts. Language is greater than the parts. They can do the parts because they have learned the whole.

Activity: Why does emphasizing language function help students learn skills as well as concepts?

Summary

An emphasis on language function in the primary grades helps develop conceptual thinking. Because most children at this age are in a preoperational thinking level, their social development is as an agent in their own pictures. So, using Viconic Language Methods™ to help students at this age translate what they hear about themselves into what they see as print about them helps develop literacy.

The more the students use their own meaning through their drawings (e.g., Gill, 2008) to produce their own patterns of print, the more the students will be able to develop a conceptual understanding of what they read and write. VLMs help children translate what they know into children's products of literacy—writing, reading, speaking, listening, thinking, viewing, and calculating. Some of these VLMs at the primary grades include students drawing their own ideas about a shared event; using picture dictionaries based on printed patterns produced by the adult along with pictographs of the print to create written, spoken, and read meaning; producing writing (with or without hand-over-hand) that is a visual-motor pattern of the content of an event; learning to watch the teacher's mouth produce shapes of what ideas look like along with watching the shapes of the teacher's hand write about shared content, and the use of relational, rich language to paint a mental picture.

Applications

- Try at least three VLMs designed for primary grade children, and evaluate your success by asking the students about what they know.
- Explain why VLMs help develop thinking for qualitatively better literacy products to a parent or another colleague.

Chapter 14

THE LANGUAGE-BASED INTERMEDIATE CLASSROOM

Learner objectives: Chapter 14

Upon completion of this chapter, the reader should be able to:

1. Explain the use of "because language" at the intermediate grades.
2. Explain the use of "I stories" at the intermediate level.
3. Explain the use of Viconic Language Methods™ at the intermediate grades.
4. Explain the use of "context" at the intermediate grade levels.
5. Explain the preoperational to concrete to formal level of language function at the intermediate grade levels.
6. Develop several intermediate grade lessons that are developmentally appropriate for concrete thinking or language function.

School is now about content,
Watch the scientist, author, and historian at work!
Learn about the world and learn about others,
Calculate, read, write, and oh so much more.

Children in the intermediate grades are usually between 8 and 11 years old, concrete in their thinking, and capable of a language level of thinking. This means that neuro-typical children, at this age, should be able to maintain a conversation about ideas for which they have knowledge. To maintain a conversation means that they can listen to what others say, follow the sound of the teacher's words, and use this level of oral language for reading and writing and calculating at grade level. With these assumed abilities, intermediate classroom teachers should be able to use children's conversational strength as pedagogy for helping children, who live in an auditory culture, learn the content. So, teachers in these grades give many oral, auditory instructions throughout the day such as lists of words on the board for homework, small group work where talking and listening is paramount, and lots and lots of talking times or discussions about content. Students read out loud for others and teachers encourage students to write from what they say. Teachers give these types of sound-based tasks because they believe that the students use the sound of their own voices for thinking.

If students are still struggling with academic tasks at this level, then they engage in more practice with the problem. For example, if students are struggling with oral reading at this level, the teachers give the struggling students more oral reading tasks. Children who struggle with spelling practice the sound names of the letters for more spelling words. And teachers give those who struggle with writing more practice writing the sounds of letters as words in print.

Even though it is logical that sound-based practices are best practices, national research (McCombs *et al.*, 2005) shows that by fifth grade these auditory methods of instruction are failing the students. Their scores in content and literacy slowly decline from fifth to eight grade resulting in fewer than one-third of the US population able to read, write, and do math at the eighth grade level. This decline may be for many reasons, but one correction is possible. If the majority of students are visual thinkers, then why use auditory methods over and over and over? Why not change the methods?

Activity: Are learners able to use a visual way of learning to be literate?

This chapter will discuss how to use the Viconic Language Methods™ in the intermediate grades to help students learn to be literate using the way they think matched to the pedagogy of the classroom teacher.[1] The VLMs that intermediate teachers report (see Chapter 16 for the research) as the most useful include the use of "because language," high levels of context, strategies for cognitive learning, and opportunities to learn new concepts or new content at a preoperational level of thinking. Each of the VLMs used in the intermediate grades will be discussed in depth in this chapter.

Activity: Why must intermediate grade teachers consider VLMs?

Intermediate literacy practices

Teachers in fourth to sixth grades expect children to learn content through literacy; literacy includes reading, writing, thinking, viewing, listening, speaking, and calculating. And, this expectation matches with the developmental notion that children with good language master an adult grammatical system by the time they are around eight years old and therefore learn to read and write with language structures at a concrete level of thinking. This means that children at this age learn science, math, social studies, history, and other content areas through the use of their language system that supports their literacy. Furthermore, a child at this level has met the social expectations of being able to share in the conversation or any other task with others.

1 Remember that Viconic Language Methods were developed based on the properties of visual languages to be imposed on English, an auditory language, so that visual thinkers are able to translate their thinking into English, an auditory language and vice versa.

Activity: What are the neuro-typical expectations of children in fourth to sixth grades, 8–11-year-olds?

If a child has a solid or strong language system that functions for conversational development, a child at this age should also have the literacy functions that match. But remember, in order for the literacy to match the child's language development, the child has to learn the literacy processes in the same way that he or she learns language. Since most of the children today think in a visual form of language, their literacy should have been taught in a visual way. With their visual way of thinking, viewing, reading, writing, listening, speaking, and calculating, the intermediate classroom provides opportunities for children to learn their science, history, social studies, and math through the same processes. Viconic Language Methods™ make the learning of language match children's thinking. In this way, children learn content through better use of language. The rest of the chapter describes some of the most effective VLMs for the intermediate grades: "because language," high context, ***strategy learning***, and preoperational thinking.

Because language

Visual language is relational in nature. Ideas interconnect. This means that connecting ideas with words like "because" should be used to help the learner understand the relationships among ideas. "***Because language***" (Arwood & Young, 2000) sounds like this:

> Please put your feet on the floor so you can sit up because your eyes need to see the print on the page in front of you in order for you to make mental pictures about the chapter.

This example shows that "because language" is relational. One idea relates to another idea creating an elaborate set of cause and effect meanings for both the child's behavior, the child's academic expectations, and the child's content.

"Because language" is good at developing these meaningful relationships for content development as well as social and behavioral expectations. These overlapping meaningful relationships create a shared referent between two or more speakers. The child is actually able to use the literacy processes to engage with others in meaningful language. The child with solid language function at this age is able to listen to the "because language" and create mental pictures of the ideas as well as follow through in spoken, read, and written language. If children do not have a solid language function, "because language" will help the student develop both cognitive and social reasons for behavior as well as for understanding academic tasks.

Activity: What does "because language" sound like? And, what does "because language" do to develop language function?

Children at this age are expected to use conversational English. And teachers expect that students are able to engage in spoken language that functions for learning academic content. In reality, many students come to school without the language able to engage in conversation. Conversational language is more than just talking to others about a topic of interest or one's own experiences and ideas. In other words, conversational language is more than a narrative (Morgan, Greene, Gill, & McCullough, 2009). Narratives allow an individual to use continuous stream of language "to talk" about ideas of interest to the speaker, independent of what other people know or care about. Conversational language expects that two or more people are able to talk about their ideas in relationship to what the other speaker or speakers are saying. In other words, conversation assigns meaning to what the speaker says as heard by the hearer or listener. The speaker is a listener and a listener is a speaker. "Because language" helps students begin to learn how the expectations between speaker and listener are more "we based" than "I based."

As "because language" implies more than the interest of the speaker, such language not only models increased language structure, but also increases the cognitive expectation of the speaker engaged with others, about others. This type of thinking or language function increases the cognitive level of the speaker from a preoperational level of being in one's own picture to a concrete level of thinking where others are in the speaker's mental pictures. The speaker thinks about others. The speaker relates to others. As language function improves, the speaker's thinking and social development also increases.

Activity: How does "because language" increase cognition and socialization?

It should be noted that increases in cognition are from learning more concepts as well as more depth of the concepts (Chapters 3–5). So, educators at this level need to be mindful that their goals of instruction are about the development of concepts over time, not the testing of skills. In this way, language function or thinking becomes the tool to mediate the development of higher cognitive and social skills.

Conceptual emphasis

Learning is both social and cognitive. Engagement is often social with students enjoying the classroom activities, while cognitive development necessitates asking students to work with literacy processes to assign language meaning to their work. If students have developed appropriate adult language structures by the intermediate grades and can easily read, write, speak, and listen at a developmental level commensurate with their chronological level, then these students are probably also thinking and viewing the world at the concrete level and have mastered meta-cognitive language strategies for academic performance. In other words, they can think about how the teacher is presenting the material and have the strategies to change what the teacher is doing into their own concepts in the way they learn best. In other words, students must be at this concrete level of language function to be able to understand socially how to use their own language to learn. However, because the majority of students are not thinking the way they are being taught the majority of students may not have the concrete language function to be able to use language as a tool for their own conceptual learning. As a result, they struggle with learning the concepts of the content.

Activity: Why do some students struggle learning the content?

In order to be sure that the students are learning concepts the way that the teacher is presenting materials, the teacher needs to know how much language the students have as a tool for learning. This chapter will highlight the practices of an outstanding intermediate teacher, Alyse Rostamizadeh, a fourth and fifth grade teacher. Rostamizadeh collected language samples on her students to determine their levels of language function. She wanted to see if her pedagogy provided the best practices for conceptual learning. As part of her pedagogy, she typically uses Viconic Language Methods. For this particular data collection (Rostamizadeh, 2009b), she wanted to see if discussion would provide a better avenue to providing to socio-political conceptualization. She used some standard methods in setting up the classroom discussions and she used her typical visual forms of products where she modeled for the students the way to make their picture dictionaries, flowcharts, and so forth (Rostamizadeh, 2009b).

The students really loved the discussion process. This means that she saw they were engaged and they showed social gains such as following her lead in producing their ideas for others to hear. But Rostamizadeh knows that children learn cognitively as well as socially and her goal is to improve her students' conceptual learning, so she recorded some of their discussions to analyze their use of thinking or functional language to determine their progress. There were at least two types of data: One type of data was to look for an increase in products: more talking, more ideas, more sentences, more vocabulary used, and so forth. The second type of data meant looking at students' language to see if they were able to *really share* in the conversational process. In other words, if the students were able to share in a conversational process, the students would show an increase in language functions: displacement, semanticity, flexibility, productivity, and less redundancy of surface structure. Did the students increase their conceptual learning? Their language would show changes in the depth of conceptual understanding. She used the chart shown in Table 14.1 to analyze the utterances.

Table 14.1 Viconic Language Methods for cognitive levels of thinking and language

	Cognitive concepts	**Academic tasks**	**VLMs: classroom strategies**
Preoperational thinking (ages 3–7)	"Mine" Agents Actions	• Find/locate • Repeat • Copy • Fill-in-the-blanks • Grammar • Conventions • Drill and practice	• Hand-over-hand writing and drawing • Picture dictionary • Cartooning • Matching • Memorization of code, answers, plagiarism, etc.
Concrete thinking (ages 7–11)	"Yours/ours" rules	• Each student does his or her own task which becomes part of the whole classroom's work • Event-based learning • Multiple projects scaffolded across topics • Multiple use of examples	• Cartooning • Multiple choice • Vocabulary pictographs of rules and definitions • Early flowcharts • Inquiry based on who, what, where, and when
Formal thinking (ages 11+)	• Formal thinking • Concepts such as homelessness, respect, war, responsibility, trust, social issues • Problem solving at the formal level • Critical thinking at the formal level	• Explain relationships among concepts • Make connections among formal concepts through symbolization • Infer concepts from symbols • Use of essays and debates	• Flowcharting • Discussion from others' perspectives (drawn multiple cartoons connected with arrows) • Explaining in writing and in drawing and in oral language the use of formal concepts • Inquiry based on why and how

Table 14.2 shows an analysis of language from one of the discussions (Rostamizadeh, 2006).

Table 14.2 Assessment examples of language levels

Participant	Probe	Student utterance	Developmental level	Criterion reference—expectation for chronological age	Language level
Madison (10 years)	What is the setting?	Maybe the setting is at their home and in the town	Five-year-old language level; literal, here-and-now, not temporarily organized	Complete understanding of the location	Pre-language
Paige (9 years)	Where is segregration?	I don't really think it was everywhere because, well, I think slavery is kind of like segregration, and it says from slavery that there was an underground tunnel to this other place where there wasn't slavery, so I think that there is kind of a place that isn't segregration	Five-year-old language level: multiple expanded relationships, not temporarily connected	Conversational switching of topics, adult grammar of language	Pre-language
Gavin (9 years)	Who is the author?	That she was either the white kid or the African American kid	Literal, here-and-now, typical of 3–7-year-old cognition	Expansion beyond the here-and-now and think of alternative possibilities	Pre-language
Trevor (10 years)	African American people are friendly	Well, what I don't get is in the book it doesn't really describe the setting almost	Five-year-old language level; does not refer to probe and structure is a sentence question	Conversational switching of topics, adult grammar of language	Pre-language

continued

Table 14.2 Assessment examples of language levels *cont.*

Participant	Probe	Student utterance	Developmental level	Criterion reference—expectation for chronological age	Language level
Courtney (10 years)	Who is the author?	She was maybe one of the friends. Or... she might have not even been in this book. She was just over in a different house watching... watching to see...she couldn't hear what they were saying, but she just kind of made up her own words	Five-year-old language level; literal, story language that words in books are meant to be heard by others, must place the author in story to understand her	Expansion beyond the here-and-now and think of alternative possibilities	Pre-language

There are a couple of interesting issues: These students are at the upper age limit for concrete thinking, but their language functions at a pre-language level with thinking more like a three to seven-year-old. Even though it is a safe learning environment, where students are engaged in something they reportedly enjoy, their language still does not reflect a concrete understanding. This finding is what the author views in about two-thirds of all school children. Research shows that children from lower socio-economic environments tend to possess lower language functioning (e.g., Qi, Kaiser, Milan, & Hancock, 2006) and this is a rural, Title I school with a significant number of ELLs.

The author also finds that students, even at the college level, often do not think about others (concrete level) or demonstrate formal critical thinking (e.g., see Halpern, 1990). Without language function and concrete thinking, the children in Rostamizadeh's classroom are at an academic disadvantage before even starting middle school or junior high school. Without schools "thinking" about how students thinking, not only are students from low economic situations not developing a higher level of thinking, but also even high end students are not critically thinking to be able to problem solve.

Activity: Why is language function at a concrete or higher level of function important for society (Chapters 3–6)?

Rostamizadeh's goal was to improve her students' thinking, not just their products. Rostamizadeh used a reading methodology that encouraged discussion of socio-political (formal) concepts.[2] Through conversation the students' conceptual understanding of those concepts was supposed to increase. Because Rostamizadeh knew her students were visual thinkers, she drew concepts during discussions about the formal ideas. But she did not ask

2 Rostamizadeh holds a master's degree in education in addition to an endorsement in reading.

the students to draw their own ideas and therefore think for themselves and use their own language (Rostamizadeh, 2009b). The students liked the process (according to a survey and anecdotal comments) and the students showed an above-average engagement in the activity. The bottom line was that the students did not have a concrete language function to be able to use classroom discussion or conversation for improving their conceptualizations. *Remember that a speaker must be at a concrete level of language function to be able to use language to develop a formal level of thinking (Chapters 10 and 11).* And, a speaker must learn new concepts in the way the speaker learns. Discussion was auditory, not a visual-motor task and therefore did not match the way the students learned new concepts.

Rostamizadeh (2009b) found an invaluable piece of data: Teachers who try to engage students in conceptual development while also emphasizing their own pedagogical effectiveness may not be effective at providing the best conceptual student learning. Student learning must emphasize the students' learning systems, not the teacher's system. The following section discusses this extraordinary finding.

Activity: At what level is a learner able to use language to access his or her own thinking so as to improve concrete ideas to formal ideas?

If Rostamizadeh had not collected language samples, she would not have found out that the students really did not understand the concepts at a concrete or formal level. Just based on the enjoyment of the discussions and the students' abilities to match or copy patterns (drawings, sentences, spoken utterances) on tests and on class activities, Rostamizadeh would have thought that the students' increased use of words and discussions were representative of "knowing." Even tests of definitions showed an increase of students' abilities to repeat or match what they had been told or read but not their actual understanding. When the data was shown to other professionals, the professionals were amazed at the students' progress in developing more products. But the students did not increase their conceptual depth of understanding.

Let's examine why the students did not increase in conceptual depth of understanding: First, Rostamizadeh's drawings of her thoughts about the subject matter as models for the students were her ideas, not the students' ideas. Increases in conceptual depth from a preoperational understanding of a formal concept to a formal understanding of a concept like the concept of segregation results from a learner being able to use his or her own language to assign meaning to the examples. This assignment of meaning comes from concrete functional language. *Modeling typically does not increase language function for greater conceptual depth because the modeling uses the teacher's language, not the students' language.* A second reason why the lessons did not show greater conceptualization was that the functional analysis of the students' language showed that they were not really conversing; Rostamizadeh was doing the connecting of the ideas with her language. For example, Rostamizadeh would ask a question such as "What is segregation?" and one student would give an idea about the girl in the book. Then another child would talk about the fence and the girl. And then a third child would use a borrowed phrase such as "I think Sally means..." and would say something not connected to what the other two students said.

Rostamizadeh would use her language to weave all of the ideas together. The students did not really show an ability to converse. They could talk but they did not refer to what others said and add their ideas to what others said. In other words, the students would have to refer to what another speaker said, add his or her own thoughts (predication), and then the next student would have to maintain this process of referring and predicating. This last ability is a part of the linguistic recursive principle; the ability to expand language within language. This principle is used by linguists to determine how well a language functions.

In the case of these fourth and fifth grades, their language did not meet the ***recursive principle***. This means that they had narrative abilities but not conversational abilities. In other words, their language was restricted to more of a pre-language function even though the use of discussion assumes a concrete thinking ability with language function. It should be noted that most educators are not aware of what constitutes true conversational ability because they are used to using their own language to guide student product development. *Only through the use of a learner's own language can a learner build from the concrete to formal level of thinking and problem solving.*

Activity: Language function at a conversational level must include the ability to be recursive. What does recursive mean? What were two reasons why the students in Rostamizadeh's classroom did not develop their conceptual knowledge about formal concepts?

Remember that at the pre-language level of function, children do not use language as a literacy tool for learning. Rostamizadeh's students did not have the language function to show an increase in conceptual learning. Rostamizadeh was surprised with the results. After all, the students talked a lot more with the explicit emphasis on discussion. What the activities did show was that the students' quantity of language showed more words, vocabulary, borrowed phrases but this type of increase did not increase the cognitive function of language or conceptualization. Rostamizadeh was thinking about her pedagogy so much that she began teaching instead of helping the students learn through the use of VLMs to match the students' thinking with their language. Figure 14.1 shows an example of a student who copied the patterns of Rostamizadeh's work for a picture dictionary definition of segregation.

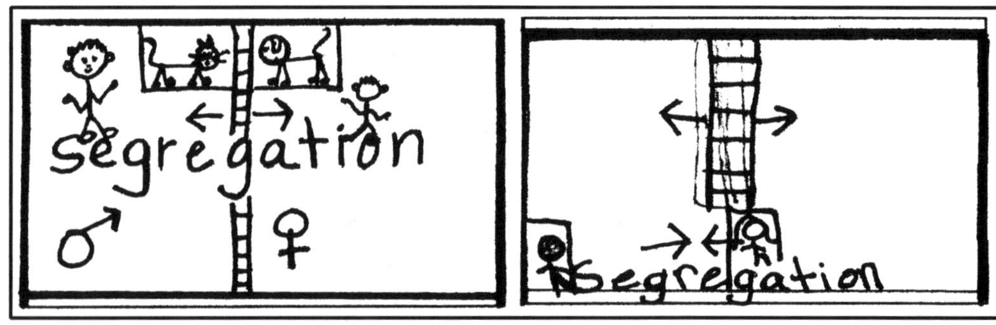

Figure 14.1 A teacher's definition copied

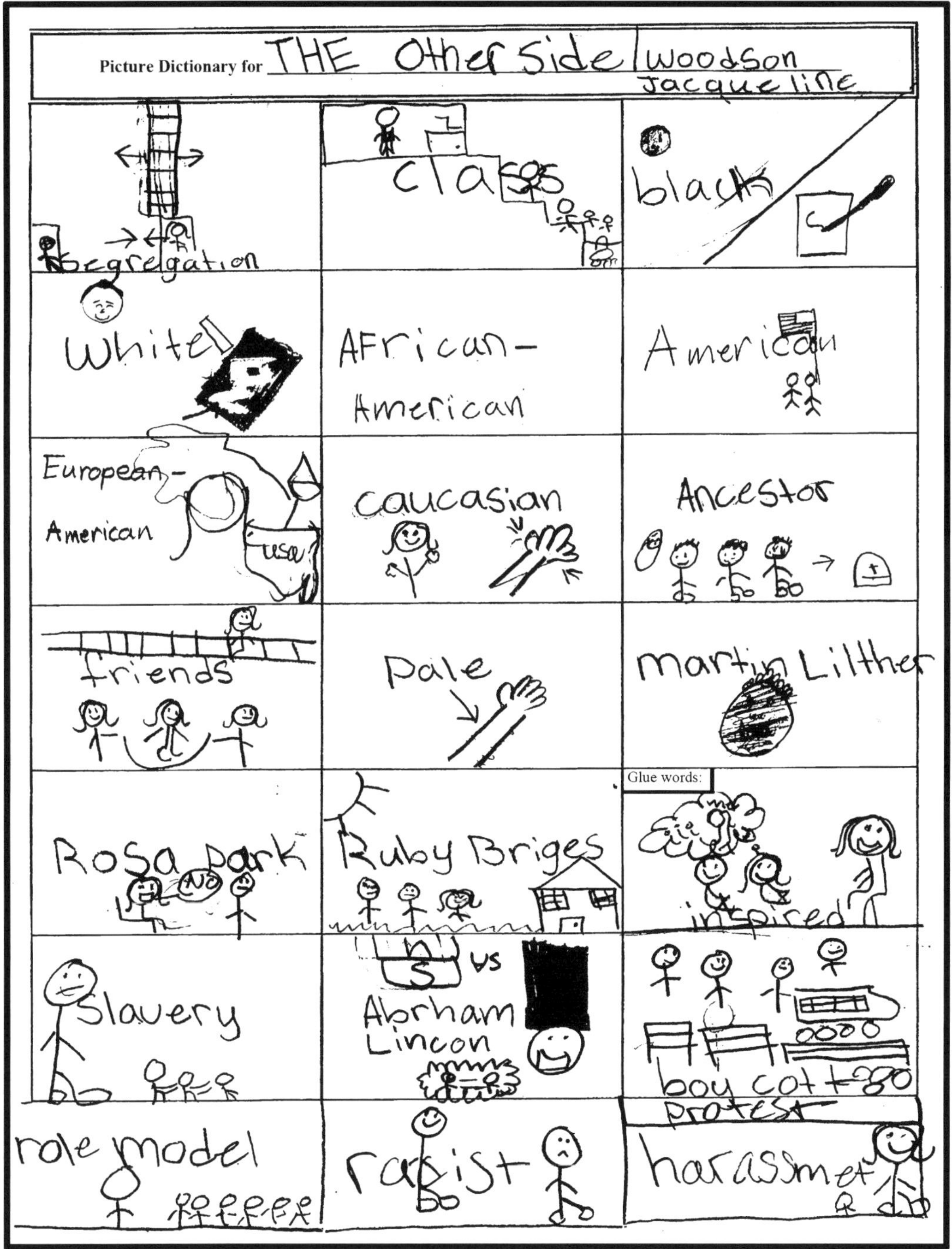

Figure 14.2 A student's picture dictionary

The type of copying seen in Figure 14.1 was also found in all students' definitions in the picture dictionaries and in all flowcharts. So, even though Rostamizadeh was providing visuals (Arwood *et al.*, 2009) for the students, the visuals were at too high a level for scaffolding them from their preoperational level of language function to a more concrete to formal level. The students were just copying, matching patterns. The students needed to draw their ideas of what the words meant and then refine using their own visual-motor drawings and writings. Discussion was an auditory function and the drawings or visuals belonged to the teacher's thinking system.

So, Rostamizadeh immediately changed the process of discussion so that students draw and write their ideas in response to others' ideas in a visual-motor dialogue instead of an oral discussion. The students showed just as much engagement but very different results. Learning new concepts must begin with language at the student's preoperational level.

Activity: Why did emphasizing the teacher's produced models not work well for increasing conceptual learning?

After discovering that even the best methods used by Rostamizadeh did not raise the students' thinking, Rostamizadeh used the students' data about their language to change her work. She had always used visuals to help students learn but when she left her theoretical basis for what she did and emphasized an adult-based teaching pedagogy, she was not using what she knew that students need. *Students need their own thinking and language systems to develop their conceptualization.* Today, Rostamizadeh's students draw their own meanings based on what they read, talk about, and then she draws her meaning and they refine their knowledge through thinking with their visual drawings of definitions or pictographs of the picture dictionaries and their flowcharts, not the teacher's visual drawings. Figure 14.2 shows a student's picture dictionary.

Figure 14.3 shows a student's ability to draw out the concrete examples of a formal set of related concepts.

Instead of assuming that the students have the language to develop their formal understanding of concepts by setting up a discussion of such concepts, Rostamizadeh changed to doing an "I story" and having the students then do their drawing followed by discussion from their pictures about their related stories. In this way, the curricular emphasis shifted from sound to sight; from teaching to learning.

This visual-motor conversation of drawing and writing follows the "because language" properties. Rostamizadeh uses the constituents of who, what, where, when, why, and how to help the students make the connections in the socio-political literature while making sure that students use their own visual-motor language. Rostamizadeh helps scaffold their thinking from preoperational levels of understanding to higher levels of thinking and language function. When a speaker uses "because language," the listener is expected not only to receive the message but also to be able to converse about it in writing or speaking. The following is an example of the same teacher's use of an "I story" with adequate language function to set up a science lesson while also helping the students understand the content.

> When I look up at the sky, I see so many different clouds. Some are big and fluffy and some are flat and spread out. The authors of our science book show a lot of pictures of these different looking clouds. Open up your book and find a picture of a cloud that looks like a cloud that you have seen in the sky. Then draw a

picture of the cloud. Put the cloud's name or type in your vocabulary (picture) dictionary. When you put the name of the cloud type in your dictionary and also draw a picture with each cloud type, then you will be able to recall the names of the clouds or their types when we have a test.

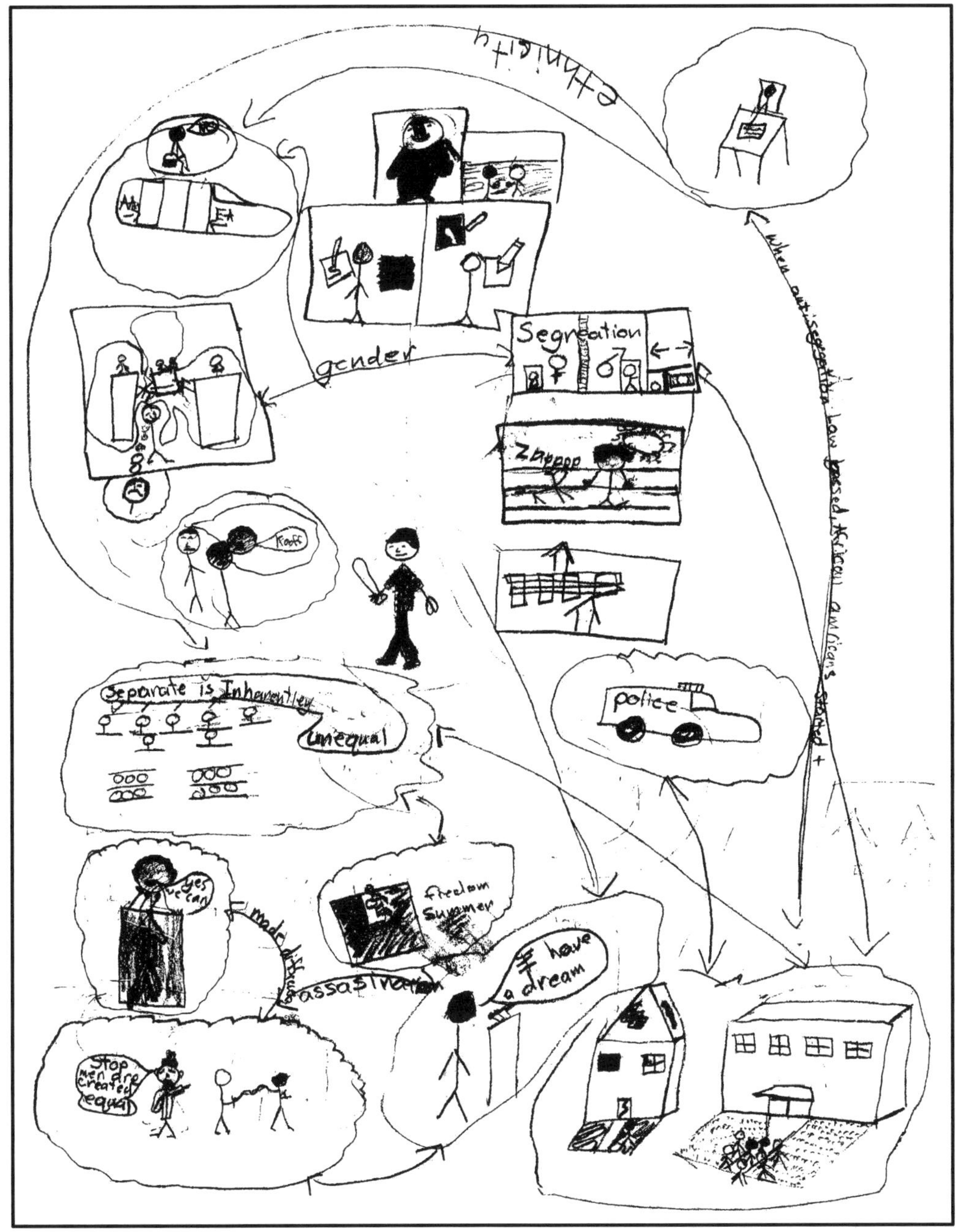

Figure 14.3 A student's flowchart

In Rostamizadeh's language, she is providing the students with a rationale of why they will want to connect their drawn pictures of different types of clouds with the written words of the different types of clouds. Notice that the actual word "because" is not used. Instead there are other cause-effect types of words such as "when" and "then." But, the principle of "because language" is used: *Connect ideas with time-based English so as to create mental visual connections.*

Activity: Explain how language function for academics must belong to the students' ideas.

"Because language" allows time words and other functors or function words like "so" or "also" to connect ideas into relationships that help build the meaning of "why" a child needs to learn something, how ideas connect for more meaning, and what the relationship is between what the child knows and is learning. *Remember that concrete language function requires the thinker to be able to understand multiple ways that ideas can be used in connection to each other*. "Because language" helps create these multiple relationships that raise the learner's ideas from a preoperational understanding to a concrete level of language function.

Activity: How does "because language" work in visual thinking to increase conceptual learning?

Students are also encouraged to use "because language" when they write and talk by showing them how to answer who, what, where, when, how, and why of ideas they are trying to share in speaking, understanding what they read, or writing to others. Instead of marking all of the structural problems within a written assignment, teachers might try using "because language." For example, a student has trouble with spelling:

> John, I sometimes have trouble understanding your paper *because* some of your ideas are not written in the way I expect to see them.[3] For example, when you write "hose" for "house" then I am unsure if you mean a "garden hose used for watering the yard" or a "house, a place where a person lives." Perhaps you would like to put the words you cannot clearly see as a mental image onto a vocabulary sheet (picture dictionary). Then add a pictograph to the words. The pictographs or pictures give you the ideas. When you write your ideas, you will be able to recall which written pattern goes with the idea you are trying to write.

Activity: How does an emphasis on who, what, where, when, why, and how help to develop functional thinking? How does seeing an idea as a picture help a person write without sound?

Sometimes young students need help writing the first correct pattern of the words. This can be accomplished by taking the child's hand in a hand-over-hand process and writing with the child or by typing or printing the exact pattern of the word for the child to copy. Students sometimes also need help in learning to make the word a mental picture. Tell the students to use their eyes like a camera. First they look at the word and take a mental picture.

3 This is a student friendly way of saying "conventional spelling."

Then they close their eyes and see if they can see the word as a mental picture. If they can see the mental word, they will probably be able to recall the mental picture when they want to write the correct pattern; if not, then try to use some bubbling (Arwood & Kaulitz, 2007; also see Chapter 13) of the words that they do not have a mental image. Helping the student understand the relationship between a method and what they do to learn is a form of "because language."

"Because language" also helps with refining content. For example, if the teacher does not understand the student's ideas, the teacher can ask for more information by using "because language." "I read that the main character, Sarah, climbed the hill; but, I am not sure why she climbed the hill. Where was she going? Why was she climbing the hill?" When the students learn to add more meaning through answering the who, what, where, when, why, and how, then students begin to show more problem solving, more concrete understanding of their concepts, and better language function through expansion, extension, and modulation of their ideas. Their language begins to take on adult grammatical structures that function in conversation. This expansion of recursive language means that students are becoming more capable of using language for a variety of literacy functions. The use of who, what, where, when, why, how makes a form of "because language" that connects a variety of meaningful relationships.

Activity: Why does "because language" help a student in the intermediate grades increase their language level of function or thinking?

High context

Because most students are visual thinkers, they are able to make more meaning when the instructional methods match the way that they think. One of the properties of a visual language (Chapters 3 and 4) is the use of ***context***. Visual thinking uses the context to create relational meaning. Context refers to the use of people (agents), their actions, and their objects and/or locations. For example, if a teacher said, "Today we are studying clouds," the students must already be able to understand what "studying clouds" looks like. On the other hand, when the teacher begins a lesson with an "I story" to create context, students are more able to put themselves into the context.

> Yesterday, I went to the airport to meet a friend who was flying in on a plane. When I arrived at the airport, her plane was still in the sky; so I sat down by one of the big windows to wait for her. When I looked out at the sky I saw a lot of really round, fluffy clouds that were very gray and I wondered if her plane could fly through those clouds.

Now the students are mentally able to see themselves looking up at clouds, even if they have never been to the airport. The teacher is the agent or person and her story allows the students to think about when they were the people watching clouds.

Activity: What does context do to help a learner?

In addition to the oral use of language to create context, the teacher can draw this introduction as a quick stick-figure drawing (Arwood *et al.*, 2009). Once the teacher creates the context, she then turns the task over to the students so they can use their language to assign meaning. "What do you think? Do you think the airplane could fly through those clouds or not?" As the teacher takes four or five student answers and writes the students' words on the board or a poster paper, the teacher adds another layer of meaning according to what the students say: "Why do you think the plane won't be able to fly through those clouds?" or "Why do you think the plane will be able to fly through those clouds?" This inquiry by the teacher helps the students make the meaningful connections (expanded semantic relationships) inspired by a form of "because language" that is contextually helpful. Rostamizadeh teaches a lot of science lessons that are loaded with visual conversations between her drawing and talking about the content and the students drawing and writing to what she drew. Then she helps them redraw and write based on what they have learned using picture dictionaries and flowcharts and essays. In this way, the students learn a greater visual understanding of the content that matches with the way they learn concepts.

Activity: How does guiding the students' thinking with who, what, where, when, how, and why help students develop contextual meaning?

This contextual use of language brings each student into the learning at a preoperational level, the level of thinking where the learner is in his or her own picture. To the students' pictures, the teacher is setting up the opportunity for the students to research what others say about the clouds. By adding this layer of meaning, the teacher is beginning to move the students' thinking from their preoperational level to a concrete level. After a few students tell what they believe about the plane being able to fly or not being able to fly through the clouds, the teacher says: "Well, I wonder how we can answer these questions?" Again the students are led to find or look for answers through the use of computers, books, and other materials in the room. This introduction to clouds sets up each student as a scientist who is researching the available materials to answer a question. In essence the teacher has provided a context for the scientific method: Ask a question, do some knowledge building, make a hypothesis, and then create an experiment to test the answer. This latter step might be in the form of an experiment or experimental types of classroom activities. Note that when the students look up their information about clouds and flying, they are asked to draw and write about their information and then to report the information back to the group in one of the literacy forms. This keeps the activity a visual-motor language activity; not just sound-based discussion and not just a copying or regurgitation of what they see in a book. This process also keeps the students in their pictures (preoperational level) while learning what others (books, media, Internet, etc.) know. Developmentally, this is the best level for learning new concepts: preoperational to concrete back to preoperational to concrete and so forth.

Activity: How does providing context at the right developmental level help students learn concepts?

The contextual lessons with an emphasis on drawing and writing are conversations between the learners and their guide, the teacher. The teacher provides opportunities for the students to be the scientist, the investigator of the answers to the teacher's questions. These types of lessons can be used for children to study history as historians, study social studies as social scientists, create writing as authors, give reports as reporters, calculate as mathematicians, and so forth. Each activity is a process of guiding the students from what they know to new levels of knowledge that raise their conceptual understanding of the content which allows them to draw, write, draw, talk, write, and so forth through layers of preoperational to concrete cognitive language function.

Activity: How do students use others' roles to provide the students with their own opportunity to learn?

Since the developmental levels of the students' language tells Rostamizadeh what the students understand, Rostamizadeh (2009a) often uses Table 14.3 to remind herself of what the language and concomitant behavior should be like for her intermediate, concrete thinking students.

Table 14.3 Language level of learning

Preoperational language	Egocentric "I" speech Blaming others—no ownership Puts the speaker at the center of the event Can match behavior, but may not be able to change behavior Language may be repetitive, trite, or cliché Underdeveloped thoughts Unconventional comments
Concrete language	Speaker relates to and with others Shared power Understands his/her identity in relation to others Extending appreciation to others' actions Moves from external motivation to internal motivation Understands the needs of others Understands consequences Begins to take others' perspectives Shares in decision making and planning Tries to gain support for and with others Connects with others; identifies with purpose of groups
Formal language	From others' perspectives Takes responsibility for his or her own behavior Shows a personal code of others and respects others' codes of ethics Uses "integrity of self" to separate his/her own thoughts from others Realizes that they cannot change the behavior of others Uniqueness and diversity are honored Shared power that benefits all involved Shows appreciation for others and for self Personally ethical, not rule governed

Activity: Why is it important to remember where students should function?

Looking at Table 14.3, it is easy to see where students are functioning when they blame others—the preoperational language level. Or, when students support others' works, they are at the concrete level. Or, when students show appreciation for others and self from others' perspectives, they are at the formal level. This knowledge reminds Rostamizadeh that her students' actions follow their thinking and their thinking should be at a concrete level most of the time. She also helps the students learn about themselves as way for the students to begin to develop learning strategies about how to be a learner or better thinker.

Activity: How does knowing the language that goes with actions help to understand cognitive language function?

Strategy learning

Learning in this book has been defined as a Neuro-Semantic Language System by which the students are able to think according to what input their systems are able to recognize and convert into concepts. Because the majority of learners think and therefore learn concepts with a visual-motor process, students need *learning strategies* that help them translate the auditory curriculum and auditory pedagogy into visual-motor thinking. Below is a list of some of the strategies that Rostamizadeh uses in her classroom along with an explanation of why these strategies work.

1. Cartooning. This is also called oral cartooning (Arwood & Kaulitz, 2007) and Mabel Mini-Lectures (Arwood *et al.*, 2009). These expectations can be for social and behavioral issues as well as content. A previous example was given for behavior. Here is an example for social development. Carl is 12 years old and continues to talk about things that are not real such as "Super heroes will do your writing for you." Because he talks this way when tasks are difficult, students do not want to spend a lot of time with Carl and Carl wants friends. Here is a mini-lecture:

   > No!...there is no super hero over here...say what is real...say what is there...otherwise people will think you do not know what is real and what is not real. When you say things that are not real, people who hear your words learn that the words that come out of your mouth are not real. When people think you do not talk about real things they also think that they cannot trust you. If they cannot trust you, they do not want to be your friend...they do not want to play with you or work with you. Say what is real so that people know they can trust you. And when people know they can trust you they might want to become your friend. The book and the paper sitting on the table are real. Let's talk about what we see in the book. Then let's make a picture dictionary about the ideas in the book. After we make a picture dictionary, then we can write our ideas.

   Another example for learning about how to make a dictionary might sound like this:

   > Open your literacy packet and take out a blank picture dictionary sheet. Put your blank picture dictionary sheet on your desk on the side you write with... that is the side you hold your pencil with. Then open your science book to page 87. It looks like this (holds up book and draws page on poster paper). On page 87 there are 20 words that we need to know what they mean. Write each

word in its own box in the picture dictionary. When you are finished writing all 20 words, pass your picture dictionary to your partner and ask your partner to check to be sure you have written each word just the way it looks.

The next activity will be to assign meaning to the words with drawings, with discussion of drawings, with role playing the meaning, and with the students putting their own meanings as pictographs connected to the written word in the picture dictionary.

2. Draw expectations for behavior with viconic oral language. This is similar to the cartoons found in Chapter 12. Rostamizadeh draws and uses oral language at the same time to create mental pictures. She then expects the students to draw before they write and to draw before they have an oral presentation. In this way her methods become strategies for the students to learn better.
3. Draw concepts to increase academic language, for both students and teacher. Rostamizadeh draws out all new concepts such as words like evaporation, condensation, mass, energy, volume, vertical, segment, fraction, and so forth. These are drawn in context of the lesson on large size poster paper. The students then write and draw in their own words and pictures into their vocabulary dictionaries to be used in other activities. This gives the students the correct patterns of the words, their concomitant definitions, and a visual-motor way to recall. In turn, Rostamizadeh expects her students to use drawing for taking notes and for learning to develop a deeper understanding like with the flowcharts. She wants them to take their own personal strategies to the next grade level as tools of functional language for better learning.
4. Use picture dictionaries to increase concept or language development, spelling, writing fluency. These are the same type of picture dictionaries that were discussed in Chapters 11–13. At this level of language function, these are really more of a vocabulary picture dictionary because the emphasis is not on learning to write the word but learning the meaning of the word. Rostamizadeh expects her students to use a picture dictionary like a learning strategy where they are learning how to take someone else's word and turn it into a meaningful concept that the students can read, write, talk, listen, view, think, and calculate about.
5. Rostamizadeh uses "I stories" to introduce all major concepts and begin the process of layering concepts for learning, from what the students know at a preoperational level to what others know (books, Internet, peers, teacher, parents) at a concrete level to finally a formal definition. An example of an "I story" that Rostamizadeh used was provided earlier in the chapter. What she helps the students understand is that they have to have lots of different ways to think about an idea before the students know the idea. In this way, she encourages the students to use their own language in a variety of ways to assign meaning so as to develop their concrete level of thinking. Rostamizadeh uses language as a learning strategy for the students to understand how to retrieve and recall information.

Activity: What are some learning strategies that can be used to help students in the intermediate grades learn to think at more of a concrete level of language function?

By the time that students are around 9 to 11 years old, they should have enough language to begin to list their own *personal learning strategies*. For example, each fourth grade student should have a personal list of strategies that he or she has written. The strategies include what that specific student needs for learning such as "If I do not have a head picture for a word the teacher says, then I will write the word down and raise my hand and ask the teacher when she is no longer talking." Or, "When I don't know how a word looks, I will ask another student to write the word on a sticky note for me." Each student should know what he or she needs to learn in a classroom so that the student becomes his or her own advocate for learning. In this way, students learn what they need to do to learn.

These learning strategies are meta-cognitive ways for students to understand their own learning systems as well as to understand what they have to provide themselves for their best learning. As students become wiser about their learning, they tend to expect more of their own education and are able to become more responsible for their own learning.

Activity: Why are cognitive learning strategies important for students' development, socially and cognitively?

Preoperational opportunity

All learners begin to scaffold the meaning of a new academic concept at the preoperational level. For examples, concepts like evaporation, condensation, animal families, and nature all begin their development at the preoperational level; at the level of what the student knows about the new concept. For example, fourth through sixth grades have curricula about formal concepts such as weather, insects, plants, integers, fractions, and so forth.

stipule
petiole
stem
axil
vein
midrib
leaf blade
leaf apex
① Pick a leaf
② Observe and draw leaf
③ Find these leaf parts

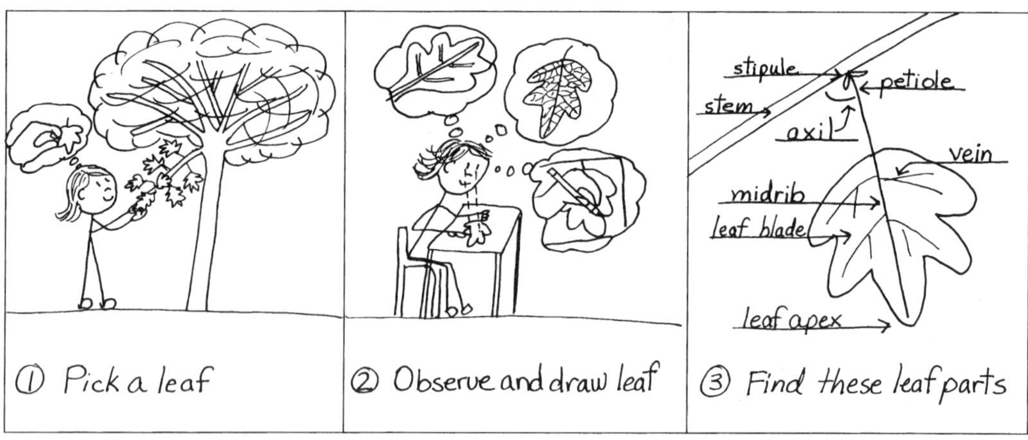

Figure 14.4 Students follow teacher's directions

In an intermediate classroom of students, it is safer to assume that new material needs to begin at the preoperational level of learning than to begin at a higher level and leave behind many students who can hear what the teacher says, spit back what the teacher says, but not understand the meaning of the material. If they do not understand the concepts of the material, the material will have to be retaught later. There are also those students who will create behavioral diversions that are meaningful to them when they do not understand the class material. These behavioral diversions might include pro-social options such as being a class clown or anti-social options such as scratching the desk tops with something sharp.

> ***Activity:*** Why is the preoperational level of concept development important for learning new concepts?

To engage students at the preoperational level, the teacher wants to be able to provide the opportunity for students to be in their own pictures of what they do, how they do it, when they do it, and so forth. For example, the earlier strategy of starting with an "I story" is one way to begin the task. The teacher tells something about the teacher's actions in an everyday conversational form: "Yesterday, when we were walking to the park to look at some of the leaves that were changing color, I was wondering, why do leaves change color?"[4] The teacher looks at the students and waits for some answers which the teacher writes on the board. The teacher orally summarizes the students' guesses.

> Well, Beth said that maybe the chemicals in the leaves change, and maybe that is true but what are those chemicals? And Matt said that the leaves get old and dried out from the summer. That may be true so we will need to see what our books say about that idea. And Mickelle said that she thought the trees go to sleep so that they don't freeze in the winter. I think that may be true as well. So, how will we figure out what really happens to change the leaves?

When the teacher turns the search for the answers back to the students, the teacher is providing the students the opportunity to become agents (like scientists) in their learning. If the teacher has set up these opportunities in the classroom, the students will know that they can suggest that the class members look in their textbooks, go to the library, to the Internet, etc. The teacher accepts their suggestions and offers some guides such as using some reference books that the teacher has brought to the class for the students to look for information for the next 20 minutes. The teacher then can use their findings to draw and talk with the whole group about the information. As the teacher draws out their ideas of the trees, their leaves, inside the leaves, and what happens as the color of the leaves change, the teacher helps the students create a vocabulary picture dictionary of all of the terms such as photosynthesis, oxygen, carbon dioxide, and so forth. Each student draws a picture of the meaning of the words that goes with the vocabulary. Figure 14.4 shows a teacher's cartoon to develop students' thinking about leaves.

The experiment about leaves requires observation and of vocabulary. Figure 14.5 is a picture dictionary that goes with the leaf lesson.

> ***Activity:*** Why does this type of lesson provide students with a preoperational opportunity to learn new concepts?

4 The teacher may also want to draw this story in simple stick figures on the dry erase board or on a poster piece of paper. An overhead requires the students to look at the teacher and her hand upside down which is too many cognitive functions and should be avoided at the preoperational level. More technological advances such as SMART Boards™ (SMART Technologies, Calgary, Canada) allow for drawing and using Internet pictures are easier to understand because the material is parallel to the teacher who is writing on the board.

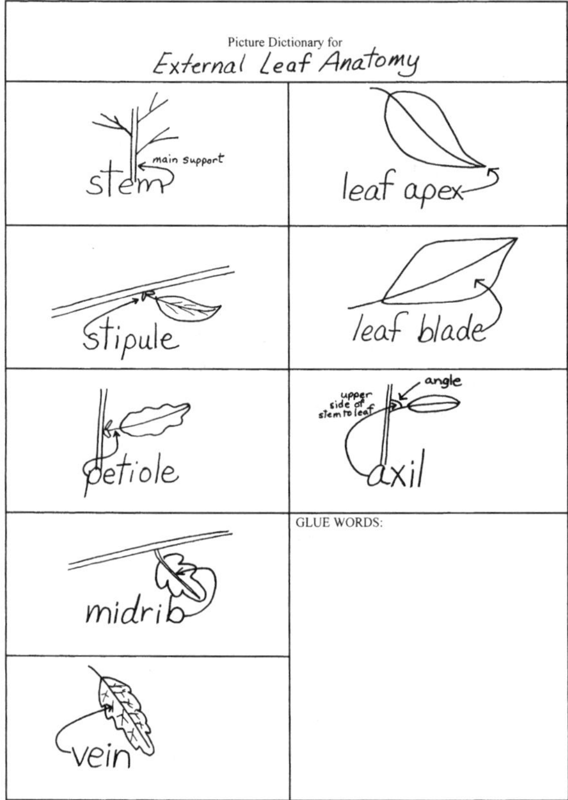

Figure 14.5 A classroom picture dictionary

By allowing students the opportunity to begin the lesson with the teacher's "I story" connected to an activity that the students complete, the students, as agents, research, draw, listen, write, read, and so forth. The students are in their own pictures of learning about what leaves look like and then what they are able to see and not see in the leaf, what the color changes mean, and so forth. Students begin with the surface anatomy of the leaf and end up learning about carbon dioxide exchange and so forth. The students become engaged from their preoperational levels of knowledge through the concrete level of learning via multiple concepts in multiple forms. Finally, they are learning about the formal concepts—concepts that they cannot see, touch, or feel. Students are learning more meaning about leaves at each of the developmental levels. The teacher uses a layering of activities that moves between what the students can do and what the teacher does to guide and organize the scaffolding. For example, the teacher began with her "I story" and then the teacher turned the task to the students; the teacher added some organized information within the whole group, and then the students draw their meanings of the words, etc. By doing this scaffolding at this level, the teacher is going back and from what the teacher and others (references, other students, Internet sources, etc.) provide at a concrete to formal level to back to what the students are able to do at a preoperational level. This developmental process cannot be emphasized enough as most schools do not provide for a concrete level of learning. Most teachers have students (preoperational in thinking about new concepts) memorize the patterns of formal concepts which means that the students are not learning concepts but the patterns.

Activity: Why is the process of learning concepts from a preoperational to concrete to formal level an important tool in teaching?

Students learn concepts the best at the preoperational level while the teacher guides them into adding information to form more depth in thinking. The greater depth in thinking results in a higher layer of understanding. This higher layer of meaning requires multiple sources of input to create the concrete level of knowledge that will support the formal level of meaning of words like photosynthesis. By learning the concrete meanings of these words, students are able not only to regurgitate for tests but also to be literate about these concepts; in other words, the students are able to talk, read, write, listen, view, and think about the concepts. Since long term memory is semantic in nature, then as students use their own language to assign meaning by drawing, writing, reading, talking, listening, viewing, and thinking about the concepts, these concepts become part of the students' semantic memories. Students truly learn the concepts!

Activity: Why do students learn formal concepts from a preoperational to concrete level of meaning?

"I stories"

There has been a significant mention of the use of "I stories" but how these stories are used is important to discuss. Rostamizadeh uses a lot of "I stories" as ways to create a preoperational opportunity for her students. For example, in teaching the concept of condensation to fifth grade students, she has several options:

> I was driving in the car last winter with a little girl that I babysit. I looked into the rearview mirror and I saw the little girl drawing on the window. She was making pictures in the water that was on the window. Have all of you been in a car when there was water on the inside of the windows? I wondered where that water came from. I remembered something from my science textbooks that when a car is warm inside but it is cold outside the car, then the invisible floating water vapor cools off next to the window, it condenses into liquid and sticks to the window.

Rostamizadeh draws this story on poster paper at the same time she tells the story. The students then put the word "condenses" into their vocabulary picture dictionary and draw what they understand to be the meaning of that concept. The class shares their definitions in a discussion as well as their pictures. Rostamizadeh then "retags" the meaning: "This water on the window is called condensation." The students add that word to their dictionary and then Rostamizadeh asks them for other examples of condensation.

Activity: How does the lesson incorporate the preoperational level of thinking?

There are many, many ways to begin this type of lesson. Here is another story from Rostamizadeh: "Wow! It was so cold this morning that when I walked outside I could see my breath! I wondered why I could see my breath better when I breathed through my mouth than my nose?" She then draws in real time so that the students can watch her hand move.[5] As she draws, the students create their own mental shapes of the concepts. In this way, the students can make their own pictures. Figure 14.6 shows a student's cartoon.

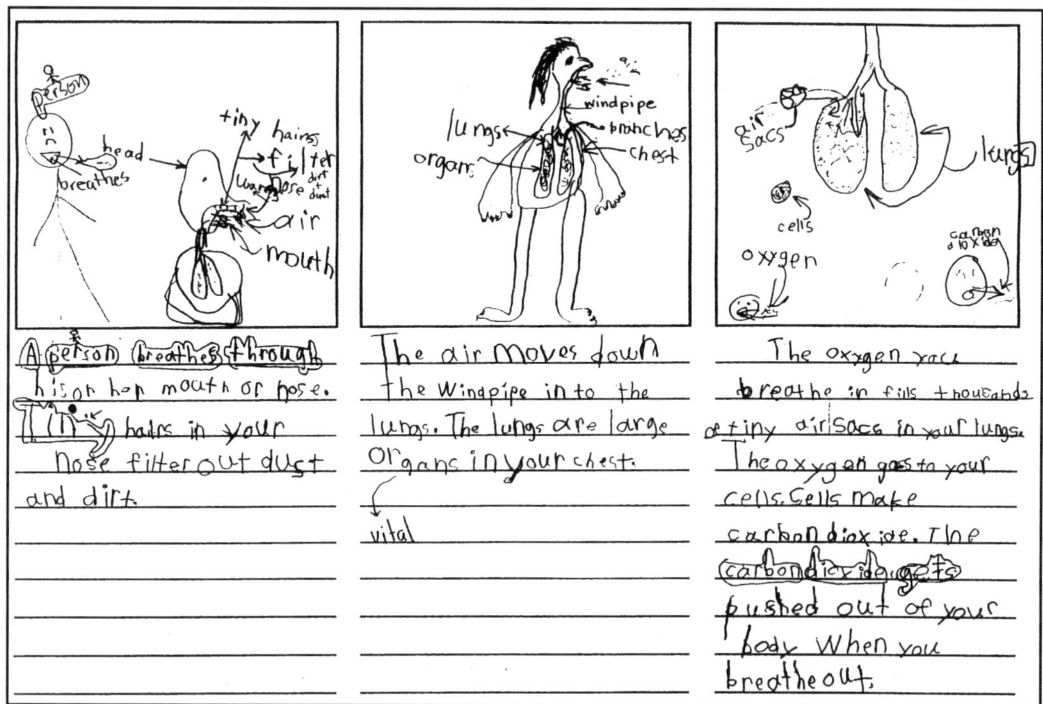

Figure 14.6 A student cartoons his knowledge of classroom material

This student also needs the concepts put into a picture dictionary so he can learn the meaning of the vocabulary as well as be able to write the words in a conventional pattern. Figure 14.7 shows the vocabulary dictionary for the student.

As students begin to understand the concepts, Rostamizadeh adds more layers of meaning. For example, Rostamizadeh reminds the students that there is invisible floating water vapor that is cool in the outdoors but warmed by the lungs so that the water vapor begins to condense and can be seen. Because understanding these formal concepts such as condensation requires multiple examples or layers of meaning to create a concrete foundation, she then leads the students to another example of condensation which she also draws out. "Remember this summer when it was hot outside and you got a cold drink with lots of ice? The cup would begin to have water or condensation (example of retagging) on it." Rostamizadeh then leads the students to other examples of what they saw on the window and what they saw with cups. Finally, she takes these multiple examples and connects them to other formal concepts such as weather, stages of matter with temperature shifts, and climate changes. The students are then guided to put condensation, temperature, vapor, water droplet, states of matter into their picture dictionaries. Figure 14.8 is a picture dictionary for part of the water unit (see p.325).

5 Remember that some students who think with visual meta-cognition create meaning for concepts from the shapes of movements (Chapter 5).

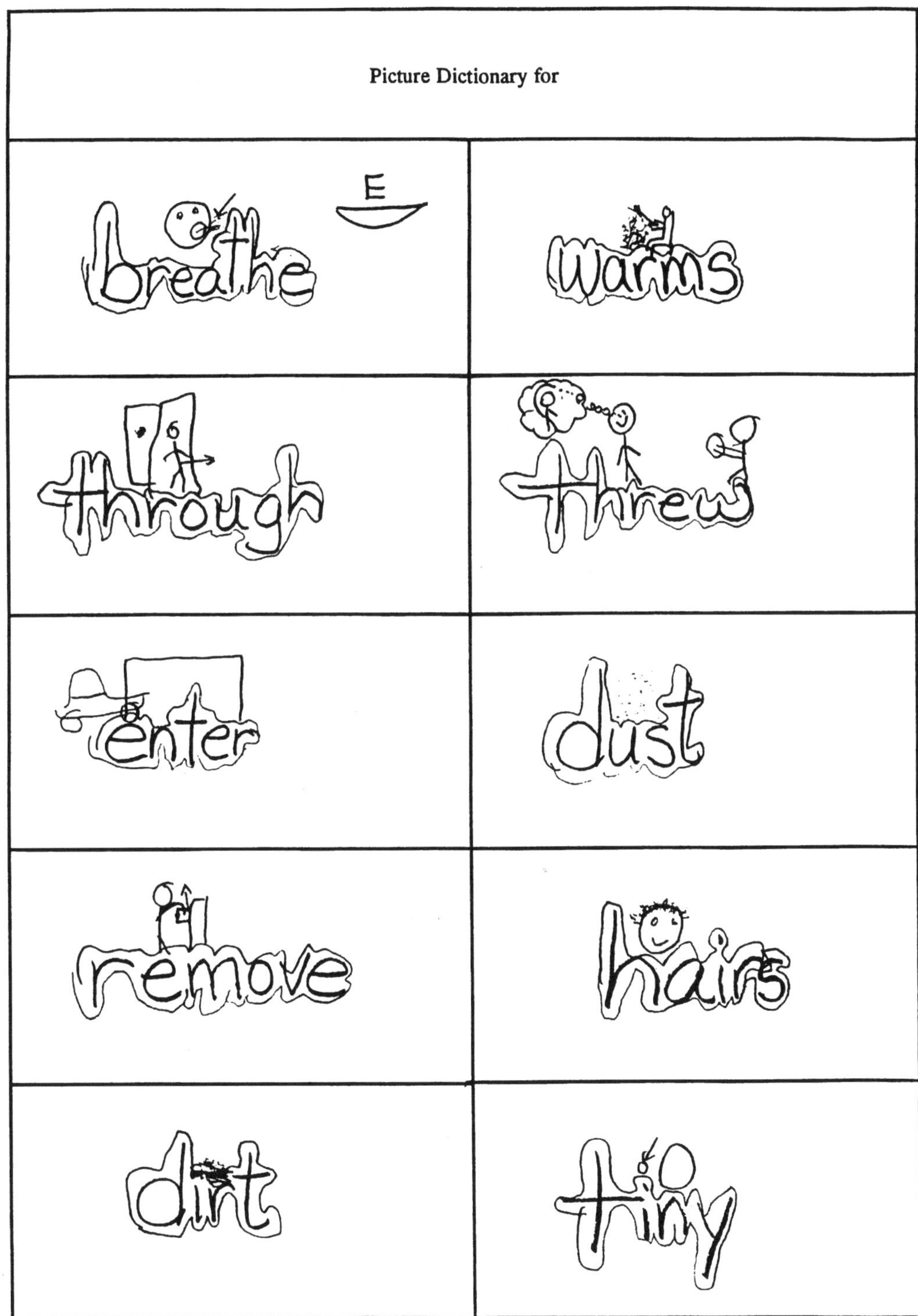

Figure 14.7 A vocabulary dictionary for "breathing"

Because concrete understanding of rules about condensation requires multiple examples and because the students must use their own language (preoperational, pre-language function) to put these meanings into long term or semantic memory, the students must write, draw, talk, and read about the concepts. For example, the students write about why water collects on the outside of a cold glass.

> When you get a cold drink, water does not leak through the glass. You know that because it happens with all kinds of liquids, like soda, and if it were leaking through, it would be sticky and the color of whatever you are drinking. So why does the outside of the glass get wet?

Rostamizadeh is looking for students to put the concepts about water vapor and condensation into their own words. Rostamizadeh uses the students' writings as authentic assessment data that tells what the students actually are learning and at what conceptual level.

Activity: Why do students have to have multiple layers of information to begin to understand a formal concept like condensation at a concrete to formal level?

Because the concrete development of these formal concepts requires multiple examples, the students must produce multiple examples from their own language learning systems. So, in addition to writing about cold liquids, the students must also write about questions related to other examples such as weather:

> When you look outside and see that there are no clouds and that it is a warm sunny day, you know that it is not going to rain. But late in the afternoon, you see big billowy clouds starting to develop. What type of clouds are these? Why do they develop more often in the later afternoon into early evening?

Formal concepts are developed from the way the overlap of concrete meanings. Figure 14.9 is a cartoon of an experiment a student wanted the class to perform based on something he took from the Internet (see p.326). As he told about the experiment, the teacher drew out the steps.

Activity: Choose a topic and write out an "I story" to help engage the students at a preoperational level of thinking. Be sure that you include a drawing of your story to account for those students who think in visual concepts (the majority of students).

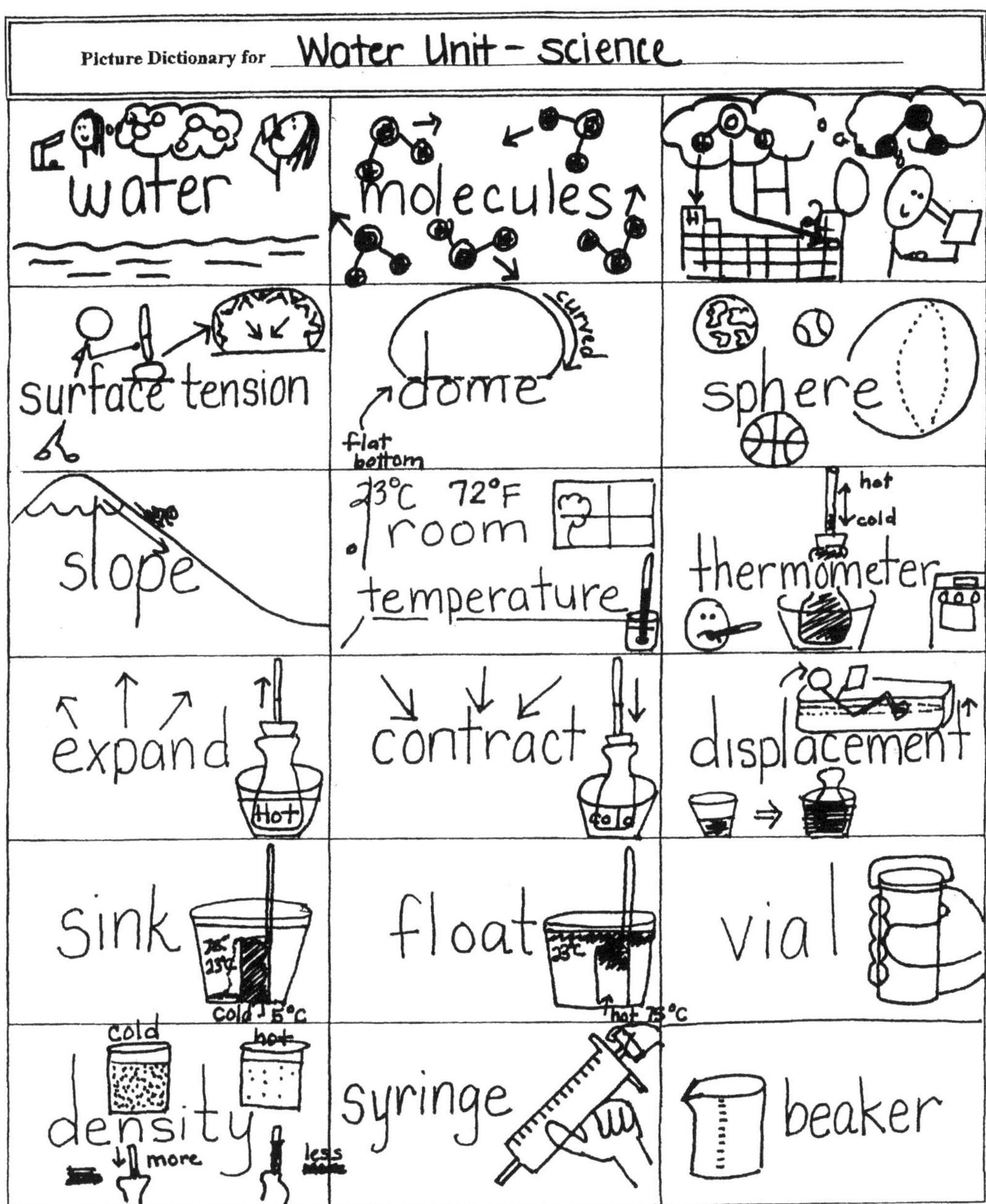

Figure 14.8 Water picture dictionary

6 cups flour
2 cups salt
4 Tbs. oil
2 cups water
knead
First, I make the dough for building the volcano by mixing together the ingredients in a large bowl. Using my hands I work the dough until smooth and firm.
open
Second, I set a 2 liter soda bottle in the center of a baking pan so I can mold the dough around the bottle to create the volcano. I keep the bottle mouth open.
red
Third, I use a funnel to fill the bottle with warm warm about $\frac{2}{3}$ full. Then I add 7 drops of red food coloring to the water in the bottle.
Baking Soda
dish detergent
Fourth, I add six drops of liquid dishwashing detergent into the bottle, followed by 2 tablespoons of baking soda.
vinegar
Fifth, while using the funnel, I slowly pour $\frac{1}{2}$ cup of vinegar into the bottle and then I remove the funnel. Then
I quickly jump back to observe what happens.

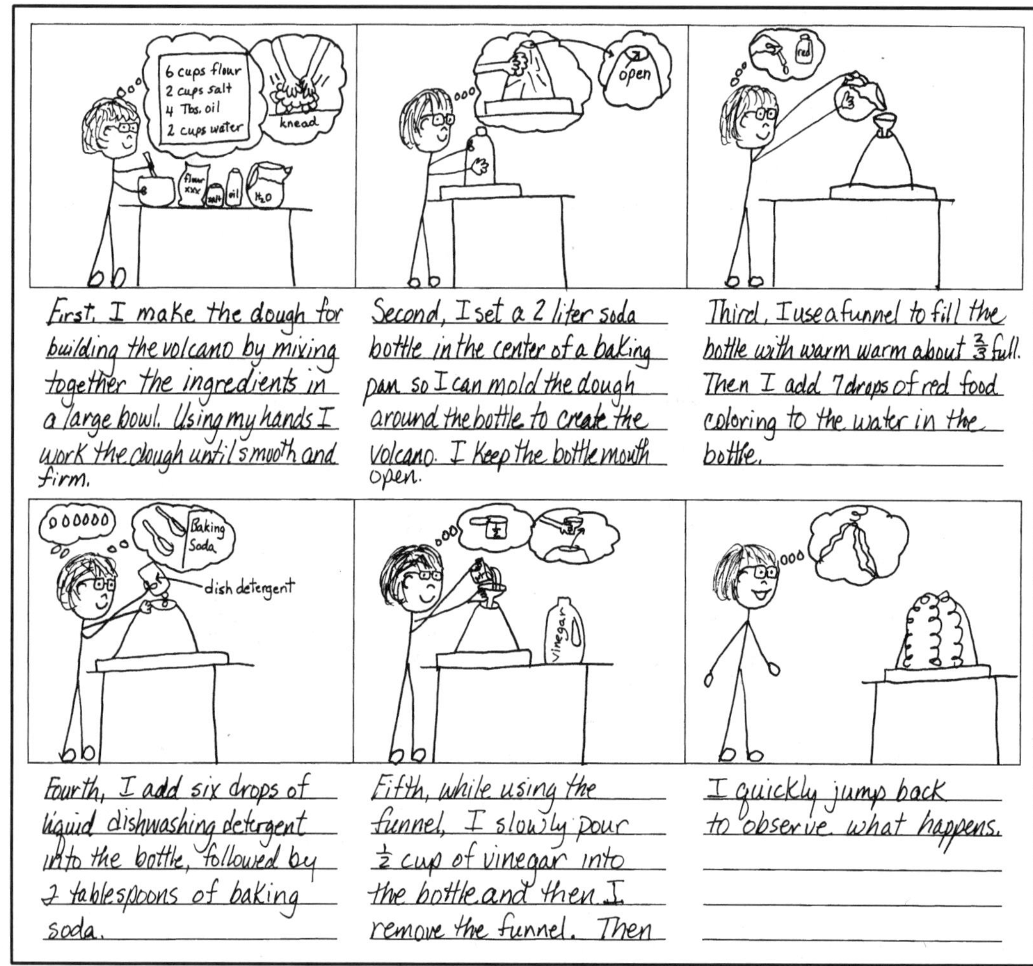

Figure 14.9 An experiment to try

Summary

Intermediate grades are typically for children between 7 and 11. Children of this age typically think with a concrete level of language function. Most students use a visual meta-cognition to learn new concepts found in the content subjects of these grades. When interviewed about her classroom, Rostamizadeh (2009a) said that there are five things that characterize how language functions in her classroom:

- Lack of language allows students to get stuck at the pattern-level of skills so we use lots of language to allow students to begin "higher order" conceptual learning.
- I was trained to use brief and limited language but that will not create mental pictures for my students so I adjust my verbal instructions from the traditional restricted forms to rich language so as to paint a picture of my expectations.

- In order to provide the best language for my students, I need to know where they are developmentally; so I listen to what they actually say without filling in the gaps for them…these types of authentic assessments tell me what level the each student is learning at.
- I always give students the benefit of the doubt when they misbehave because I most likely did not explain my expectations in a way that they could understand which is why I look at their behavior and then add language to help them mentally see what I meant. By being more visual in my language, I do not need to use external rewards and punishers.
- Students love to learn and I have found that the richest language comes from starting with the content (social studies, science) and teaching the "skills" (reading, writing, math) from there. Literacy comes from having something to say, read, write, and talk about. I also realize that literacy is about thinking and viewing so I use lots of language both for social and academic purposes.

Chapter 15 provides the reader with applications of language function at the next level of development.

Applications

- Observe an intermediate classroom and determine how well the students are learning the concepts by asking them questions about their learning.
- Develop several lessons that begin at the preoperational level, add concrete layers, and result in formal conceptual learning.

Chapter 15

CONCRETE TO FORMAL THINKERS

The Language of Higher Order Thinking

Learner objectives: Chapter 15

Upon completion of this chapter, the reader should be able to:

1. Explain how language for individuals who are thinking at a formal level must consider the use of time.
2. Draw out a cartoon of how to plan a task.
3. Explain how to use space to compensate for time.
4. Explain how to contextualize content for better learning of higher order concepts.
5. Explain how formal concepts require multiple ways to integrate concepts.

I want to know how to think from your perspective
When I sit for an exam…
Knowing how I think is knowing who I am.
Knowing who I am lets me know who you are.

Chapter 13 discussed how to provide Viconic Language Methods™ for children in the primary, early elementary grades; Chapter 14 described Viconic Language Methods™ used for those in the intermediate grades of four through six. This chapter is designed to provide language support for those individuals who are beyond the intermediate grades. By sixth grade most students are at least 11 years old. This means that they should be able to think with formal cognition, both socially and academically. Socially, a formal thinker is able to take another person's perspective and critically think or problem solve from what is good for the whole class, whole family, or whole society and so forth.

Decision making at the formal level means that the thinker is able to use language as a tool to access the most symbolic meanings connected with words that cannot be seen, touched, or physically experienced such as the concepts of respect, liberty, government, integrity, chlorophyll, meiosis, ethics, and so forth. This chapter will discuss how to apply Viconic Language Methods™ for those individuals who are older than 11. This chapter includes those students at junior high, high, secondary, and post-secondary schools.

Beginning to learn formal concepts

All learners begin to scaffold the meaning of a new concept at the preoperational level of thinking. For example, concepts like government, liberty, evaporation, and meiosis cannot be physically seen or touched. Students can say these words, imitate the definitions of these words, and even match patterns on a multiple-choice test without understanding the conceptual meaning of these types of words at a formal level. For example, an adult is able to hear a word such as "shibui," can imitate the pattern "shibui," can act on the word when it is put into a sentence such as "Shibui the door," and even use the word in a sentence, "I shibuied the door." But these are all patterns because the adult does not know the conceptual meaning of "shibui." So, for the adult to learn the concept of "shibui" the adult needs more information.

Starting with the patterns, layers of information are added until the adult has a formal understanding that "shibui" was a non-sense word, created to demonstrate the use of applying grammatical rules as patterns. Shibui has also been the name of a type of wallpaper and a spa. Anytime a learner is acquiring the meaning of a new concept like "shibui," learning begins as a pattern to which layers of conceptual meaning are added. The lowest level of conceptual meaning is the preoperational level. At the preoperational level, a concept relates to what the person knows based on the person's own experiences. The adult who was asked to "shibui" the door knows that "shibui" has something to do with door. The beginning of conceptual meaning always starts with the sound input of the senses that overlap the patterns to form concepts at the preoperational level. Chapters 13 and 14 provided numerous examples of what the preoperational level of thinking is like.

Activity: At what level does conceptual learning begin?
How does a learner acquire a formal concept?

The layering of information actually adds to the clarification process of understanding a concept. So, the meaning begins with the input of patterns that integrate to being to form preoperational concepts. These concepts integrate with new input to form a deeper conceptual understanding. At the next level of understanding, the concrete level, the adult, or learner older than 11, knows that "shibui" was made up (neologism) to represent an example. At the formal level, the adult might be able to say:

> Arwood used the term "shibui" in reference to a door to demonstrate how adults are able to imitate acoustic patterns like shibui and even use patterns like shibui in grammatical sentences, but still not know the meaning. I can see why it is important not to just teach students patterns, but to be sure they are learning conceptual meanings.

The formal level is more than an example; it is a definition, an example, and an application.

Activity: What is the formal level of thinking like?

Anyone over the age of 11 is expected to be able to acquire formal thinking. For the majority of thinkers who use a visual meta-cognition in an auditory culture, VLMs can be used to help the person translate the auditory words like government into visual forms of understanding. For example, "pragmaticism" is a real word, but the reader may not know anything about the pattern, "pragmaticism," unless the reader has had some extensive American philosophy classes. At the preoperational level, the thinker knows what the spoken word sounds like and what the word "pragmaticism" looks like in print. The preoperational thinker is able to copy the written pattern, "pragmaticism." If the thinker has learned that "pragmaticism is a term coined by Charles Peirce," then on a test of multiple choice questions, the preoperational thinker can even match the pattern "pragmaticism" to its founder. When given many examples of how the word "pragmaticism" functions, the learner may be able to give an example of pragmaticism: "When a teacher considers the whole child and not just the outcomes, then the teacher is utilizing some of what Peirce believes." Finally, with more layers, the thinker, who is more than 11 years old, has layered sufficient information to acquire a formal understanding of the word, pragmaticism. "Pragmaticism is a term coined by Peirce to explain how the whole is greater than the parts as applied to many different situations such as the military or the child." The formal thinker will be able to provide numerous examples of this principle as well as apply the principle of pragmaticism to novel situations.

Activity: Why does a concept begin at the pattern level of language acquisition? What are the levels of conceptualization that occur after the pattern level of acquisition? What is the formal level of concept attainment like?

Therefore, in a classroom of students, it is safe to assume that new material needs to begin at the preoperational level of learning to meet the needs of all students, at any age or grade level including adults. Since most students who are older than 11 are learning formal concepts such as chlorophyll, civil war, Constitution, freedom, meiosis, DNA, and so forth, classroom activities must provide multiple examples of these types of concepts to create layers for a concrete understanding, before moving on to definitions and applications at a formal level. Keep in mind that the students are very good at imitating the patterns of what they read or hear without conceptual meaning. But memorizing patterns does not provide access to conceptual learning.

When material is not learned conceptually, teachers must reteach. Remember that a learner can recall patterns as long as the patterns or their devices, such as mnemonic devices, for recall are being practiced. Once the patterns are no longer being tracked or practiced, there is nothing in the brain to connect to for later recall. Concepts, on the other hand, create multiple places for connecting in the brain and therefore multiple places of recall. The higher the conceptual thinking is for a learner, the easier it is for the learner to recall the material. Beginning with conceptual thinking and providing layers of meaning is worth the effort because it allows the students actually to learn the material for later use and application.

Chapter 14 provided examples of how the learners must receive multiple opportunities to learn the formal concepts.

> ***Activity:*** Why is conceptual learning better than rote memorization of patterns?

If students are not learning material that can be used later, they will lack reason for engaging in classroom activities. Chapter 14 provided some examples of how students may use behavior to divert their inability to attend to the material. To make classroom material the most meaningful, the following issues must be considered:

1. New content must begin at a preoperational level, even though the learner is older than the preoperational cognitive stage of development.
2. The classroom environment must provide multiple activities for application of the concepts to create a concrete understanding. Concrete understanding requires multiple ways of seeing or thinking about an idea.
3. The teacher must provide opportunities for definitions, applications, and dissemination at a formal level after the student has had concrete examples of the concepts.

> ***Activity:*** What is needed to create a concrete understanding of a concept in a classroom? What elements are needed to make sure that formal concepts are learned at a formal level?

To engage students at the preoperational level, the teacher wants to be able to provide the opportunity for students to be in their own pictures of what they do, how they do it, when they do it, and so forth. For example, the learning strategy (Chapters 13 and 14) of starting with an "I story" is one way to begin the task, even for individuals at the middle school to college level. The teacher tells something about the teacher's actions in an everyday conversational form: "Last night I was watching TV when I saw a commercial for a new car that has eight gears for an automatic transmission. I wondered, 'What does that transmission look like?'" If this is a class on auto mechanics, the teacher can then begin to draw out what the gears would do. If it is a class for high school science where the students are studying gears or mechanical energy, the teacher might ask the students, "How do you think eight gears would work?" After several guesses that the teacher writes on the board, the teacher says:

> Let's find out what this means. So, look in your books and see if you can find out how gears work. We will then take what you find out and draw out a simple machine that includes at least two gears. From there we will build a model that eventually will have eight gears.

The idea is always to put the students into their own pictures (preoperational concept development) and then into the teacher's pictures (concrete concept development) where all of the various models of what the students find and what they draw creates a concrete understanding. (For more examples of how the layering between preoperational thinking and concrete occurs with language function, see Chapters 13 and 14.)

> ***Activity:*** How does an "I story" help provide the beginning of learning formal concepts?

For a student to learn a formal concept at a formal linguistic level, the learner must be able to develop the meaning of the concept from the preoperational level through the concrete level to the formal, linguistic level. *Linguistic function* (see Chapter 11) of a concept means that the thinker is able to use the concept with maximum displacement, semanticity, flexibility, productivity, and with the most efficiency (minimum external redundancy). From previous chapters, the reader knows that a thinker with linguistic function for a concept like "an automatic transmission with eight gears" is able not only to say the words and explain what the transmission is like but also to talk about how eight gears is a new technology, and then the linguistic thinker should be able to provide some critique or analysis of the product. In other words, the formal learner who has a linguistic understanding of these concepts is able to talk about the ideas, not just show a diagram or model which shows a maximum ability to use language to explain the transmission and gears (displacement). The formal thinker is also able to use the words (jargon) about transmissions and gears that well-educated mechanics use (semanticity) in a variety of situations (productivity) and in a variety of ways (flexibility). Furthermore, the formal thinker is able to use grammatical language which matches expected time and sound based properties of English. More about these principles will be provided later in the chapter.

Activity: What are the linguistic principles of displacement, semanticity, flexibility, productivity, and efficiency (limited external redundancy)?

Linguistic thinking

Linguistic thinkers are able to use the tools of literacy to raise their own thinking to a formal level. However, learning in an auditory culture often prevents a thinker from using language tools for learning at a formal level. Educators must provide the rules about how to think with a more visual way of understanding the formal concepts of an auditory culture. Visual thinkers who are learning in an auditory world must be able to translate what they know cognitively to a visual language function, to be able to think at a formal level. This translation is based on what properties a visual language, like American Sign Language (ASL) or Mandarin Chinese, utilizes to represent visual thinking. The following section offers an explanation of how those properties help translate visual thinking to auditory English.

Contextual sensitivity

While English, an auditory language, uses words as the unit of analysis, other languages such as Chinese, a visual language, use relationships among ideas as the unit of analysis (see Chapters 4–6). So, in English, a teacher is able to bring a new set of words to the classroom without any sensitivity for the context: "Today we will discuss Newton's First Law." Without any background, the listener or student must wonder: Who is Newton? Does First Law refer to a type of law or a time of a law? What was the law all about? And so forth. The speaker of English words assumes that the listener will write down the spoken words, mentally use the sounds of words to wonder about the meaning, and then wait for more spoken words to answer these questions. However, people who think with visual ideas do not think with spoken words; they think with what they see or have seen. Without *context* (context was defined in Chapter 4) to provide background meaning to the topic of Newton's First Law, the visual thinker may not have enough meaning about Newton's First Law to think, "Today we will discuss Newton's First Law." The thinker may not process the words and therefore be viewed as a student who does not listen. Or, the visual thinker may recall mental images or concepts about Newton, a place in the Midwest. These visual images may be detailed like the real setting once seen by the learner. However, the teacher is not talking about a place so the learner has the wrong mental pictures, also known as misconceptions. The teacher is not talking about a Midwest town named Newton; the teacher is talking about a person who conducted physics experiments. As long as the thinker has these visual mental ideas of a Midwest town, the thinker typically does not realize that the mental pictures of a Midwest town do not match the meaning of the teacher's spoken words unless the teacher is drawing out her meaning of Newton's first law. Such misconceptions look as though the learners do not understand the material, are not listening, are not paying attention, or don't care.

Activity: Does a person's mental pictures always match another person's spoken words?

In order to be sure that a teacher in an auditory culture uses language that will match with the mental pictures of a visual thinker, *the teacher will want to provide context that connects the relationships among thinkers and their pictures*. For example, Dr. Joanna Kaakinen (Arwood & Kaakinen, 2004, 2008, 2009; Arwood *et al*., 2002) draws concepts for the students of college nursing courses so that the students can see what she talks about. Figure 15.1 provides an example of a finished board that she has drawn in real time with her students.

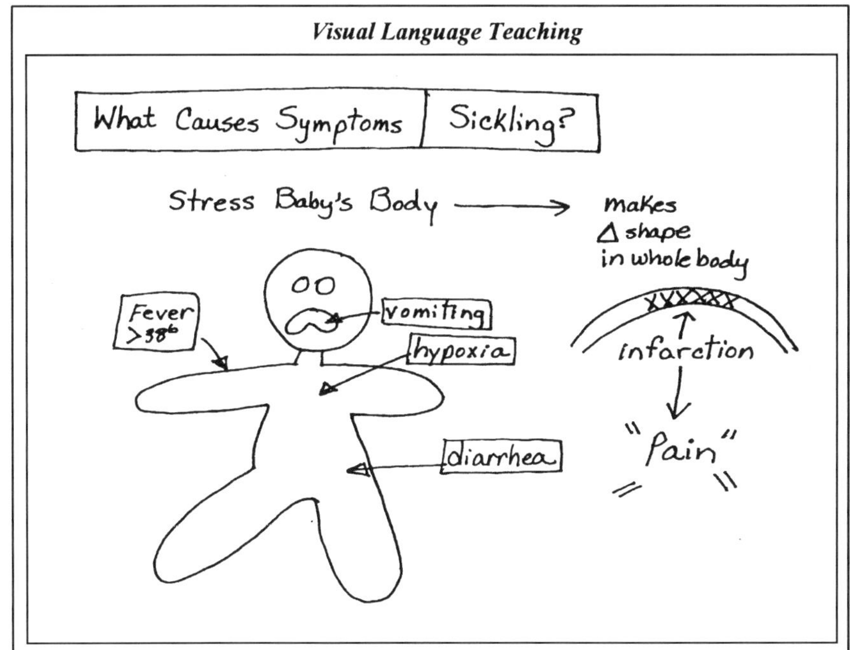

Figure 15.1 An adult example of a drawn set of concepts
Source: Reprinted with permission from Arwood, E., Kaakinen, J., & Wynne, A. (2002). *Nurse educators: Using visual language*. Portland, OR: APRICOT (p.9)

While drawing in real time, Kaakinen provides the students with contextual meaning for the content. As context always provides people or agents doing something, these real-time drawings include people, the teacher, the student nurse, the patient, and so forth. By putting a person into the picture, the drawing is preoperational in nature. The person could be a nurse, a scientist, an author, a historian, a thinker, a football player, etc. Even very young children are able to identify with a person who does something. Figure 15.2 shows the difference between the same content utilizing words and then utilizing pictures showing the person.

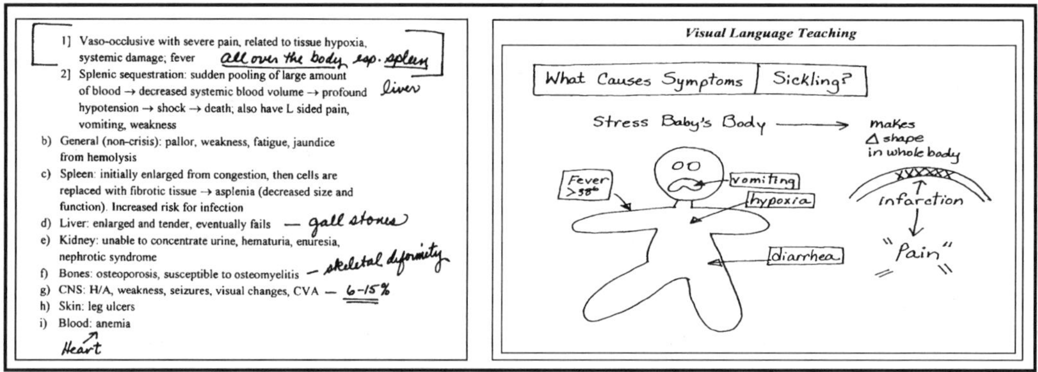

Figure 15.2 Comparison of auditory teaching and visual teaching.
Source: Reprinted with permission from Arwood, E., Kaakinen, J., & Wynne, A. (2002). *Nurse educators: Using visual language*. Portland, OR: APRICOT (pp.8–10)

Putting a person into the picture makes the lesson preoperational in level and creates context for easier understanding of the concepts. The context provides ways that ideas relate to one another. With a person in the picture, the concepts are about agents, their actions, and their objects or the places of the event. Arrows are drawn to show complex relationships. Once a drawing is made, the teacher can zoom in on a picture to bring a part or piece of the picture out such as the inside of a leaf from a tree or an artery from a leg of a person or a thought bubble from a philosopher and so forth. These drawings contextualize the language for the learner.

Activity: How does context provide additional meaning?

Context can also be created from the drawing of pictures before reading, writing, or other literary tasks. For example, Norman Stremming,[1] a high school teacher, used drawing to bring Shakespeare's *Merchant of Venice* to a preoperational level before the students read (Stremming, 2009). In this way, 97 percent of his students said that they enjoyed the class more with the visuals, and he noticed that the students were able to understand the material better. Figure 15.3 shows the final, on-the-board, product from pre-drawing the content to create context for the students.

1 Norman Stremming, Ed.M, MAT, is a gifted teacher in an urban school district at the ninth and tenth grade level.

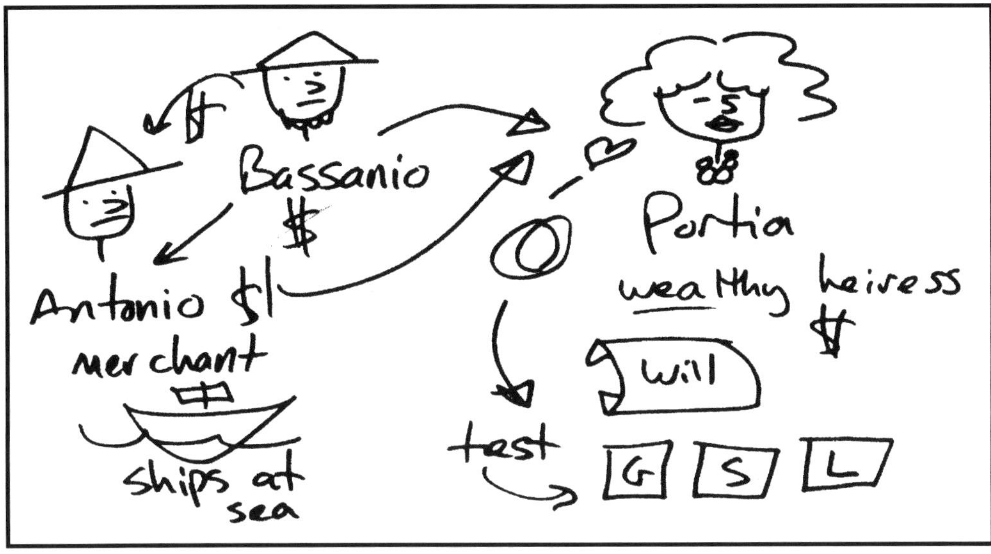

Figure 15.3 Drawing high school literature

Once context is provided for students, then the classroom lessons are more sensitive to those thinkers who use a visual language function.

> ***Activity:*** How does creating context make content easier to learn?

Creating multiple relationships

Culturally, the context provides relationships among people and their events. Drawing creates context, but the drawings will not stand alone without the whole story told in words or written and told to create the connections of the relationships. For example, visual cultures emphasize doing business as a relationship among people. Each person has a role within a business, a family, or an organization and, within the context, each person's role or purpose of the role is understood. For example, adults such as teachers may serve in an authoritarian role and so children learn that role at home and bring it to school where teachers are treated as "authority figures" in charge of the student's every act. The relationship is more important than the learning because the authority knows best. This relationship is expressed through both verbal and non-verbal acts such as how a person walks, where a person walks, talks, sits, etc. The position or *aspect* of each person's hands, feet, and relationship to others has meaning for a visual thinker. The authoritarian teacher has a place to stand and sit and the student has his or her place to stand or sit. Every event is a setting of people within a space of actions that relates to each other. *This context relates how everyone is connected.*

Mental pictures represent how one person thinks about all of the relationships. Every act is related to every other act and the whole synergy of the group is more important than the individual's needs. For the use of "visuals" within a classroom to be effective, they must provide the context which includes the story of the relationships among the people and their visuals. Stremming (2010) draws multiple visuals across lessons that the students write and draw about. This provides the layers of the concepts to develop the formal level of thinking. The next six figures (Figures 15.4 to 15.9) provide examples of the teacher's board drawings about the US branches of government.

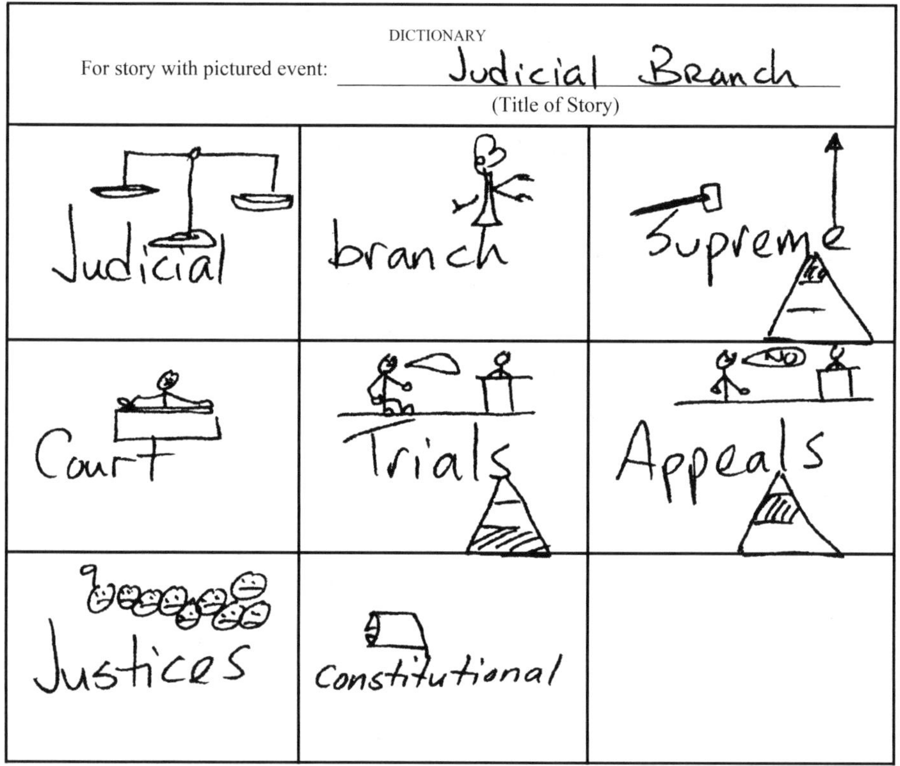

Figure 15.4 Picture dictionary about the Judicial Branch of the US government

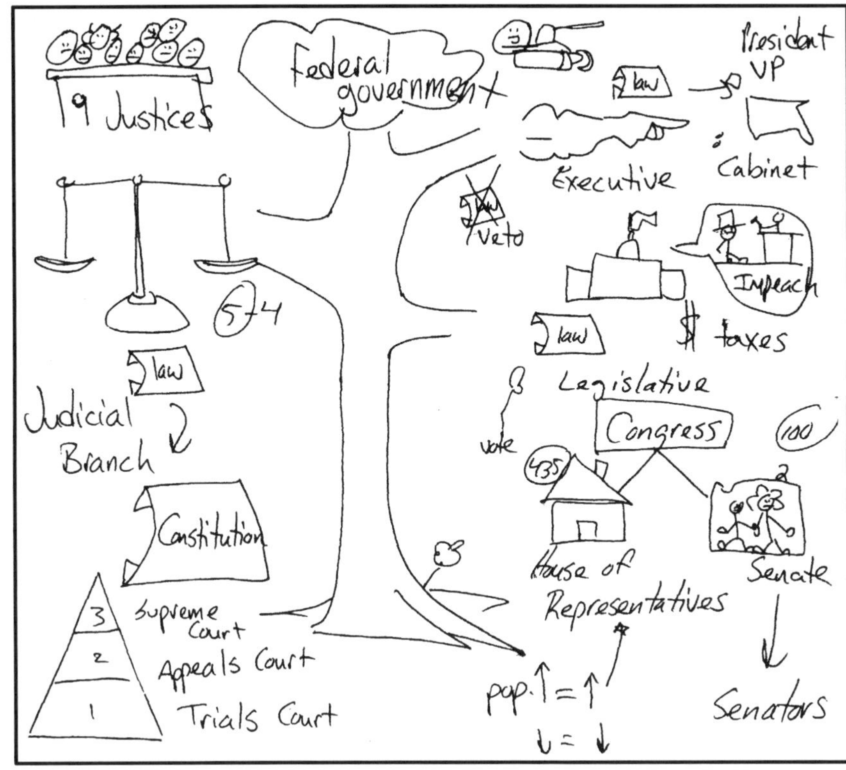

Figure 15.5 Flowchart of the interconnections among the various branches of government

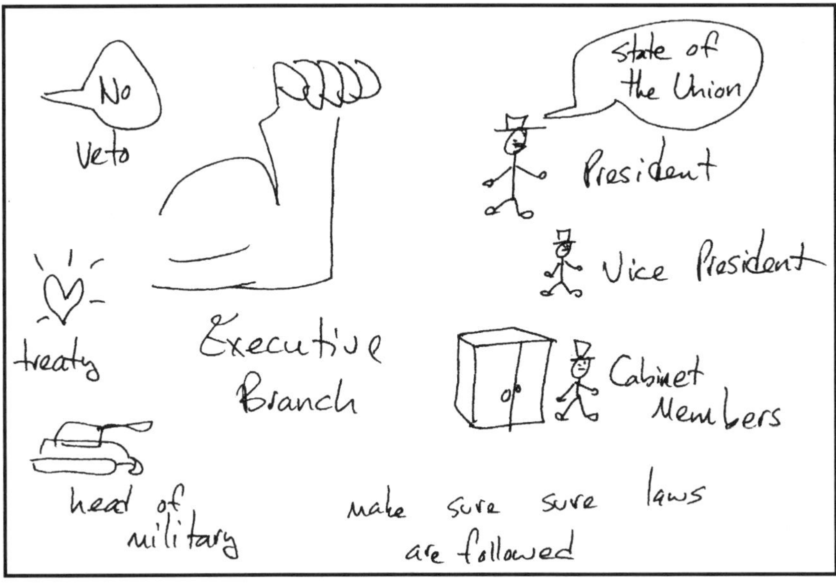

Figure 15.6 The make-up of the Executive Branch

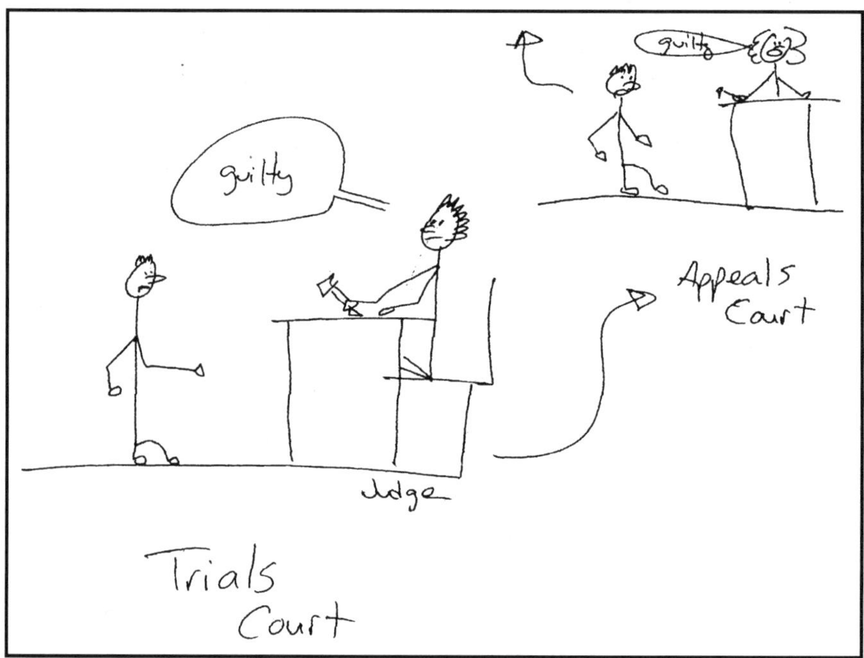

Figure 15.7 One aspect of the Judicial Branch, the court system

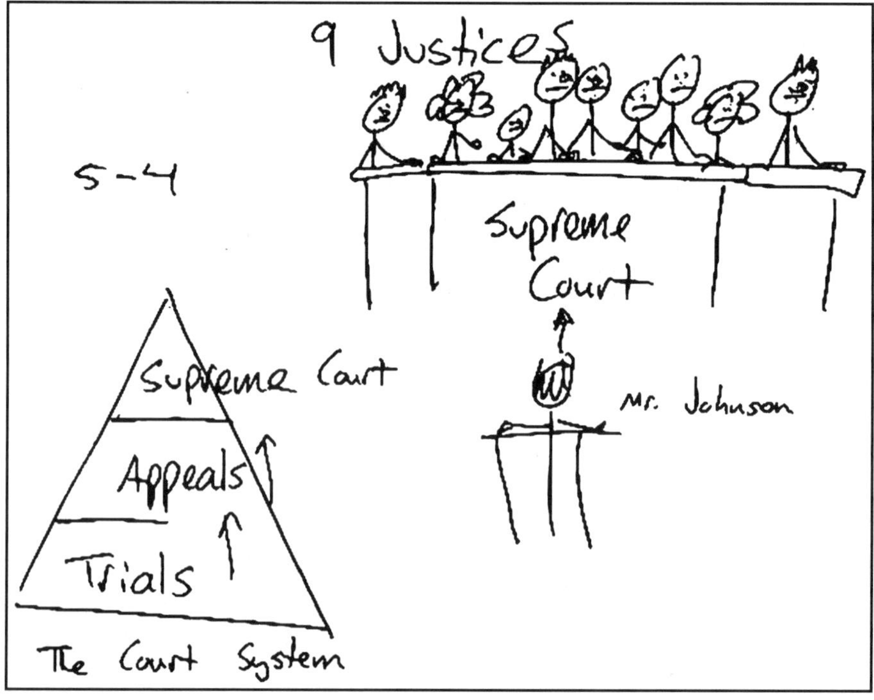

Figure 15.8 The highest court of the Judicial Branch, the Supreme Court

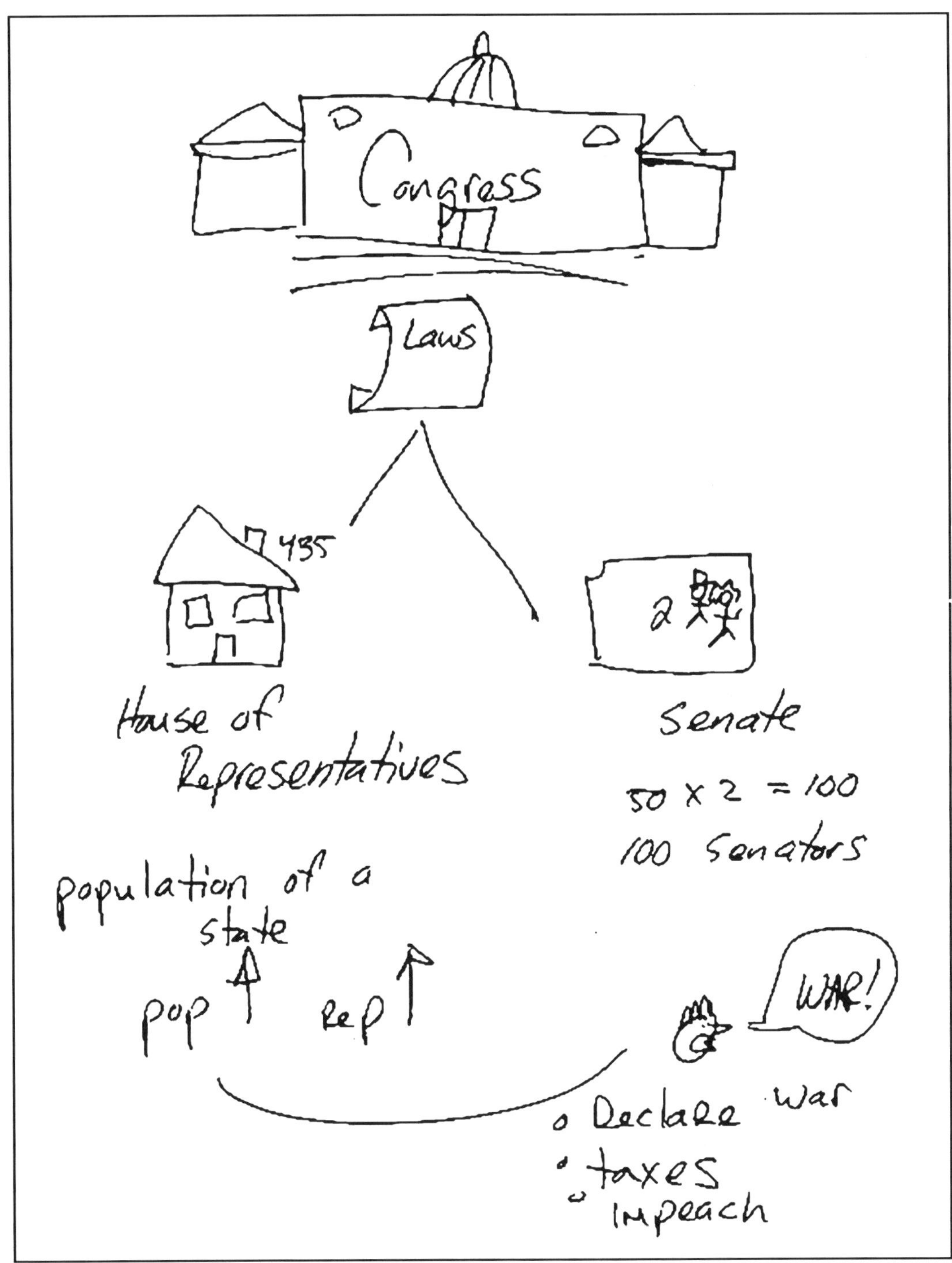

Figure 15.9 The relationship of the US Congress

Activity: How do thinking, context, and multiple relationships connect?

Without an understanding about how visual thinking includes the relationships among ideas, a visual way of thinking in an auditory culture can result in problems of communication. For example, if a visual thinker does not use enough words to explain the content of his or her mental pictures or to tell the story that goes with the pictures, the listener lacks sufficient meaning to interpret the visual thinker's graphics. For example, a college teacher drew a diagram on the board. The diagram had letters such as "r" or "m" and lines connecting other letters. The instructor turned to the class and said, "This is it. This tells the whole story." One student who needed more meaning raised her hand and asked, "Could you explain the diagram?" The instructor responded, "There is no need for an explanation. This is everything you need to know. One picture stands for a thousand words." The instructor may be right about one picture, his picture, taking the place of a thousand words that he already knows, but what are those words? When the students do not know the meaning of those letters within the instructor's diagram, the students do not have any meaning. Listeners cannot be expected to "mind read." What is the instructor's story that goes with the diagram? *Pictures are ideas or concepts that represent one's own thinking, not the conventional meaning of the language shared among members of the culture.*

Activity: Why does a person's drawing or diagram require the use of English words to explain the meaning to another thinker?

In an auditory culture, roles, relationships, and the aspect of a situation mean very little so visual thinkers must provide the story that goes with their graphics, pictures, and visual representations. The instructor's thinking that he represented with lines and letters meant very little to the students. These lines and letters are not conventional symbols; that is, they do not have a ***shared referent***. If a teacher is to draw out ideas, the ideas need to be in context by adding a story which includes a person, the person's actions, and the objects and/or places of the event. The whole story needs to relate the drawing of the concepts to the standard convention, English, in order to share meaning adequately. Likewise, the teacher must draw in ***real time*** in order to provide a visual layer of meaning to go with the teacher's words. In this way, the students gain both the visual-motor thinking of the concepts and the standard English meaning through oral English.

Activity: Why does the visual thinker need to provide a story or explanation (oral or written) to go with the visuals used in a classroom?

Not all visuals are the same

Pictures mean something different to different people (Arwood *et al.*, 2009) and all mental visuals are conceptual but not conventional. In other words, each person would create a different mental head picture for the same idea based on the person's own perceptions. This instructor who drew the diagram marked with letters thinks he has drawn something meaningful for those sitting in his classroom but, in reality, he has only drawn what is meaningful to him. The students are waiting for the teacher to assign meaning with language. The instructor's concepts are his experiences of perception and the language has to be assigned to the instructor's meaning for the students to share in the experience. *In other words, language provides the contextual meaning for the students to be able to share in the meaning of the instructor's concepts.* The diagram has meaning only if the context is added to the visuals through the use of language. *Language is the shared set of conventional symbols.* As a concept increases in meaning, the thinker needs more words and pictures to explain the language that goes with the visuals. Sometimes, as concepts become more complex, educators think they need to use fewer words, but when it comes to understanding the meaning of a concept, more information is needed. If students are to regurgitate what they hear or read, then less works better. But to raise a student's learning to a higher order thinking requires more language for more concepts for higher conceptual thinking. Formal concepts like "gross national product" or "principle of recursion" need a lot of words, to create enough meaning to develop a formal concept that goes with the drawings or diagrams of the instructor.

Activity: Why do more complex concepts need more words and more pictures to explain the shared meaning?

When using visuals to add meaning to the context, the teacher will want to be sure that the visuals match the language level of the students. For example, a single object on a card such as a ball (Arwood *et al.*, 2009) is out of context and therefore is quite abstract. This type of visual is formal and actually more difficult for a person with little background or language than a complete story about how two teams were playing baseball when a dog ran onto the field. Context that is provided with stories, spoken words, and drawn in real-time increases the meaning of the visuals and simplifies the cognitive level for easier processing. *Making materials more contextual helps reduce the difficulty level of learning new concepts.*

Activity: What is meant by contextual meaning?

Contextualize the content

Teachers can add meaning by contextualizing the content. For example, teachers can provide explanations in story form for content by using primary sources, by creating "I stories" (Chapter 14), as well as by using community experts to bring their disciplines to life in the classroom (Arwood & Young, 2000). For example, a fifth grade teacher used to challenge his students to bring experts that they might know to the classroom. Students borrowed all sorts of people. Students provided for a cardiologist who arranged for dissection of human hearts and a parent who created a corner of the classroom as a natural wetland. Some students brought in professional athletes they contacted such as a basketball player who came and talked about the connection between school and sports. Another student contacted a professional chef who came to class and showed how math is used in cooking. Students were encouraged to write to university authors for critique and so forth (Arwood & Young, 2000).

Even though these are all rich experiences, the reader needs to remember that the physical experience does not become a semantic memory for future recall without language being used to tell the story of the physical experience. *Language is a cognitive tool that creates a level of thinking that works at the linguistic or formal level of thinking.* Language at the linguistic level provides the learner with a tool for understanding complex ideas.

For example, a field trip to the Liberty Bell in Philadelphia has little cognitive meaning without first providing the students with the language through drawing and writing and talking about what the people did, when, where, how, and why that related to the bell. Again, by putting the people into the task and relating the ideas, the classroom teacher makes the task easier (preoperational). The extra tasks about the people and what they did, where they did what, and when they did what, provides the concrete level of development which helps the students create mental visual thoughts that are meaningful when they look at the Liberty Bell. *The linguistic level provides the cognition for* ***symbolization****, the act of making formal concepts from previous concepts.* Formal thinking is characterized by the linguistic function of symbolization. Only at the formal level does a person really understand how the physical symbols only represent the underlying cognitive function of language.

Activity: Why is symbolization an important function at the linguistic level?

Symbolization occurs as a result of a thinker using language to assign formal meaning to thoughts. For example, a 13-year-old knows what a bell is because he *rings* a dinner bell at his ranch. At Christmas, he hears the carolers *ring* bells during a song, and his ears *ring* after he goes to a loud concert. And, for his eighth grade graduation, he received a class ring, a piece of jewelry. These multiple functions of the concept "ring" allow the learner to begin to use "ring" in a variety of formal ways that are *symbolized.* For example, when the teacher talks about the tree rings, he knows that this does not mean there are bells in the tree. He also realizes that "ring" is about objects, not just actions; so, he realizes that this is something that has to do with the tree. As soon as he sees a picture of the inside of a tree's trunk with the words about the tree rings, he sees what the teacher is referring to because there are circles in the tree trunk much like the class ring he wears. He is learning the concept of ring at a formal level which allows him to problem solve flexibly. He uses his own language to think mentally, "I wonder how the tree makes those rings?"

The learner uses language to raise the meaning of "ring" to a more formal concept. This process symbolizes the concept ring for higher order thinking and conceptualization. Language creates formal meanings of concepts through linguistic function. Linguistic function includes cognitive symbolization that separates the human thinker from other animals. Such symbolization is more than just making an artifact such as a piece of jewelry, a tool, a dance, a picture...*symbolization requires the assignment of language to share the meaning of higher order thinking with others.* Providing multiple examples of the concept, ring for example, creates a process of contextualization that a formal thinker is able to use for greater symbolization.

Linguistic thinking with visual thinking in an auditory culture requires the increase of context in multiple relationships that are more complex visually at increasing levels of conceptualization. These visual functions compensate for the time-based property of English.

Activity: What does contextualization do for raising the level of meaning of a concept? How does symbolization increase the meaning of a concept?

Time-based concepts

Individuals who are older than 11 years should be able to use the properties of English in a formal way. One of the most important properties of English (Chapter 4) is the use of time. To use English as a time-based language, formal thinkers must follow the conventions of the auditory, English language, if they are to function within the culture's symbolized expectations. Therefore, English speakers are expected to be able to use the sound-based property of English, time. *Time refers to a set of related concepts (semantic field) that denote the way a person thinks about time.* Time can travel through a person (Arwood, 1991a, 1991b) such as "I am late for class." Or, a person can travel through time: "I need to hurry up so I won't be so late to class."

Because English is a time-based language, time should be adequately used for thinking and for planning and organizing. In Chapters 10 and 11, the reader was introduced to how time was measured in a person's use of language. Note that as most learners today do not think with an auditory, time-based form of language, the majority of thinkers also struggle with developing a linguistic function of time concepts, even though the dominant culture still uses time as a value.

Activity: What is time? Why are time concepts difficult for the majority of learners today?

In order to help a learner develop a formal understanding of "time concepts," the teacher must apply the same VLMs as stated in Chapter 14: add context, make time concepts as visual in meaning as possible, create meaningful relationships, and provide visual opportunities to understand the concepts at the appropriate developmental level.

Add context

Turning the time concepts, which are auditory in the English language, into visual properties requires the use of space instead of time. Spatial concepts do not have directionality or temporality. Whereas time is multidimensional, a person moves through time or time moves through the person or both, space is unidirectional. A person can go through space in one direction at a time. Like a movie, in space, a person is able to move from one frame of the film to another frame of the film in a chronological order. This person is covering more and more space. Previous chapters provided many examples of how to move from space to space by cartooning. However quickly the person moves and however quickly the frames move do not matter. The person is in space and moves through space, not time.

Activity: How does space compensate for auditory time?

A visual thinker organizes and plans based on the space that past tasks occupy. So, understanding that combing hair takes the space of the minute hand on a clock moving from one number to two numbers away is the space of 10 minutes. All activities take up space. To understand the space occupied for a task, the thinker must understand the context; what comes before the occupied space and what comes after the occupied space. For example, a child may know that when the bell rings at the end of the day, it is time to go home. But what does it look like to "get ready" to go home? What tasks in what frame of space does "getting ready to go home" take? Without the context for "getting ready to go home," the student at any age, including college, may not take home his or her homework, assignments, books, and so forth. For the student's backpack to arrive at home, the student must be able to see the relationship between one space of the bell ringing, to another space where the student picks up the backpack, to another space where the student walks out of the last class to the space of walking down the hall to his locker. Context is required to understand the space that an event or task occupies in relationship to other tasks that occupy other spaces. Seeing this context as an event in which the student occupies a certain amount of space provides meaning to visual thinking.

Activity: Explain how a task takes up space.

In an auditory thinker's system, multi-tasking means thinking about different tasks while doing a specific task. Thinking is in the sound of words such as "While I punch these forms, I will also staple the second set." However, a visual thinker is able to do the task within context of what the visual thinker mentally sees, one space and one task at a time. It is difficult to see one set of physical input while seeing a different set mentally. This is why it is believed that most people today cannot adequately multi-task (e.g., Ballenger, 2009). Thinking in pictures that take up space means that the learner is able to think about the space the learner is in, one picture at a time. Therefore, multi-tasking may not be possible.

For visual thinkers, adding context helps put the learner into the space that he or she is in. Then moving the thinker through multiple pictures as the pictures relate to choices increases the opportunity to engage in multiple tasks within the same space because the learner is given the visual thinking that goes with the multiple acts. For example, cartooning out the steps of an experiment allows a visual thinker to see himself doing the tasks shown in the experiment. Adding the words to the experiment helps the visual thinker create meaning for the experiment so that answering the lab questions has meaning that can be recalled later. Each step of the cartoon of the experiment is a space on the face of the clock. The first step takes 15 minutes and so forth. By putting the times on the clock face, the student begins to see "how much space" a task takes. This cartooning adds context and the context (people, their actions, and objects) requires a certain amount of space that can be measured. These measurements provide the learner with a visual structure of the space that is filled during the experiment. Once the thinker has the pictures for multiple experiments about a given concept such as "evaporation," then the learner can begin to put his or her own language to the experiments so as to think about ideas that are not necessarily seen or heard. The learner begins to symbolize the concept of "evaporation" which means that the learner can also begin to think about other, related ideas. For example, "Is evaporated milk made through evaporation?" With this mental language added with mental pictures, mental words, mental spoken ideas, then the learner is able to begin to think about multiple concepts in relationship to one another. This is the beginning of multi-tasking. For example, as the learner is doing one experiment about evaporation, he is thinking how he might do another experiment about evaporated milk. The greater the knowledge the thinker is able to access with language, the more likely the person is able to think about other tasks. In order to multi-task, a thinker must be able to have a formal way of thinking about time: How to plan with time, organize with time, and use time for assigning meaning to tasks as events that take the space of time. And, to have a formal level of thinking with time, the learner must also have conceptualization for the multiple tasks also at a concrete to formal level of language function.

Activity: Why is the measurement of space important for a visual thinker to begin to understand time?

Make time relational

English time functions like this: "When you go to school in the morning, don't forget to take your homework so that your teacher can grade it." Almost every word has a time basis. Words like "when" and "in the morning" directly assign time meaning, while verbs in English simultaneously show time such as "go," "don't forget," "to take," and "can grade." And then there are the time markers for change such as "to school" and "so that." This leaves "you," "your homework," "teacher," and "it," which are nouns, as the only non-time-based words.

Spatial concepts are relational in nature. The space that one person occupies is different than the space another person occupies. So, when English is made more relational it sounds like this:

> Put your homework into your backpack and put your backpack on the hook by the backdoor so that when we get ready for school tomorrow morning and walk to the backdoor to leave for school, you will see your backpack and remember that you need to take the backpack to school so that when you get to school you can take your backpack to your locker, open the locker, set the backpack down on the floor, take out your homework for your first period, and then put your backpack into your locker. You will close your locker and then walk to your first period with your homework in your hand. When you get to your first period classroom, take the homework that is in your hand and put it into the teacher's basket that is for homework. The teacher will take your homework out of the basket and look at it to see if you did the work correctly. After she finishes looking at or grading your homework, then she will record your grade so that she has a grade in her grade book that she can give you.

This type of relational language is spatial in that it connects the student and what the student does in relationship to the teacher and the teacher's need to provide a grade for the student (see oral cartooning and Mabel Mini-Lecture in Arwood & Kaulitz, 2007; Arwood *et al.*, 2009).

Activity: Practice using relational language.

This relational language in the previous examples might need to include the reason for grades related to credits, related to graduation, related to obtaining a job or going to school, and so forth. The author has worked with many young adults who have traveled through general education without a diagnosed disability but who still do not understand the relationships among homework, grades, credits, graduation, job, money, emancipation, etc. Unless auditory time is made into a spatial construct of taking up space in relationship to others and what others do, then a visual thinker may not understand the basic issues of planning, organizing, multi-tasking, and problem solving with English, a time-based language. Everything that speakers of English do is related to time and without a visual mental set of concepts about time with which to work, a person who is a visual thinker will struggle in an auditory culture. When the auditory culture has a significant portion of the population who is unable to function in time, the culture and language must change. During the process of change, there are economic, political, and educational effects. People often work and study harder while money is harder to make because of the lack of ability to multi-task, to plan a job, to cost out a job, to follow through with efficiency on a job, and so forth.

Activity: How does time turn into space? Why is relational language more spatial than temporal or time based? How does a person who thinks with visual mental cognition but who does not have the tools for using time affect culture and the language?

Create the picture of space

Learning to think in spatial dimensions instead of time must be explicitly taught in an English speaking society. For example, telling students "to keep their hands to themselves" does not talk about space but about the event of doing something in time. From a time perspective, the words mean "never" to touch others. But a visual thinker, Johnny, looks at his hands and mentally sees his hands when the teacher says, "Keep your hands to yourself." In other words, Johnny hears that he has hands and so he does. Johnny continues to touch the walls or others around him, so the teacher says, "Johnny, keep your hands to yourself." Johnny looks at his hands by his side and smiles and reaches up and touches the boy in front of him. The teacher is angry because Johnny is not responding to her words. In actuality, he did. He saw his hands by "his side" which is what "to yourself" means. Johnny and his hands are in Johnny's space. Johnny does not think in the *time* of "keeping." For Johnny to learn about the space of the action, the teacher needs to teach the visuals that go with these words explicitly.

> When you are walking across the room, you keep your hands by your side so that you do not touch someone else or touch other people's materials, or materials on the walls. Keeping your hands by your side makes walking around the room safe for everyone to move. When we move around the room and are safe, then we can make head pictures about what other people might be thinking about. If we keep our hands by our bodies, then others can move around without their thinking pictures going away; but, if we touch someone then their thinking pictures will go away or change and they won't be able to learn. Our job in the classroom is always to think, to make pictures so that we are learning.

How much language is provided to make a picture of how the learner moves through space in a safe and respectful way depends on the age and the development of the learner. Sometimes students do not know that they have a bubble of space around themselves because they have not been explicitly taught about that bubble in an auditory culture. The teacher and parents must explicitly teach about the bubble because English, as an auditory language, assumes a distance developed through the time it takes to reach a person. For example, the teacher must teach visual thinkers that they do not want to pop their own mental bubble by reaching out of that bubble and touching others. Sometimes older students need a reminder that for everyone in the class to feel safe, the class members need to move around with their hands down, their lips closed, and thinking of the class content, making pictures about the topic, so that they are respectful of others' thoughts. Reaching into someone's bubble or space while they move around will make that thinker's head pictures go away. *Explicit teaching about space is necessary if a visual thinker in an auditory world is going to develop the language tools required for formal thinking to compensate for the lack of internal time.*

Activity: Why does an auditory culture have to teach explicitly about the space a thinker occupies or the space events take or tasks require?

Chapters 13 and 14 provided examples of how ideas may be cartooned to understand how a person fills his or her own space; but space is also a set of dimensions that includes more than the horizontal cartoon. Space also includes the vertical and diagonal dimensions. Students between 7 and 11 are learning how to stay within their space bubble (horizontal) as they move around others' space bubbles. They are also learning how objects such as letters fit within their space. For example, the teacher writes words on the board. The students are sitting on their bottoms on their desk seats. The students' bottoms are horizontal or parallel to their desk tops, and their trunks are horizontal to the board. Horizontal cognition is the easiest level of ***spatial development*** (Arwood, 1991a). But, the students' trunks do not do the writing; their hands do the writing. So, when students raise their hands to put them on the desk top to write, the students have crossed the horizontal plane of their bodies to the board. Now the students' hands are perpendicular to the board or vertical. Writing letters requires this extra step of thinking how to make the shape of the letter go a particular direction. Add to this extra spatial dimension the notion that letters have directionality, such as an "s" faces right, and that the teacher wants the letters written from the top of the paper down, the student who is writing by letter only is engaging in three-dimensional thinking: first, body to paper to board; second, hand to eyes looking at board to writing on the paper; third, letters are directional to the paper to the board to the body to the writing.

Most auditory thinkers use the meaning to write: "I want to write the word was. If I write the letters in reverse, the word will be saw." But students who are visual thinkers are using the shapes of the ideas for thinking about the way an idea looks. Because letters are not ideas, they often struggle with making their writing make sense. If picture dictionaries of ideas are provided, students are able to learn the meaning and write ideas, not letters. Chapter 3 provided the reader with another aspect of creating the picture of space, grounding. When thinkers are working with meaningful information, their bodies are relaxed; they are grounded in the space they are in. This grounding allows their arms to be free, their writing to be clear, their mental pictures to be clear. Therefore, if students are crawling up on their desks, rolling around on the floor, leaning back against the book shelves or any of the other many postures to connect to a large surface (their bodies are horizontal or parallel), the teacher needs to realize that the material is being presented with too many dimensions, too much cognitive translation for the student.

Activity: How do the dimensions of space affect student thinking and writing?

Creating formal semanticity of time

Time concepts are like all other concepts. Time concepts are acquired gradually and are layered. At the formal level of time, a linguistic thinker is able to use time as part of the conversational aspect of language: The speaker says something and then the listener becomes the speaker and says something about what the first speaker said and then the second speaker comments on what the first speaker said the second time and so forth. This very exchange, in English, is temporal in nature and allows for higher order thinking through symbolization. However, many visual thinkers like the technology of texting and other restricted forms of language because the interpretation is really left to the reader, not the writer. This works well for restricted forms of language: Language function that is limited to the "here-and-now" about the speaker or sender is restricted. However, this restricted type of language does not capture the time elements of formal English. Formal English allows for the function of maximally displaced formal concepts such as understanding Ancient Egyptian culture. Ancient Egyptian culture is not about the here-and-now. To understand about the people of Ancient Egypt and to be able to communicate in writing and speaking about Ancient Egypt, a person must have acquired the formal understanding of time that is not in the here-and-now.

Activity: How does the semanticity of time occur?

This ability to understand time means that the visual thinker realizes how much space 2000 years ago occupies. For example, to a visual thinker, 2000 years ago might mean that there were more than 100 generations of people, each generation occupying an average of 20 years of space, per person. The author has worked with high school students, college students, and young adults who do not have a formal concept of 2000 years. They literally think that Ancient Egypt is someplace now that they cannot see or just before the last generation. To symbolize time, like formal concepts of 2000 years, the visual thinker must be able to create visual meaning (semanticity) of the space of the time. This is like an event calendar instead of a time-line or date-line. Each event occupies space. For example, a child who is getting dressed looks at the clock before dressing and after dressing. The event of getting dressed took 10 minutes of space on the clock face. But after school, the child measures how much space math homework occupies, and the child finds that math homework takes 20 minutes of space and so forth. This is called clock time.

Activity: What is clock time?

Even visual thinking adults who are expected to meet deadlines or create a time-line for a project that has multiple components struggle with a formal understanding. For example, a contractor agreed to do a small project nine months in advance. The project had to occur during a specific set of three weeks but the project would take only about five work days to complete. So, the contractor had time in advance to plan the time, to organize his workers, to set aside five days within a window of three weeks. He could not do the task. The project dragged five weeks beyond the third week. The contractor came in to measure one cabinet three times. Each time, he took 10 minutes to measure the cabinet but, he took about 30–45 minutes to come to do the measurement. And measuring the cabinet is all he would do. He could do only one thing at a time. He was harried doing the project as he was also doing a large project at the same time. He could not figure out how to set aside large chunks of time from the other project to do the small project. After the project was more or less finished, there were many mistakes including water damage from a sink not being connected correctly that caused thousands of dollars of damage. This contractor's actions are too often typical for much of today's workforce in the US. He did not have the cognitive language tools to plan the project, organize the tasks, and do the work. As a result, a very kind and competent person made huge mistakes costing insurance companies, owners, and others, time, money, and emotional stress. Because this thinker did not have a formal way to think about time as layers of overlapping spatial concepts or events occupying space, he lacked the maximum meaning (semanticity) of his space or time and therefore lost his flexibility and productivity.

Activity: How does not having an understanding of the space that time takes result in problems in the cultural ability to use time?

At the formal or linguistic level of thinking, the thinker is able to show maximum flexibility; an ability to use formal concepts, including time concepts, in a variety of ways to think critically and problem solve. Because the contractor was no longer flexible, his productivity slowed down and actually became less than useful.

This contractor needed visual methods of learning how to draw out a job within the scheduled space of events so that he could see what needed to be done within a space of an hour or six hours or three weeks. He needed to have the mental pictures of where he was at what time or space of a day during the space of three weeks doing what job. He needed to measure the space of the tasks, such as how much space it takes to drive to the spot to measure a cabinet so he could see how he was "wasting the space" or time that he was to occupy. Because he had more than one job to do, he needed multiple drawings like cartoons to show how he could not be in two spaces at the same time of the day but would have to have others working while he was doing something, and so forth. These types of cartoons of space for learning about time can be part of education (Arwood & Kaulitz, 2007; Arwood *et al.*, 2009). By drawing a person into the space of a day cartooned out with the clock for each activity of that day, a person begins to see the space that time takes. Figures 15.10 and 15.11 show how a task such as turning a paper in to the teacher really consists of several steps working backwards from submitting the paper to beginning the paper. This task is drawn from the plans of someone else. In order for most visual thinkers to develop their own plans cognitively, they need to draw from the completed project backwards, then do the tasks based on what they see (Arwood & Brown, 1999, 2001)

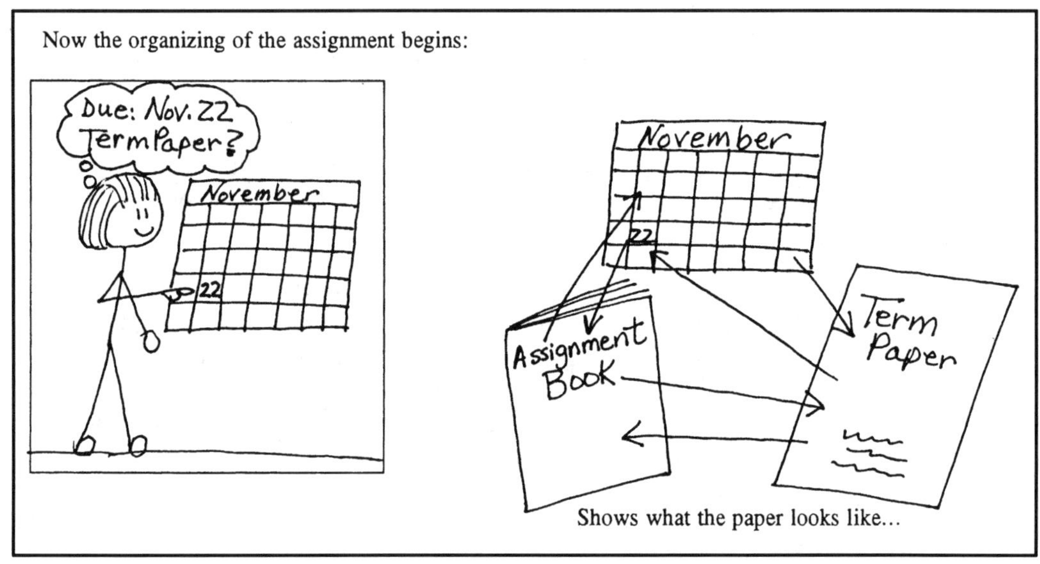

Nov. 22nd Turn paper in to the teacher. The completed paper looks like this! It is organized and contains a bibliography, table of contents, and title page.
Term Paper
Nov. 19/20
Cartoon sections of the paper.
Nov. 15, 16, 17 & 18
Edit paragraphs of each page (use cartooning).
Nov. 9, 10, 11, 12, 13, 14
Word process from the 3 x 5 note cards or reference cards.
topic
Library
Nov. 1
Draw out the steps of the given assignment
Nov. 3
Visit the library or Internet and obtain information
Nov. 4, 5, 6, 7, 8 Create note cards with different sources on each card

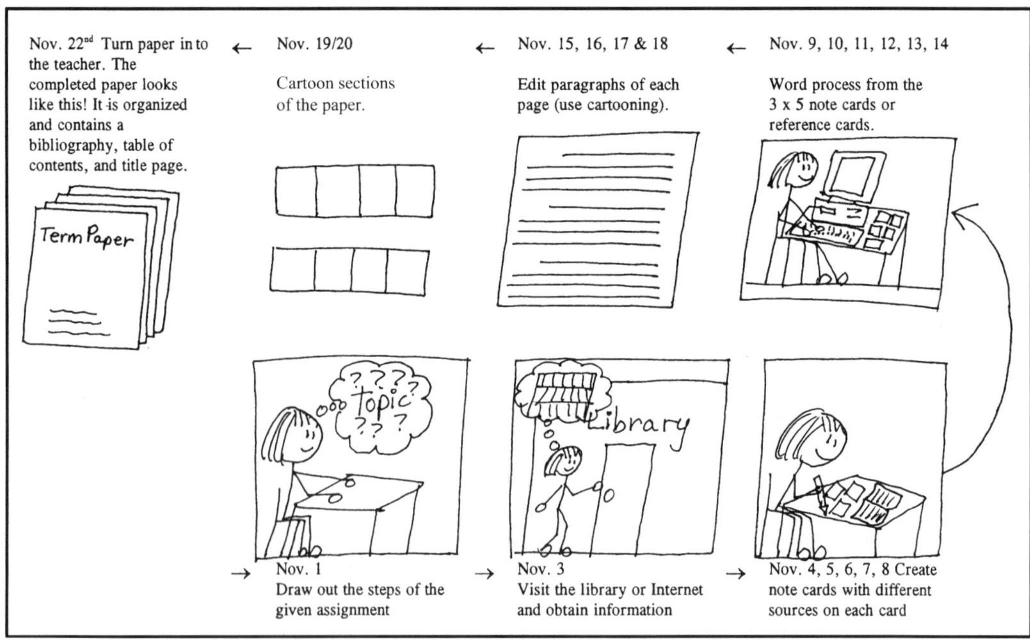

Figures 15.10 and 15.11 How to clock time for completing a task.
Source: Adapted with permission from Arwood, E., & Brown, M. (1999). *A guide to cartooning and flowcharting.* Portland, OR: APRICOT (pp.48–49)

Activity: How does drawing the space of time help a person see what space the person is in? How does planning require the visuals to translate oral language into efficient visual thinking?

By planning out the space of events, a person who is a visual thinker can acquire the formal semanticity of time. For example, a visual thinker once told the author that he has the sound of time in his head. He worked at a movie theater and could hear the clicks of 35 millimeter film in his head. He knew how much space a movie takes within that 35 millimeter film. So, for the rest of his life, he could space his time according to the clicks that occupied the space of a standard reel of movie film. As a result, as long as he "knew" how much space an event took because he had done the event before, he was good at planning the time a task would take. He had, by chance, developed a way to fill the space of his thinking with clicks that would occupy the space of time. Another person talked about how he learned how much space most everyday activities took because he lived within the structure of the US military. For 25 years, he was used to doing all tasks by the 24-hour clock time that was spelled out by someone else. When he left the military, he knew how much space on a clock most activities took. However, if the task was a new task, he had trouble deciding how much time the planning would take. Therefore, he often waited until someone else demanded the task be done.

Activity: How does time relate to linguistic function?

Summary

Society expects individuals older than 11 years to function with linguistic thinking. Linguistic thinking involves formal symbolization of concepts that cannot be seen, touched, or heard. Such concepts include words such as justice, liberty, rudeness, meiosis, conjunction, government, evaporation, and envy. Linguistic function allows for maximum displacement which includes an understanding of time for planning, organization, and multi-tasking. Semanticity is formal at this level which means that the thinker is able to use language for maximum symbolization. At this level, language functions in a linguistic way as a tool for higher order thinking. Language is flexible and productive so that the person is able to multi-task and problem solve for efficiency without stress. This also means that at the formal level, the individual is able to think about others from their perspectives.

Most of the legal component of society is concrete in nature, but the dominant culture expects that people are able to use literacy processes of thinking, viewing, listening, speaking, reading, writing, and calculating at a formal level to communicate with the time-based conventions of English. Because most people think with visual cognition, it is important to translate (Viconic Language Methods™) auditory English into visual thinking to get the majority of society able to function at a concrete to formal level for planning and organizing tasks or activities as well as developing an understanding of tasks or activities from others' perspectives.

Applications

- Draw out a multiple cartoon about how to plan an activity and then cross-reference it with another person's expectations of what the cartoon should show.
- Develop multi-tasking by drawing out cartoons of activities.

Chapter 16

EVIDENCED-BASED RESEARCH FOR VICONIC LANGUAGE METHODS™

Learner objectives: Chapter 16

Upon completion of this chapter, the reader should be able to:

1. Explain the qualitative research method of triangulation.
2. Provide examples of research on Viconic Language Methods.
3. Explain the data that comes from language sampling for understanding language function.
4. Explain how knowledge about the brain and learning fit into literacy programs.
5. Explain how a cultural perspective affects data interpretation.
6. Describe a paradigm shift that affects education's and society's view of learning.

Seeing makes a difference—
But who, what, where, when, why, and how do you know?
Evidence is in the learning as language shows,
Data creates the measure of knowing.

Educators expect today's educational practices to be grounded by some sort of "evidence" that the methods "work" as measured by "research." This chapter discusses the evidence available for Viconic Language Methods™. This evidence comes from several sources: logical deduction based on scientific research about the brain and the mind triangulated with what is known about languages; research-based studies over a period of 30 years; and effectiveness studies as stipulated by professionals who use VLMs on a regular basis.

Triangulation of data: brain, mind, and language

Triangulation is a research methodology that utilizes an examination of the trends and interplay among three or more sets of related qualitative data. For VLMs, three sets of knowledge-based data were integrated:

- Neuroscience knowledge that describes the way the information is received by the sensory system and processed for language functions (e.g., Butler & Hodos, 2008).
- Neuroscience studies that show the limited ways that sensory input integrates (e.g., Calvert, Brammer, Bullmore, Campbell, Iversen, & David, 1999; Dana Foundation, 2007) to connect to form language and thinking (e.g., Calvin, 1996; Carruthers, 1997; Damasio, 2003).
- Studies on language that show *not* all languages function with the same properties of English (e.g., Arwood, 1991a; Carroll, 1956; Gal & Irvine, 1995).

From this body of knowledge the following logic was used: As sensory input develops the brain and brain development results in higher order functions such as thinking, language is the result of the brain functions. So, language functions develop as well as the brain develops. This last argument is supported by studies (e.g., Goodwin, 2003) that show damage to the brain in specific sites does adversely affect language. Therefore, language, as a brain function, reflects the sensory input and processing of the learner. In tact brain function results in expected or typical language function. Likewise, analysis of language function indicates how the brain processes develop for conceptual thinking. Conceptual thinking or language function is a brain-based development, learned through the neurobiological system.

Activity: What is meant by "triangulation"? What is the logic part of triangulation?

If language reflects brain function, a sampling of language should provide an understanding of how a person uses language for thinking, viewing, reading, writing, and the other literacy processes (Arwood, 1991a). Even though specialists have used language samples (e.g., Lund and Duchan, 1983) for four decades (Launer & Lahey, 1981) as a valid method to assess the development of language structures of syntax, morphology, and basic semantics vocabulary, it should be noted that most people who analyze language have an in-depth knowledge of language structure, not language function. More recently, the same language sampling methodology (Arwood & Beggs, 1989) may be used to determine the way a person's language functions (Arwood & Kaulitz, 2007).

Examining language function, although often found to be more preferable than a structural analysis (Hux, Morris-Friehe, & Sanger, 1993), requires an in-depth knowledge of language function. Language function is a cognitive process which reveals how well the brain works. This knowledge of how language represents thinking provides the evaluator with a wealth of professional knowledge from which to perform an analysis of language function, as interplay between learning and thinking.

Activity: What knowledge would one acquire from analyzing language function?

Language functions (Chapter 3) *are tools of the mind.* So, to understand the relationship between how language and the brain work, an understanding of how language interfaces with the mind must also be investigated. Data from brain research provides the basis of the brain function. Research about language provides the basis for how language functions, culturally as a social product of learning, and cognitively as a linguistic product of learning. Because language represents brain function, doing research on how language functions provides knowledge about how the mind, brain, and brain-based learning of concepts intersect.

Activity: What are the three types of data being compared to understand language function?

As explained in earlier chapters, language function is a product of the learning system. Therefore, data about how learners use language helped inform the author about how language represents the mind, a product of brain function. There were several sets of data that the author collected to determine how individuals, who are expected to think with English, an auditory language, actually learn to be literate. Prior to collecting this data, the author accepted the premise that individuals who have lesion-specific brain injuries (e.g., Goodwin, 2003) have corresponding losses of language. Therefore, individuals who demonstrate problems with learning literacy processes, such as reading or writing, should show differences in their language function. Understanding language functions in turn helps explain how the brain, mind, and language interplay.

Activity: How does the use of logic provide validity for the premise behind research?

Research-based studies on language function

The author collected data from several different groups of individuals over the span of about 15 years to determine how individuals who do not think with the auditory language properties typical of English actually think. Some of the data is described in this section. One type of data came from sampling two groups of adults (Arwood 1991a, 2003) who experienced language learning issues at some point in their lives, but managed to become college functioning adults. The first group consisted of nine adults (Arwood, 1991a) between the ages of 21 and 42 who were interviewed for about three hours using the same informal questions about thinking and learning, their responses transcribed, and their responses analyzed for how they think. The data were analyzed using triangulation: Their introspective understanding of how they think in relationship to how different types of semantic language functions work. Table 16.1 shows a sample of the data to one of the questions: When someone talks, how do you think about what the person says? What each person said is put in relationship to how the English language functions.

Table 16.1 Transcription of adult data

Subject and transcription to question	Analysis based on English functions
Subject 1: Well, I don't hear what is said, I see what is said... Like right now, I don't hear what you say, I see what you say.	English is an auditory language; this person does not think in auditory sound.
Subject 2: I don't think exactly like the others, like in pictures; I can see the real thing in my head... (and) I have a rolodex in my head. I take what you say and it goes into my brain and then to use it I pull it up on a rolodex or picture. Like when I think of you teaching, I can see you at the board drawing out classroom management. I see everything you draw. My notes are your pictures. I can close my eyes and see you say what you said, verbatim, word for word on September 21st blah, blah, blah. But, I want to remember something from that class, I spin the rolodex, and up it comes. (What do you mean by "it"?) What I can mentally see.	English uses the sound of words as they are created mentally. This person does not use the sound of his own words but the exact sound of others. He is phonographic in ability and his pictures or photographs are indexed like a rolodex that allows him to pull up what he heard. This does not mean he understands what he phonographically or photographically stores.
Subject 3: I think, um, I see, what your mouth moves (lots of repeated, redundant language), I see it and up comes a movie of Scarlet O'Hara and Gone with the Wind...(question is repeated) Well, I just don't get it. (Do you know what I am asking?) No, I don't know what sound words mean... I only know the pictures of what I read. I read everything. I mean like I read whatever I can get my hands on. I read about glaciers and sex, and everything (Do you have to read something to understand the meaning of complex ideas?) Well I see your mouth move but I guess I do not know what you are saying.	This person is using the shape of the speaker's mouth to develop mental visual pictures as movies matched against ideas that she has read. Later in the interview she explains how reading is not sound-based but she sees the shape of the words and they create mental pictures that are real and more like movies.

The aforementioned data about how each person learned concepts (from the nine participants across 20 questions) was then analyzed in comparison to the academic and/or social difficulties each participant had in an auditory English culture. Table 16.2 shows the comparisons for the aforementioned three subjects.

Table 16.2 Adult subjects compared with success and strategies

	Diagnosis/academic problems	**Success**	**Strategies/coping**
Subject 1: Does not hear what is said	She had trouble learning to read sounds, struggled with education expectations. Does not always understand what people say on the phone. She was diagnosed with disabilities (second grade with mental retardation; fourth grade as having dyslexia; middle school as learning disabled) but learned on her own how to use her visual, not auditory thinking, system.	By college, she had no diagnosis. She worked and paid for her college education. Had a high Cummulative Grade Point Average (CGPA) (overall mean of grades or marks), took care of her grandmother while being a full-time student, held several jobs at a time, and took calculus types of classes for "fun." Graduated with her degree in five years and took a job as an educator where she was successful as long as she used her visual strategies, not her old coping mechanisms.	Her coping mechanisms included watching people's mouths, having others write what they said such as in lists of what to do, and reading with ear phones on so as to block her own voice while looking at the textbook. Her visual strategies that she developed as an adult included: reading with mental pictures, not sound; using her photographic memory mentally to see the shape of words so she could write and not require others to write for her; and learning to take class and book notes as pictures.
Subject 2: Did not use sound of others for learning	He had no diagnostic labels. As a student, he depended on a specific student (female) all the way through Catholic elementary and high school. When he went to college, she was not there and he struggled until he finally dropped out and lost his football scholarship.	He raised a family; and, after raising several children, began to earn his college degree. He was just beginning to learn strategies that matched his thinking when this data was collected.	He was learning not to copy others' works but begin to draw and then write his own ideas. He had depended on others to write his papers. He would talk, they would write. With taking visual notes, drawing his ideas, and using the computer to write from his drawings, he was able to do his own work.

continued

Table 16.2 Adult subjects compared with success and stategies *cont.*

	Diagnosis/academic problems	Success	Strategies/coping
Subject 3: Did not use mental pictures but converted the shape of motor patterns into mental visuals	She dabbled with anything that others did… drugs, sports, drama. In school she was seen as eccentric, talented, and gifted, and yet also a "brat" as she talked a lot and read voraciously. She often did not complete work, follow through with expectations, or socially act as expected. Both her parents and this young woman did not understand that her anti-social behavior was a result of her lack of understanding what others say and expect (also a sound-based task).	She had scholarships for academics and was an athlete but she did not want to learn new strategies. She was a con artist and when asked about being a con artist, she said she respected those who could see that she was a con artist because then she had to try to act differently. She ran into academic problems related to working with others, lying, stealing, and doing drugs.	Of the nine adults, this is the only one who decided not to learn visual strategies to meet her visual thinking system. And, she is the only one who continued to use her coping mechanisms, which eventually did not pay off academically or in getting and keeping a professional job.

Analysis of these data from the nine individuals suggests that social issues and academic issues were directly related to their use of cognitive thinking strategies or language function. If they tried to cope using auditory thinking methods such as drilling with more sounds to read or using sound to imitate what others said, then they continued to struggle with social and academic tasks (Subject 3, for example). On the other hand, when eight of the nine subjects used cognitive language strategies that matched the way they conceptually think, they were highly successful in an auditory culture.[1] *This data provided the evidence that when language function matches the way a person learns new concepts, then academic tasks and social tasks can be learned.*

Activity: How does analyzing language about learning help determine the way that people conceptualize?

Learning to be successful academically and socially is better when a person is able to use strategies that match the person's system of learning concepts for reading, writing, and so forth, than when a learner tries to cope with the sounds of the assumed English perspective. *Enhancing these individuals' strengths worked better than working to eliminate deficits.*[2] For example, instead of drilling on sounds for spelling (Subject 1) or imitating the sounds of what a person says (Subject 2) or copying what others say (Subject 3), strategies for seeing

1 One of the subjects did not choose to use the strategies. She wanted to be different and yet could not be successful by not trying to conform with learning strategies. More about her will be provided later in the chapter.

2 All of these individuals described many sound-based strategies that they had used over and over as they went through school such as practicing spelling again and again and still missing the words on the spelling test or later in a writing task.

the shape of words (Subject 1) as well as the ideas of what a person says (drawings for Subjects 1 and 2) helped these subjects read and write with conventional visual translations of English. These strategies converted English, an auditory structured language, into mental pictures, a visual cognitive function. It should be noted that this data provided information about not only how language functions in these group of people but also what happens when education does not consider the way the person learns concepts. More about this latter data will be provided later in this chapter.

Activity: How does language reflect the understanding of academic tasks in relationship to how a person learns concepts?

Thinking with language-based function

This same data collection process was completed in 2003 with six different adults (Arwood, 2003). The six adults responded to a call for volunteers to "talk" (same set of interview questions) about their language and their learning system. Five of the six adults were identified as using visual strategies and one of the adults was identified as using an auditory learning language system (*TEMPRO*: Arwood & Beggs, 1989). Again they were video-recorded, audio transcribed, and then analyzed. The five individuals with visual thinking systems all used some sort of mental visual graphics for semantic memory and the one auditory thinker reported that she has "no mental pictures" but the sound of her own voice which matches with the auditory language assumptions of sound-based English. All six adults used their mental functions, whether visual or auditory, to learn and perform literacy tasks. The five visual thinkers talked about academic pressures to learn to match what they heard or saw (phonographic and photographic patterns) instead of being given other ways to learn concepts in education. All five of the visual thinkers expressed specific literacy problems in school just like the previous nine adults. None of these individuals had been diagnosed with any learning or language problem at any time, nor did any of them receive any special assistance in the schools.

These visual thinking adults talked about how each of them had to learn to use visual strategies instead of the auditory sound-based coping mechanisms to become successful, despite the education emphasis on sound. For example, instead of writing down the professor's words verbatim (auditory coping mechanism), one adult talked about how he had learned to draw pictures that represent what he sees in his head as the professor moves his or her mouth. His iconic drawings then become his language function or cognitive thinking for learning the concepts. Figure 16.1 shows an example of his notes.

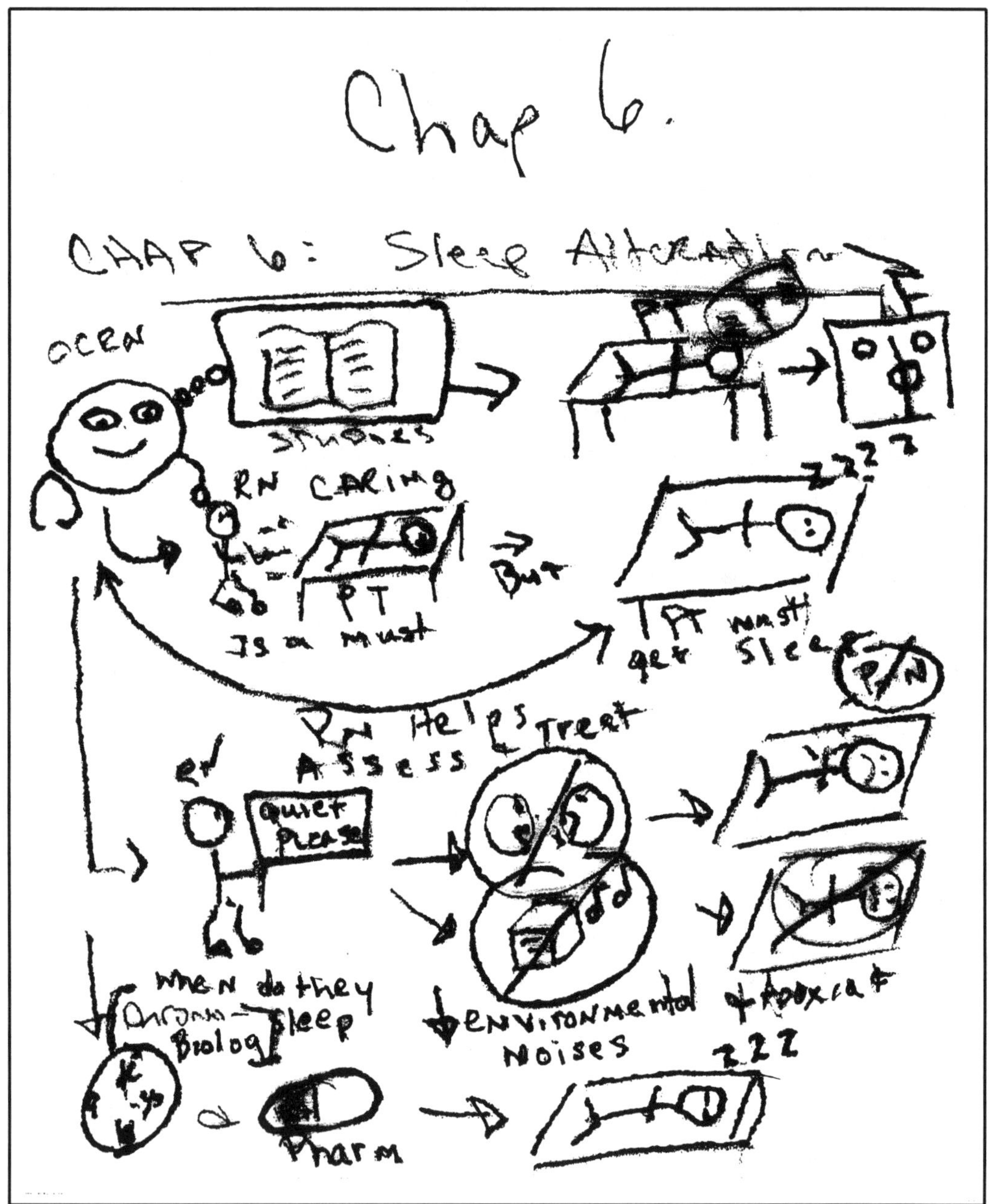

Figure 16.1 Class notes

In contrast to the visual thinker, the one auditory person said she had always been the "average" person in school, receiving mostly As, some Bs. She said school was "easy and a social experience." She found the "sound" activities in literacy such as games with sounds and letters "fun" but "unnecessary;" she never really understood why the other students couldn't hear the sounds in phonics instruction or for spelling. She never really thought about how to read or write: "You look at the letters and say the sounds in your head and that is the word." The other five students looked at this auditory thinker in disbelief, because they do not hear the sounds make words. When asked why these five adults thought they had become good students and made it to college even though they each struggled with sound activities in the lower grades, each one shared experiences about how they learned to read at home, before they went to school. This means that they also had sufficient language to support learning to read. When asked about how they learned to read, they all said something about how a family member would tell the story of the book, then point to the words and say the words. These adults said they learned the way the words looked that went with the pictures of what they know about the story.

Activity: What do most of the adults interviewed use for thinking?

Did these adults struggle with academic issues because of the way they were taught to read, write, listen, and so forth? In other words, are there other valid ways to learn to read and write than with the utilization of sound-based approaches of phonemic awareness, phonetic fitness, and oral fluency used since the 1950s, in English speaking countries? This latter question has a logical answer. There are other languages such as Mandarin that have orthographic representation that are not auditory (see Chapters 3–6). Obviously, the human mind is able to read the characters of Mandarin even though they do not use sounds and letters for decoding. In fact, they use the meaning of the idea rather than the sounds that make up a pattern that must have meaning. Logically, the human mind is able to use print on a page as a set of visual shapes of meaningful relationships, not just as a set of auditory sound-letter constructs.

The author compared the introspective data of how these adults think, along with the case studies of hundreds of other children and adults with whom she had clinically worked over the years, against the cultural properties of languages like Chinese and English. The results showed that the language function reflects the thinking which reflects the learning of the language processes (see Chapters 3–6).

Activity: How did these studies show a relationship between learning concepts, how language is used to become literate, and how one learns to be literate?

Culturally, English is an auditory language, but the human mind does not have to use the auditory properties of translating oral English to orthography for teaching a person to decode the meaning of print. Linguistically, English is characterized by the relationship between the sound of oral language and orthography as an alphabetic language, but decoding for meaning can be based on concepts, not just patterns, especially as children learn more than patterns of language (Chapter 2). Concepts are cognitive functions of learning a language (Chapters 1 and 2) while patterns are imitated sets of sensory recognition. Thinking, the ability to use concepts, requires the use of the way concepts develop, not the way that English is described. Language function reflects the acquisition of concepts for thinking.

Activity: What is the connection between English, the language, and the auditory cultural perspective? How does language represent thinking? How does thinking represent the acquisition of concepts?

Brain-based learning and language

This type of information from the aforementioned two sets of adults along with other data from other children and adults who struggled in school were triangulated against brain research to see how the brain-based learning fits into the actual introspective data of those who struggled in school literacy programs. Again, the triangulation process of comparing brain research about academic tasks to language function to the data about visual thinkers results in some interesting data. Following are some examples. The author attended a session by a neuroscientist, at the Learning Brain Conference in Washington DC, May 2009. This particular speaker stated that those individuals who have no pictures in their heads have different brains, and he showed brain images to reflect these differences. Interestingly, he also showed some transcripts of what these people said to a stimulus in which the subjects were asked to describe what they think when someone talks about "a beach." He then compared the data from those who had visual pictures in response to the task with those who did not have mental visual pictures in response to the task.

From a linguistic perspective, it was obvious to the author that the language function for the two groups was very different when he showed the transcripts of the language. Those who had "something different" with their brains and could not use pictures used the more complex auditory, time-based English language structures. On the other hand, the people with the mental pictures described what they could cognitively see. Their language showed many qualifiers such as colors but the language lacked the function of time and was more like a series of qualifiers about something they could mentally see. From the presenter's perspective, people who think with visual cognition are the norm for creativity. His interpretation of the data was predicated on the notion that to be creative involves being able to see the mental picture. And it should be noted that, according to the author, most people think with visual images. So, most people would be creative in the way that he described as the norm.

On the other hand, a sound-based language user can also be creative by producing the mental sound of English to imagine a beach. However, to imagine visual images, an auditory thinker needs more oral language (mentally or physically) to refine the concept of a beach: What type of beach (black, brown, rocky, etc.; auditory categorization)? What time of day (evening, morning, etc.; auditory time-based referring)? What is the purpose of the beach (playing volleyball, chasing seagulls, fishing, swimming; maximum productivity)? Where is the beach (maximum displacement; for example, Hawaiian black sand beaches are different than the brown sand beaches in Oregon)? And, why imagine the beach (maximum semanticity sets the level of the task at one of the cognitive stages such as is the thinker going to be on the beach or paint the beach)? Therefore, without the details of the sound of English to narrow down the possibilities (language functions), the concept "beach" has little meaning. Words, lots of words, provide more creative response by the auditory thinker. If the visual thinker hears "beach" and thinks of only one picture, that is preoperational in nature; multiple still pictures would be concrete in thinking; and multiple movies or sets of pictures in contrast to one another would be formal.

Activity: What is the difference in imagination or creativity to words for visual thinkers and auditory thinkers?

The auditory thinker who asks all of the questions in order to imagine a beach is also creative but is actually functioning at a higher cognitive level of language function than the visual thinker who has a very creative detailed single specific picture of a beach. The auditory thinker realizes that there are a lot of concrete examples that feed into his or her imagination and that a formal imagination would require borrowing information from lots of sources. This neuroscientist had the brain images and the transcription, but he had not triangulated his data against what is known about language function in terms of learning and thinking. Researchers who are going to interpret brain-based research need to consider the tool for interpretation, language: How does language function? How is language acquired? What is the relationship between language, the brain, and the mind? What is the difference between language structure and language function?

Activity: How does auditory thinking use language to be creative?

Another example of how brain research needs to control for language function or consider language function during analysis of the data has to do with the notion that the human brain does not multi-task well (e.g., Manhart, 2004). For those who think with visual cognition and with only one movie at a time or in frame-by-frame pictures are not going to be able to think about multiple activities at once. This type of linear thinking may be efficient for specific single tasks, but is also concrete, not formal in seeing how others' tasks relate to the thinker. A visual thinker, who knows a topic well, is able to display multiple screens of movies mentally. For example, one biochemist learned as a graduate student that she needed more filing systems for her visual pictures so she mentally began to index the various pictures of different types of biochemistry on her fingers. She could look at her finger and all the visuals related to that particular set of thoughts could be retrieved. She could then multi-task in her biochemical classes without losing track of the organization of content. This person is thinking at a formal level of biochemistry and later earned her doctorate and became a professor. Again, she could multi-task as she could teach, run a home, and engage socially in the community. She had the language tools for thinking at a formal level, a level of thinking that necessitates multi-tasking in an auditory culture.

On the other hand, a person who is using sound-based cognition can, in fact, use the mental voice along with time markers to keep track of multiple activities or tasks such as overseeing multiple workers doing different tasks, as all activities are in time, not space. Auditory English is designed to "think" in time-based language: "I will play my violin while I watch the baby play with her blocks." "I am baking a cake while the clothes are in the dryer so I can be cooling the cake while I am folding the clothes. And while I fold clothes I am mentally going to start writing the new article for work." Yes, this type of activity may take more energy but the human brain can do it with the aid of language to tell the brain what it will focus on. Understanding how language moves a thinker into multiple activities at one time is a function of semanticity and results in better productivity, displacement, and flexibility. And, most research (e.g., Walker & Hulme, 1999) shows that cognitive function is easier when tasks are meaningful and at a lower level of concept development. So, multi-tasking is probably a function of the language level, the cognitive level, and the use of literacy for thinking. The brain research needs to consider the use of language for thinking at the various levels. And, knowledge of language functions will help to interpret the brain research. For example, meaningful tasks are typically viewed as cognitively easier and the brain interprets those meaningful tasks differently (e.g., Decety, Grezes, Costes, Perani, Jeannerod, Procyk, Grassi, & Fazio, 1997). Knowing that the brain recognizes differences in meaning supports a Neuro-Semantic Language Learning Theory.

Activity: How does the idea that the human mind does not multi-task contribute to a better understanding of the function of language?

An increase in language function logically increases a person's ability to think about multiple activities: Likewise, cognition that is at the concrete or higher level uses language to think about ideas in multiple sets of relationships. For example, to understand a formal level of the word "respect," a person has to have multiple ideas integrated together into the formal concept. Without the ability to "multi-task" about a concept, individuals remain at a lower cognitive level. To think formally would necessitate the ability to think about multiple ideas at a time. For example, when adults are asked what they see when a person says "respect," those who have a lot of knowledge about "respect" see multiple sets of pictures about different types of respect. Those with little language may not see but one example of "respect." Those with an auditory thinking system may be able to give a formal definition: "Respect refers to the ability to think about others in relationship to one, one's actions, one's self; discernment for others; courtesy to others and their objects." Again, by using a triangulation of information about language, the use of language and thinking, and what the brain research tells, it is evident that the higher the language functions, the better the thinking.

Activity: Why does formal thinking require multiple sets of ideas to be integrated?

As mentioned in Chapter 6, brain research (e.g., Shaywitz *et al.*, 1998) shows that individuals who struggle with reading sounds with letters have differences in the brain. Well, if the majority of people are culturally visual thinkers, it is logical that perpetuating reading, writing, and literacy programs that try to use deficits as the basis for learning to be literate are going to clash against conceptual ways of learning. The result of this clash is in the data. Early programming of sound in the primary grades shows an increase in sound-based decoding skills but with lower thinking levels in the upper grades, as these programs do not emphasize thinking. It is apparent that there is a shift in thinking with more people using a visual form of thinking, but there is not a shift in what is assumed to be the basis of learning to think, read, write, view, listen, speak, and calculate (literacy processes). Since the available data does not show an increase in thinking, it is logical that perhaps different literacy programs aimed at language functions (Chapters 13–15) provide an approach consistent with the way most people learn to think. Knowledge about learning to be literate (Chapter 6) in relationship to the brain and language function opens the door for thinking about more effective ways to provide literacy programs for children and adults. Research about how children think to form language functions also contributes to this triangulated knowledge.

Activity: What do sound-based programs provide for learning to be literate? Do these programs match with the way most people think?

Thinking with language research

Since the late 1980s, the author has shared the adult data in many different venues and people always want to know: How many people are like the 15 adults? As reported in earlier chapters, approximately 85 percent of the English speaking population in the US and Canada think with some form of visual cognition. This percentage of data evolved over several studies. The first set of data was collected, in 1982, by the author who collected, transcribed, and analyzed language samples on all students in an elementary school, first to sixth grades, that enrolled only those with literacy problems (52 samples were collected from students, ages 6 to 13.5, with IQs on formal tests between 80 and 120). The author had wondered if these students had the language to support their reading, writing, calculating types of programs. Upon analysis of the data, 100 percent had visual systems which today corresponds with data from Yale (Shaywitz *et al.*, 1998) and Harvard (e.g., Galaburda & Livingstone, 1993) about reading problems (dyslexia) being an auditory processing issue. *Logically, if students cannot use sound to process ideas, using sound to teach literacy processes results in learning problems, learning to read with sound. Furthermore, how well children are able to read orally (sound-based) is predominantly the way that reading is defined and tested (see Chapter 6).*

Activity: How could teaching a child a task, in a way that does not match the way a child thinks, result in a learning problem?

The first set of data was taken on children who all had diagnosed learning language difficulties. So, what was the percentage of students who had visual thinking strategies in a typical elementary school? So, the author was given permission to collect samples, transcribe the samples, and analyze the data of students at a nearby elementary school, first to fifth grades (approximately 350 students of which 270 samples were collected; students with IEPs or who did not show up on the day of assessment were excluded). The samples from students in the higher third to fifth grades revealed about 40 percent used visual thinking. The students in K–2 grade showed about 60 percent. At the time, this number seemed high. Furthermore, the idea that perhaps the ability to use auditory English in an oral way was a developmental issue, as more of the children had visual ways of thinking in the lower grades, seemed important. However, today the same data is interpreted differently. Knowing that as many as 85 percent of today's adults think visually, this data showed the changes taking place. The original data was collected in 1985. It has been a full generation since that data. Those primary students are now adults. Brain research is beginning to show that input changes thinking (e.g., Begley, 2007; Gazzaniga, 1999; Merzenich *et al.*, 1999; Simos, Fletcher, Bergman, Breier, Foorman, Castillo, Davis, Fitzgerald, & Papanicolaou, 2002).

The adults in the authors' study did better academically and socially when they worked on enhancing their visual strengths, not their sound-based system. Brain research shows that the brain develops as input is provided (e.g., Begley, 2007) so the brain could be trained in sound or sight. Merzenich *et al.* (1998, 1999) show that children can learn to discriminate sound and that brains can be trained for sounds. But, if language is a significant tool of the brain, why not train the brain to use its strengths rather than its deficits? Neurobiologically, the visual strengths would have more meaning than the weaknesses. Brain research shows that meaningful tasks are easier. So, teaching children to learn to be literate in the way they think seems to be a logically easier task. Evidence-based data for this assertion is found in the last section of this chapter.

Activity: How could some of the brain research be interpreted differently than from a sound-based cultural perspective? Why would working on visual ways to be literate be easier for some students?

If teaching affects learning, maybe the author's language studies based on sampling are related to teaching, not learning; even though the data sets of the adults showed that they had to compensate or cope for learning to be literate in a way that did not match their visual thinking. To see if the difference between auditory language function was related to brain function of auditory processes (not just teaching), Bahls collected data on some college students (Arwood, Bahls, & Crabtree, 1986). Of the students who volunteered, she was able to match nine adult students who thought with visual cognition on several variables—grades, social economic status, work, position in family, family history, English as L1, and gender—with nine who thought with visual strategies. The language between the two groups was strikingly different, especially in the higher functions of displacement (use of time), flexibility (understanding of question), productivity (clarity of understanding what the speaker meant), and semanticity (use of specific vocabulary to refer and predicate). Furthermore, none of the individuals with visual thinking had been diagnosed with special needs and all of them showed a problem with being able to have the auditory clicks of sound sped up. The brain stems of those with visual strategies could not process the increased speed whereas those with auditory language were able to process the increased speed. This matches with today's brain research that shows that individuals with learning issues have difficulty with processing speed of language (e.g., Miller, Kail, & Tomblin, 2001). However, this is the processing of auditory English, not the processing of English that has been translated into a Viconic Language Method such as oral cartooning. The author has found that children with learning problems actually process the oral cartooning (see Chapters 13–15) very quickly which means that the cognitive task of turning the sound-based words into oral pictures by an adult reduces the cognitive difficulty. Therefore, it may not be the speed but the unit of analysis, sound-based words versus mental pictures that may be the issue. Brain research to support such a method would be useful. From the work with Bahls, it is apparent that language function is different for those with differences in processing, so it seems logical that using different methods to teach language functions of literacy based on how individuals learn concepts (language function) would be sensible.

Activity: If thinking reflects differences in the brain, then teaching according to thinking differences makes sense. Why?

Because the author was the only one analyzing the language in these various studies, she decided to see what the validity and reliability were for doing the same type of functional analysis of language (to determine if the language showed a visual or auditory type of function), if others were trained to analyze the samples. Six speech and language pathologists were trained to collect language samples on five of their children diagnosed with language disorders as the primary disability. Then, by using a third-person coordinator, the samples were blindly sent around for each of the clinicians to analyze whether or not the children in the samples were able to use English as an auditory language, with time and sound-based propositions (see Chapters 4 and 5). In this way, the speech and language pathologists had contributed 30 samples from children with known language disabilities. But they were also told there would be 30 samples from those without known disabilities from a previous study and they would not know whether they were analyzing a sample with a child with a problem or not. They were never sent their own samples and they received only 30 to analyse, so they did not know how many did or did not have learning language problems. The reliability for being able to determine how many could use auditory propositions, language functions of sound-based English was 0.96 for these clinicians. In other words these clinicians were able to agree 96 percent of the time as to whether or not students could produce auditory propositions. Out of this process, the *TEMPRO* (Arwood & Beggs, 1989) was established as a valid and reliable way to analyze language function: Visual language function meant that the speaker creates visual concepts from the overlap of visual perceptual patterns, and auditory language function meant that the speaker uses the sound of his or her own mental speech patterns to create the meaning of auditory concepts. The auditory concepts were expressed as auditory propositions, arguments connected by time functions.

By examining the way that time was used in English, either individuals were visual in their thinking in that they did not connect their ideas with time-based English or they were auditory in that they did connect their ideas with auditory propositions.

Activity: How does examining the way language functions determine if a person is thinking with time or not?

Since the *TEMPRO* was established, the author has completed several studies to update the percentage of individuals who think with visual or auditory processing based on their language function, as a representation of their learning system (brain function). The studies since 2005 have been mostly written quick writes of the same question used in the *TEMPRO*: "What do you do on a typical day?" These quick writes have been completed by Dr. Joanna Kaakinen and the author with people attending nurse educator conferences in different locations around the US. Writing is different than oral language in that the person is able to edit the work as well as see what is written. So, the participants are told to write quickly for two minutes and not to erase. In this way, there is an attempt to approximate the flow of oral language and to be sure that there is some internal reliability in that the author is the only one analyzing the samples. The author analyzes the language immediately for whether the language uses auditory temporality like English or not. Typically, the author does not know any of the participants. Because the participants write and then turn in their papers, there is no opportunity to follow up with the participants on any inconclusive evidence. For example, a person might say, "Well, I usually go to work" in response to the question, and the evaluator in an oral sampling process can then say, "Tell me more." But when a person writes that type of answer there is no follow up; so, there is not the same content validity as there is with the oral *TEMPRO*. However, the results are still quite good. For more than eight groups of people, totaling more than 800 participants, there has been a consistent

86 percent in each group whose language suggests they think with visual cognition. And, there is another 4–5 percent whose samples are inconclusive, leaving about 9–10 percent who show auditory writing, and auditory language function.

Activity: Is language function related to the way a person learns concepts?

This percentage seems high but many teachers find similar results. For example, Bonnie Robb found 1 student out of 125 over a five-year study of children in her first grade who used an auditory thinking system (determined by using an oral sampling process: Arwood & Robb, 2008). Alyse Rostamizadeh, who teaches fourth to fifth grades, says the numbers are that high in her classroom as well. The bottom-line is that the numbers of people who use more of a visual way of thinking rather than an auditory way of thinking have actually increased over the last two generations.

From the analysis, then, the differences were compared to what is known about other types of languages. From this triangulation, it is apparent that languages reflect the way that a person is able to process input to form language just like different languages reflect the way that specific cultures think. This leaves the study of English language most interesting in that the language will change to reflect the changes in thinking. Culturally, time has a monetary assigned value in English speaking cultures; but, if the thinkers don't recognize the cognitive aspect of time, then the value of time becomes unimportant and the economic cost becomes significant (Chapters 4–6).

Activity: What does a TEMPRO provide a researcher in terms of language function?

One more recent finding in brain research needs to be talked about and that is the notion that human brains are not wired for reading. This is an accurate interpretation if reading is defined as an auditory function of putting sounds with letters, alphabetically, to say the sounds of the printed pattern (oral fluency based on phonetic and phonemic principles) (see Chapters 5 and 6). On the other hand, if the person sees the ideas as a set of relational shapes, the ideas use more of a visual way of reading that is not sound based. This would only be able to be analyzed when the brain images can accurately reflect the use of seeing the whole picture on the page, not the letters and sounds of words or word phrases. This type of research is yet to become viable. Again, this type of set up in brain research will need a control for language function or thinking on the part of the subjects.

Holistically, language represents the brain's function for cognition. Learning to think as part of literacy is a result of the interplay between how a person neurologically creates concepts represented by language function. Language function can be ascertained from introspection studies, corroborated by language sampling of auditory function, and considered in view of brain research interpretation of data. From this triangulation of knowledge, it seems logical that because most people think with visual cognition, a strength-based approach using visual language characteristics to interpret spoken sounds into mental pictures is feasible. Likewise, a visual approach to teaching the shape and look of print for writing is easier to match to visual pictures mentally than using sounds that cannot translate to visuals. Previous chapters described applications called Viconic Language Methods™. This section provides some data about the effectiveness of VLMs.

Activity: Does using VLMs for those who think visually make sense?

Evidence of the efficacy of VLMs

Twenty-four professionals who had received VLM training and had been using VLM strategies for more than five years were asked to answer four questions (Arwood, 2010). The questions were sent electronically and participants did not know who was invited to answer the questions. The following are the questions:

1. Which of these VLMs do you use (cartooning, oral cartooning, hand-over-hand shaping of words (bubbling), picture dictionaries, context creation by "I stories," adjustment of materials to create more visual context such as adding stories, examples, drawing concepts in real time while explaining an idea)?
2. What is your estimate of how many children and/or adults you have used these types of strategies (VLMs) with over the years?
3. What is one thing you want educators (teachers, support specialists, related services) to know about VLMs?
4. What one strategy has worked the best for you?

In analyzing this data, there are some assumptions. Obviously, these 24 educators and support specialists have already had success with VLMs or they would not have continued using them, as visual methods are not the norm and it is certainly easier in the mainstream of culture to do whatever everybody else is doing. Second, for the author to have contact access to these adults means that these professionals have stayed in touch with the author after initial learning of how to use visual methods to translate English (Viconic Language Methods™). So, those who have tried VLMs without success were not sampled. However, it should also be noted that over the years, hundreds have reported success back to the author when trying different VLMs and their data is not included here. Finally, it should be noted that these VLMs are not being compared to other methods. However, most "research" in education does not compare methods or programs. Most research is nothing more than data gathering. The one interesting fact about this sample of professionals is that all 24 sampled have been trained with a master's degree plus post master's training in the state-of-the-art methods and have chosen to change to use more visually based strategies to help their students learn to be literate and to develop content knowledge as well as behavioral disposition skills. Therefore, for these adults, VLMs appear to be the choice over sound-based auditory methods for literacy. And literacy is assumed to be the basis for learning content.

Activity: What is the basis for determining the efficacy of translating auditory English into a visually based language (VLMs)?

Of the 24 professionals who were sent an electronic request for answers to the questions, 18 responded. There was no follow-up request or check to see if the other six received the request. The 18 respondents represented seven different US states, private practice, public schools, and private schools. The respondents included classroom teachers at primary, intermediate, middle school, and high school levels; speech and language pathologists; reading specialists; special educators; ESL specialists; and administrators. There was no incentive provided for completing the questions. All professionals were asked if they wanted their words to remain anonymous or if they wanted to be quoted or given credit. Six said that they preferred to be cited; 15 said they didn't care; and three did not want to be referenced. A summary of the data is found in Table 16.3.

Table 16.3 Summary of efficacy of VLMs

Question 1: The types of VLMS used...this was to be sure that the professionals did in fact use VLMs	All 18 indicated that they used the majority of the VLMs listed; "I stories" and cartooning were most often mentioned as being used most of the time.
Question 2: Total number of adults and/or children worked with VLMs for the X professionals who responded	Many guessed...but the total was 6250. It should be noted that 5 reported that they trained all of their staff over 20 years (total) which means there are a significantly greater number who have successfully used VLMs.
Question 3: The one thing you want educators to know about the use of VLMs	Most said something about learning...this one respondent summarizes much of what was said: I'd like them to understand that seeing something is not processing that information or hearing something is not the same as processing that information. I'd like them to understand that repeating it, often is a red flag that the information did not get processed and imitation and regurgitation of information is a red flag that language processing didn't occur. (Susan Reeves, West Texas Rehabilitation Center, San Angelo, Texas) Sindi Sands of Vancouver, Washington, summarized the learning-language connection with: In order to determine what is developmentally appropriate for our students, we need to change our thinking. Brains are not all the same and when we make that assumption we look at our children as being deficit or not measuring up when they struggle with the auditory formal kind of teaching we have done for so long. If we look at children as having differences in their brains, then we can look at their strengths and work from their strengths.
Question 4: What one strategy has worked best for you?	The top three responses were: hand-over-hand anything; picture dictionaries; drawing in real time (cartoons and flowcharts). Several people commented that they did not need to use rewards and punishers or token economies when they used these methods because their learners' needs were being met.

So, are VLMs effective? Well, for the professionals in the study, they chose to add VLMs to what they already knew. As part of their training, they also have learned to eliminate as much of the sound-based activities as possible. If the VLMs did not work, there would be no reason for these professionals to have continued to use them. This logical analysis does not provide the reader with a standardized design study in which the sound-based methods are compared to the visual methods, but if the majority of thinkers use visual cognition for learning to be literate, why use anything that is sound-based to teach them to be literate?

One other piece of data is important to mention: All of these educators who responded were well trained with state-of-the-art sound-based literacy approaches and programs but found that they obtained much better results when they used visual methods (e.g., see Arwood & Robb, 2008; Rostamizadeh, 2009b). Therefore, they made a conscious decision to do something that their colleagues were not doing.

Furthermore, the increase of sound-based programs and curricula in a sound-based culture has not shown success for the majority of the population: If less than 33 percent of eighth graders in the US are able to read, write, and do math at an eighth grade level (McCombs *et al.*, 2005); it would seem that such methods by their own use have not worked well in spite of copious data collections for specific sound-based literacy approaches. Logically, the professionals in the aforementioned study who used VLMs had the choice to use VLMs or stay with their previous sound-based training. They chose to change and have continued to use VLMs and to refine their visual methods over the years by attending more workshops and training on VLMs. Obviously, more than 6000 students have benefited from the use of translating English into visual methods. And, these students received the visual strategies, not as a default option of curricular or state-of-the-art adoptions, but because their educators had been trained in both and chose a different approach that matched what the professionals knew about language, brain function, and learning to be literate.

Activity: Why does education not compare data from different types of programs? Why is it logical to change to trying something that is logical and works for others than to continue to develop programs with the same sound-based assumptions?

Like the adults stated who had been video-taped and transcribed: They do not see the sounds and do not process the sounds. As one of the adults in the second group said, "I don't hear anything you say. I know you are talking. And, I do hear sound; but I do not know how the sound goes with what you are saying." Like all of these successful adults, she had learned a lot of oral language from her family and had learned to read the way print looked before she went to school. She was being trained to be an elementary teacher so she was asked, "How will you teach phonics?" She replied, "I can't. Right now, I am teaching math in the upper elementary and plan to stay with math." A few years later, she took a job with third graders. She was asked about the phonics; she said:

> I practice in the mirror what the sounds look like and then I stay with the script. I do the program exactly like it says to do it. And, then I teach the students how to see what is on the page, make sense of the page by making mental pictures, and then how to write using picture dictionaries.

This teacher is viewed as a fabulous teacher, but like so many teachers who have shared with the author, she does the programs and then spends time teaching visual ways for students to learn. Some teachers have told the author that they just don't have time in the day to do the "learning" piece because they feel they must spend time on the sound-based programs. What happens when some of the traditional sound-based methods are used while the teacher is adjusting what she or he does to make the methods perform better by using visual methods? Obviously, the data is not conclusive and validity must be challenged. The neuroscience shows that the brain can be trained in sound, but language function is greater than the parts of these sounds. Efficacy of using methods based on data of those who think with visual concepts triangulated against what is shown in brain research and what is known about language function appears ethically valid: Use the strengths of the learner.

Activity: What is the logical reasoning behind using VLMs for the majority of people to become literate?

Two-tier research model versus four-tier research model

The two-tier model is from Western Psychology, which supports the input-output form. Therefore, almost all research in English speaking countries follows the same interpretation bias. If sound comes into the person who hears okay, intervention must work on sounds if the person has not learned to produce sound-based literacy tasks. So sound training for all literacy aspects is encouraged. However, the four-tier Neuro-Semantic Language Learning Theory provided in the first chapters of this book is a four-tier model that investigates the conceptual and language levels of the brain function. As an example of application, Carnegie Mellon scientists (Just, Carpenter, Keller, Eddy, & Thulborn, 1996) have developed a wonderful method of exploring brain-based images of "nouns." The concept of a noun is a product of the two-tier model where parts of speech are labeled. The person speaks the words. The linguist analyzes the products and categorizes them (auditory task) by what the linguist sees (input-output). The Carnegie Mellon scientists (Mitchell, Shinkareva, Kai-Min Chang, Malave, Mason, & Just, 2008) looked for how thoughts (concepts) stimulated by words alone were accurately identified using brain images. They found that the storage could be put into three groups: (1) how a person physically interacts such as kicking it, etc.; (2) how it is related to eating such as biting or tasting; and (3) how it is related to shelter or enclosure. Note that these three categories are all related to language functions, not language structures. With the two-tier model, the use of products to interpret this data limits the meaning of the data to nouns are grouped by category. With the four-tier model, the interpretation of this research suggests that concepts are related to cognitive functions that involve neuronal circuitry such as using the arms or mouth for functions representative of the perceptual meaning.

This type of research at Carnegie Mellon will help move the paradigm of thinking underlying research and education from teaching types of two-tier models to a more conceptual learning model that involves multilayers of meaning. Table 16.4 shows a comparison of how the paradigm shift might develop.

Table 16.4 Academic problems compared with strategies

Emphasis	Outcomes	Philosophy	Theory	Culture	Measure	Source
Teaching	Development of skills (stair step)	Part to whole—behaviorism, constructivism, biophysical	Assumed norm-referenced bell-shaped curve	Two-tier model	Testing scores to find deficits	Mind
Learning	Acquisition of concepts (spiral)	Whole is greater than part-pragmaticism	Neuro-Semantic Language Learning Theory	Four-tier model	Assessing strengths	Brain

Note that the paradigm shift also changes the thinking from labeling the parts of the educational process to the whole purpose for education: To develop strengths in using language for conceptual thinking that promotes critical thinking and problem solving. Brain research supports such a shift.

Activity: What is the difference between the Western Psychology two-tier model and the proposed four-tier model?

Summary

Research on any topic is only as good as the questions asked; the theory used for interpreting the data; the logic used in the analysis; and the open mind of the individuals utilizing the data. It is the author's hope that she has raised some questions for the reader and has offered some alternative ways to look at the current plethora of sound-based auditory data that some call research. Furthermore, shifting toward a more strength-based, learning approach to education will, it is hoped, offer more opportunity for readers to think about alternative ways of meeting the needs of visual thinkers in an auditory culture.

The author would be remiss not to point out a conundrum: Literacy is language based so to be literate one must learn the concepts of the language in the way the person thinks (language functions). But, if education supports only an auditory way of thinking in its curriculum, what choices do the learners have? They can fail to become literate. They can struggle through the process of being taught, disliking school and eventually settling for a lesser level of education than they want. They can struggle through the process of being taught but learn to be literate outside of education by families who pay for outside of school. They can learn the bulk of their literacy before they go to school by learning to read, write, and talk so that school activities are games that don't make sense but do not hinder their development.

The answer to this puzzle rests not only with the learner but also with society: As literacy is language based, what happens if the vast majority of people are integrated into the workplace and are expected to achieve a certain level of literacy but don't because their education system does not promote literacy as a language function? Not only does the literacy "dumb-down," but also the language changes. Language changes to match the way people think, not the way the culture functions. Cultural values are expressed through the language.

So, if the status quo continues, with no attempt to understand the relationship between learning and language, language becomes more visual with more relational aspects. This change results from the thinkers representing their learning. And their levels of learning are dependent on the culture not promoting the complexity of the language for higher order thinking. But socio-political economics are auditory in nature (time-based with low context use of words). English speaking countries expect their citizens to work with formal concepts in multifaceted ways. This mismatch between culture and thinking could account for some major socio-political changes in some of these English speaking countries.

It may be difficult to address, but it appears to the author that some choices about how to address issues of literacy are important: Do these English speaking countries begin to lose their socio-political economic strength because literacy levels do not represent the auditory, time-based value and therefore the majority of citizens function at too low a literacy level? Or, does education begin to translate auditory language like English into visual-motor conventions with formal visual thinking and thereby retain the socio-political values of an auditory, time-based, economic culture?

Applications

- Using the described paradigm shift, what are some educational changes that may be warranted?
- Think about a time where there was a misunderstanding: was there anything that might have been language-based or cultural that contributed to he misunderstanding?

Appendix A

Arwood Neuro-Semantic Pre-Language Assessment Protocol (ANSPA)

Section I: Pre-language assessment

Pre-production or silent stage—observe the child during three different activities such as free play, working to do a task with a parent or educator such as winding up a new toy, and during routine activities of daily living like eating. Check for patterns of behavior. Record those patterns of behavior.

	Activity 1:	**Activity 2:**	**Activity 3:**
Productive use of hands—e.g., reaches			
Productive use of eyes—e.g., gazes to connect people and objects or actions			
Productive use of feet—e.g., walks, stands			
Productive use of body—e.g., sits, orients toward speaker			
Productive use of mouth—e.g., talks, uses C-V-C jargon, imitates			

<table>
<tr><td colspan="4">Interpretation:

Activity 1:
Activity 2:
Activity 3:</td></tr>
<tr><td colspan="4">How does this child learn best? Apply the Neuro-Semantic Language Learning Theory to the recorded behaviors.</td></tr>
<tr><td>Sensory input</td><td>Perceptual patterns</td><td>Concepts</td><td>Language</td></tr>
<tr><td></td><td></td><td></td><td></td></tr>
<tr><td>Interpretation:</td><td>Interpretation:</td><td>Interpretation:</td><td>Interpretation:</td></tr>
</table>

Section II: What do you have to do to see a change in the child's behavior?

....

....

....

....

....

....

Appendix B

Arwood Neuro-Semantic Language Learning Pre-Language Assessment Protocol

Section I: Pre-language assessment

Pre-production or silent stage—observe the child during three different activities such as free play, working to do a task with a parent or educator such as winding up a new toy, and during routine activities of daily living such as eating. Check for patterns of behavior. Record those patterns of behavior.

	Activity 1:	**Activity 2:**	**Activity 3:**
Productive use of hands—e.g., reaches			
Productive use of eyes—e.g., gazes to connect people and objects or actions			
Productive use of feet—e.g., walks, stands			
Productive use of body—e.g., sits, orients toward speaker			
Productive use of mouth—e.g., talks, uses C-V-C jargon, imitates			

<table>
<tr><td colspan="4">Interpretation:

Activity 1:
Activity 2:
Activity 3:</td></tr>
<tr><td colspan="4">How does this child learn best? Apply the Neuro-Semantic Language Learning Theory to the recorded behaviors.</td></tr>
<tr><td>Sensory input</td><td>Perceptual patterns</td><td>Concepts</td><td>Language</td></tr>
<tr><td></td><td></td><td></td><td></td></tr>
<tr><td>Interpretation:</td><td>Interpretation:</td><td>Interpretation:</td><td>Interpretation:</td></tr>
</table>

Section II: What do you have to do to see a change in the child's behavior?

(This is the intervention piece of the assessment…you may do this after analyzing the child's behavior or after a collection of language.)

Section III: Language sampling

Attach a sample and then analyze according to the following questions. Be sure to use examples.

1. Does the child address others and expect others to respond?
2. Are the child's utterances appropriate for the context?
3. Does the child use the utterances to share the meaning of the context?
4. Does the child use consistent age-appropriate forms (productivity)?
5. Does the listener have to interpret the child's meaning?
6. Is the use of displacement in the here-and-now?
7. Are the child's utterances flexible?
8. Are the child's utterances semantically accurate (semanticity) in meaning?
9. Are the child's utterances succinct in meaning or redundant?

Section IV: Interpretation—answer the following questions and provide examples

1. How does the child learn concepts?
2. What does the adult need to provide the child to meet the child's learning of concepts?
3. How does the child's behavior change in response to what the adult provides in the way the child learns concepts?

Glossary

Access—the way that patterns overlap and integrate to form concepts; access to the neuro-semantic learning system.

Acoustic patterns—these are patterns from the ears; these patterns do not include or represent meaningful ideas.

Actions—the acts performed by people or agents; part of the semantic relationship between people and their acts.

Agency (agents)—basic concepts about people and what people do.

Alphabetic—a property of English that refers to the use of changing the sounds of the spoken language into written letters.

Anti-social—behaviors or acts that do not contribute to the initiating of healthy relationships.

Articles—these parts of speech are used in English before nouns: a, an, and the.

Assigns meaning—the act of giving a shared meaning to a verbal or non-verbal act in either a non-verbal or verbal manner.

Associations—semantic error that results from connecting semantic features or patterns into meanings that are not conventional.

Auditory—a type of processing where the visual input from the eyes is connected simultaneously with the input from the ears; auditory concepts mean that a person is able to take the sounds of other people's language and integrate at the same time with what the person is able to see to form mental concepts that are in the thinker's own sound-based language.

Auditory languages—refers to those types of language that assume the listeners and speakers are able to understand the sound-based unit, the spoken word, from integrating both sound and sight simultaneously; English is an auditory language and can use multidirectional processing for the development of time concepts (see **time**).

Auditory misperception—a semantic error which results from not being able to process the auditory patterns; a production of an intended word but is really a pattern of perception, not a word; for example, flustrated for flustered and frustrated.

Auditory proposition—when two or more arguments are temporally connected with one more additional argument, then a larger concept is developed called a proposition; as English is an auditory language, the creation of propositions is an auditory, time-based language function.

Because language—the use of connecting ideas so that complete propositions are created; for example, "She is rolling up the window *because* she wants to be sure that you are safe from rocks that might fly up from the wheels of the other cars and hit you in the face."

Calculating—a literacy function that uses both patterns and concepts for solving numeracy problems.

Cessation—a language function that indicates either verbally or non-verbally that an action is to stop.

Cognition—also known as thinking or thoughts; typically divided into four stages: sensori-motor, preoperations, concrete operations, and formal operations.

Cognitive development—refers to the stages of thinking that children pass through sequentially: sensori-motor, preoperational, operational, and formal. Also, refers to the levels of concept attainment for an idea such as table. For a two-year-old, table refers to an object's function; for a five-year-old, table refers to a household object used for various actions. For a 10-year-old, table refers to a type of furniture; and for a 15-year-old, table does not always refer to an object, such as "tabling a motion." A person's cognitive development for specific concepts can be at any level at any age.

Communication—an observer or listener finds meaning in the non-verbal or verbal messages of another person; activities shared for a purpose among organisms or animals, even at a cellular level.

Concepts—ideas or thoughts that result from the overlap of perceptual patterns thus forming the third level of neuro-semantic meaning or conceptualization.

Conceptualization—the process by which concepts increase in meaning to form more understanding.

Concrete cognition—typically the third stage of cognition between 7 and 11 years old, characteristic of rules and examples from which to make decisions which can be used at any age.

Concrete operations—also known as the cognitive stage of concrete that typically occurs between 7 and 11 years and that represents tangible rules about others and their relationships to the learner.

Conjunction—these parts of speech are used in English to bring together or conjoin to or more words or phrases; for example, "and" is a conjunction in "Sally and John walked together."

Consonant-vowel-consonant (C-V-C)—English is referred to as a CVC or C-V-C language, meaning that most words are formed from altering consonants followed by vowels followed by consonants. C-V-C structures refer to the "sounds" of the English language, not the written or orthographic letters. For example, "mail" has two vowels when it is written but the two vowels (a and i) are really just one sound so it is a C-V-C word in sound properties.

Consonants—the sounds of a language that are produced by changing the airflow of the nasal and pharyngeal airways or the articulation of airflow; provide the discrete meaning of the airflow pattern; distinctive to the place and manner of sound production for speech.

Context—the verbal and non-verbal relationships that create the shared environment among speakers for language; English requires words that use low context for usage; that is, words can stand alone whereas Mandarin uses concepts that are relational so speaking Mandarin uses high context (semantic relationships) (see **high context** and **low context**).

Conventions—acceptable language structures and functions that two or more people agree upon in meaning; all languages consist of conventions.

Conversational function—the ability to share meaning in a reciprocal fashion of referring and predicating a message or proposition.

Corpora— a large sample of spoken language that is recorded and transcribed.

Critical thinking—the ability to make choices of reasonableness that reflect the pro-social development of a society; to share those choices with others to problem solve through mediation of thought from multiple perspectives.

Cross-modal—the use of multiple inputs to develop meaning in language such as the eyes provide meaning from what is seen while the ears provide meaning to what is heard; language symbolization requires some form of cross-modal development whether from within the same sensory system such as light and movement with the eyes or from two different senses.

Decoding—the ability to decipher patterns into meaningful clusters; could be acoustic patterns as in the sounds of words or could be visual patterns as in the shapes of ideas.

Denying—the act of not allowing meaning to be real; a basic language function that develops in the first two years of language use such as a mom telling her son that it is time for a nap and the son saying, "no, no, no…" over and over. The nap will happen but the son does not want the reality of a nap to happen.

Determiners—these words define the specificity of meaning of people, places, and objects (nouns); for example, "the" table "determines" a different meaning than "a" table.

Displacement—an expanded language function also known as a linguistic function that develops as cognition increases the meaning of ideas further and further away from the physical source; for example, ideas such as liberty are more displaced because they are non-tangible than an idea about a kitchen table which is tangible.

Distance receptors (senses)—the two sensory receptors that can receive input away from the source are the eyes which receive light and the war which receives sound; note that the eye, unlike the ear, also can receive input from an immediate source by the shape of movements.

Echolalia—acoustic patterns that are imitations of delayed or immediate input.

Encoding—the process of turning patterns into spoken or written ideas; patterns can be acoustic as in sequencing sounds or visual as in sequencing shapes.

English language learners (ELLs)—refers to people who speak another language than English first and therefore are learning English; sometimes children who are learning English as their native language are also referred to as ELLs.

Event-based—an event consists of a story with agents, actions, objects in relationship with each other to develop a preoperational context.

Existence—a early language function that indicates that something exists.

Existing—a language function of whether something is here or not here that develops within the first couple of years and later interpreted as cause and effect; for example, a child runs up and shows a toy (existence) and then runs around and looks for the toy when he or she can't see it (non-existence).

Expanded language functions—language is used to expand on basic functions of agents, actions, and objects for more complex meanings (semanticity), for greater variety of language use (productivity), for greater use of language in a variety of settings (flexibility), and for more efficiency (limited redundancy).

Expansions—sentence structure complexity increases such as "the dog is big" becomes "the big dog belongs to my sister."

Extending—a simple language function of increasing the meaning of a basic semantic relationship; for example, an agent becomes "boy."

Extension—process by which meaning is adding to underlying thoughts; for example, a child thinks a dog is all animals with four legs so she calls a cat, a dog and her mom adds (extends) the meaning by telling the child that a cat has whiskers and meows while a dog does not have whiskers like a cat and how a dog barks. Also, the child may think of the space the child is in as part of the world or an extension of the objects of the world; Mom's arms, the sofa; the bed; and so forth.

First language (L1)—this is the home language or the language the child first hears and uses; native language.

Flexibility—an expanded language function, also known as a linguistic function, that refers to the way that a person is able to use language about the particular topic in a variety of places.

Formal operations—also known as formal thinking or formal cognition, which typically does not occur before age 11 and represents the most linguistic function in meaning; most abstract in ideation.

Function of language—the cognitive way language represents thinking, problem solving, and planning according to cultural and social norms.

Functors—in English, these are the words that are non-specific in meaning such as the small words (e.g., so, as, in, on, of, the) that "function" to determine the meaning.

Gaze—eye movement and focus shows recognition of people (agents), their actions, and their objects; pre-production child uses gaze to indicate a semantic relationship among people, their actions, and their objects; gaze can also be acoustic for children, especially those who are blind, visually impaired, or severely impacted by autism spectrum disorders, to indicate same semantic relationships.

Gestural sign—also known as g-sign which is a conventional movement or posture of the body that people agree in meaning such as pointing.

Global language—refers to the most translated second language for most commercial and economic uses; often considered a world language that is used by many different people on different continents, which becomes elevated to a language that dominates for communication efficiency.

Gloss—an interpretation of meaning that assumes the listener's meaning as part of the speaker's words; for example, the speaker says, "My dirt bike" and the listener glosses the meaning to be "This is my dirt bike that I like to ride."

Grammar—the structures (syntax, morphology, semantics, and phonology) of a language that includes the rules for the native speakers of that language.

Graphemes—these are the written units of meaning.

Greeting—a type of specific language function that is a speech act among two or more people; culture determines the semantic rules for how to meet another person acceptably.

Ground—the process by which a person thinks, consciously or subconsciously, about the person's body in connection to the space around the person; for example, in order for a young child to write with a pencil, he must keep a significant portion of his body still or grounded so as to move the arm independently.

Hand-over-hand—the process of putting the adult's hand onto the learner's hand in order to help the learner with the exact patterns to form drawn concepts, correct written patterns, finger spelling patterns, or sign language patterns.

High context—some languages are field sensitive in that the culture requires speakers to create meaning among people and their purpose for speaking and the setting; Mandarin speakers are field sensitive and therefore the language is a high-context language.

Indicates—a verbal or non-verbal meaning (indicator) that represents an act such as looking up at a hot air balloon suggests to others that the person is "looking" at something.

Infinite grammar—language rules of structures provide for an infinite set of possible combinations.

Inhibition—a neurological process which provides feedback to lower central nervous system structures that the input is old; a psychological process by which impulses are limited.

Integration—a sensory-perceptual process of the neurology that allows for interconnecting of patterns to form higher functions within the cellular systems.

Intend—a function of language that provides purpose for meaning (intentions or the act of intending).

Interpret meaning—listener is expected to determine the message and intent of the speaker.

Language—conventional form of communication; the fourth and last level of the Neuro-Semantic Language Learning Theory; represents the underlying thinking processes as cognitive functions and the surface forms as imitated structures.

Language functions—the underlying cognitive understanding or thinking that language represents; basic language functions occur in early cognitive development (up to seven years old) and then are expanded and extended into more complex thinking where conversation is easily shared as a language function (seven and above).

Language sampling—the process of recording consecutive and representative natural language from a speaker and then transcribing the speaker's words so as to analyze the speaker's level of language structures or language functions.

Language structures—the surface forms of language that linguists study; for example, there are many types of structures in English such as words, phrases, sentences, parts of speech, syntax, phons, morphemes, and so forth; structures are easily taught through imitation, repetition, and practice.

Layer(ing)—the process by which the meaning of a concept increases in depth by adding more patterns or related concepts.

Learning strategies—intentional cognitive rules used explicitly to translate input form into meta-cognitive processes that match the way a person's neurobiological system creates concepts.

Lexical tags—specific words within a person's lexicon (see **lexicon** and **tag**).

Lexicon—an individual's meanings for concepts or ideas; for example, people who live in Oregon often call tinsel for a Christmas tree "freezing rain" because their meaning for tinsel is related specifically to experiences with freezing rain where they live; therefore, their lexicon for what decorates a Christmas tree is different from a person who lives in the desert. Each person has a unique lexicon because no two people have the same experiences.

Limited language structure—frequency of language structures is less than expected; in many cases, the structures are two or three words in length and rarely are used.

Linguistic function—most complex use of language to extend the meaning of concepts and to expand the structures of language into formal thinking; language grammar is adult-like by age eight, but underlying thinking of function continues to extend meaning in space, time, quality, and quantity semantic fields which results in increasing the symbolization of language into linguistic function where maximum displacement, semanticity, flexibility, and productivity occurs for best efficiency (succinct surface forms with limited redundancy).

Listening—the ability to understand what others say; either by hearing or seeing their meaning.

Literacy—the language functions and structures of reading, writing, thinking, listening, speaking, viewing, and calculating; the processes by which language acquisition is used for reading, writing, thinking, viewing, speaking, listening, and calculating.

Lots of language structures—this implies that the speaker is able to talk a lot but the function of the language is limited to surface level of the structures; language functions are restricted.

Low context—some languages are not field-sensitive in that they do not use the setting and all of the relationships of the setting to create meaning in preparation for oral language; English uses low context.

Mark (marking)—to assign a meaning to an idea such as to mark or to name a person or an object or a place; for example, the lady said the house was huge means that she "marked" the size of the house for others so that they know she thinks the house is "huge."

Misconceptions—the act of understanding something in a different way than most people expect; often the result of not acquiring the perceptual patterns necessary to form specificity of concepts.

Misperceptions—production of sound according to the way the speaker hears the sounds; patterns are produced by what is perceived to be the correct form.

Modulate (modulation)—to change the meaning in a language such as to add morphemes to words; for example, add "-ly" to terrible to change an adjective (terrible movie) to form an adverb (she was terribly sorry).

Morphemes—the smallest meaningful unit of language that speakers are consciously aware of such as adding an "s," a bound morpheme, for plurality in English; or, the use of "dog," a free morpheme that can stand alone. Dogs is two morphemes; dog + s.

Morphology—the study of the smallest meaningful units (morphemes) of a language.

Native speaker—whichever language a person speaks first makes that person a "native speaker" of the first language.

Natural language—the function of language according to expected societal conventions; representative of semantic acquisition.

Negating—an early language function occurring within the first couple of years of language that negates what someone says; for example, "That is a big dog" and the child negates it by saying, "No, dog little."

Neologism—this refers to the creation of new words; may result from putting new sound sequences together (phonological neologism such as "the dan" for man); changing morpheme sequences such as copheliter for helicopter; and/or arranging words for a semantic neologism such as "put ons" for socks.

Neuro-atypical learner—person whose development does not follow predicted outcomes; whose socio-cognitive learning (functions) is different than expected.

Neurobiological learning system—the central nervous system pathways that allow for incoming information to create tracks of learning for later recall and retrieval.

Neuronal circuits—several connections of cell clusters of nuclei occur to form concepts.

Neuro-semantic—meaning in the central nervous system (brain and spinal cord) comes from the development of input at four levels (sensory, perceptual, conceptual, and language) as defined in Arwood's Neuro-Semantic Language Learning Theory.

Neuro-typical learner—person whose development does follow predicted outcomes; whose socio-cognitive learning (functions) is similar to what is expected.

Non-existence—a language function that suggests something is not present.

Objects—acted upon by agents or people within a setting or context.

On-topic—speaker or hearer stays with the referring and predicating process shared with another person.

Off-topic—a semantic error in understanding the functions of referring to what is shared between two speakers in a conversational task.

Overlap patterns—as sensory input increases and the body recognizes the input of these patterns, they begin to overlap increasing the depth of meaning to form a concept; concepts also overlap and form more depth in conceptualization.

Parts of speech—a way to categorize a language by surface structure such as nouns, verbs, prepositions, adverbs, conjunctions, and articles.

Pattern recognition—at the second level of neuro-semantic organization, the receptor organs and brain stem along with higher mid-brain structures are able to detect (recognize) whether or not input is old or new.

Patterns—see **perceptual patterns**.

Perception—the second level of meaning in neuro-semantic development; formed from the overlap of sensory input as perceptual patterns; also considered the process by which a person's body recognizes the sensory input as meaningful. As all people have unique input, all perception is valid.

Perceptual patterns—neuro-anatomy recognizes the organization of the sensory input in the neuro-semantic development as patterns of perception or perceptual patterns.

Performative—some English words actually perform a speech act such as worry, promise, vow, kill, marry, and divorce; these performatives create a meaning that is greater than the individual words.

Perseveration (perseverative behavior)—the repetition of an act or behavior as the result of patterns of input not integrating into concepts; provides the neural system more and more patterns at the same level.

Phonemes—the smallest meaningful unit of sound; phonemes consist of parts of sounds or phons; often organized by place of production and manner of production as distinctive features.

Phonics—a set of rules designed to explain the relationship between the gap of spoken English, an alphabetic language that has evolved quickly, and a standard written language that has evolved more slowly.

Phonology—the study of the sounds and sound sequences of a language.

Portability—in linguistics, this concept refers to the ability of speakers to talk, read, write, and speak about an idea that is at a distance from the source of the idea; the way a language allows speakers to take an idea to another place; to move about with ideas; to share ideas with others who do not necessarily have direct experience about an idea; for example, modern-day speakers are able to talk about Ancient Egypt.

Possessive pronouns—these words are used to refer to belonging to someone or some group or agency, such as "her" is a possessive pronoun in the phrase "her dog."

Pragmaticism—a term coined by Charles Sanders Peirce to mean the whole is greater than the parts so that a child's complete story is greater than the words within the story; it is not the same as pragmatism.

Pragmatics—the study of the rules for how language and a person's behavior relate; for example, turn taking is a unit of pragmatic analysis. Pragmatics is the study of how language functions to represent social development.

Predication—language function that connects two or more ideas into a bigger idea; words like "also," "however," "even though," and conditionals such as "if, then" lend themselves connecting two or more arguments.

Pre-language function—thinking occurs about people, their objects, and their actions before a child actually develops a full grammar; this period of functioning is pre-language in nature.

Preoperational cognition—second stage of thinking for most neuro-typical children between three and seven years; characteristic of thinking the world revolves around the person which could occur at any age.

Preposition—a part of speech that places attribution to a phrase such as the word "on" is a preposition in the phrase "on the box" that provides the meaning (attributes meaning) for where something is placed as in, "She put the book on the box," or, where something is located as in, "The bowl is on the box."

Pre-production period—this period of language development occurs when a child is learning the meaning but does not yet have the structures to express the child's ideas; same as silent period with English language learners.

Productivity—an expanded language function also known as a linguistic function that refers to the ability to create a variety of utterances about the same topic.

Pronouns—when an object or person is referred to in a non-specific way, such as "she" is a pronoun to refer to a specific person, Sally.

Propositions—messages formed from connecting more than two arguments or ideas together with complex time-based language; also auditory propositions.

Pro-social—acts or behaviors that contribute to the initiation and maintenance of healthy relationships.

Reading—is a process by which a reader uses his or her language as a tool to interpret the meaning of the ideas on a page.

Real time—the activity takes place in front of the listener or the observer; real-time drawing occurs in front of the learner, not before class.

Receptors—anything that receives, as in the human organs that receive sensory input; eyes, ears, nose, mouth, and skin.

Recursive principle—the ability to expand language function within language structures; to add meaning by completing predications of multiple propositions such as "The girl, who is my neighbor, forgot to roll the cans out to the street (two sets of arguments) for the city waste management folks (connected by predication to another set of arguments) which means that I will have too much garbage this week" (connected to a third set which forms a proposition that infers: if cans are not emptied, then there is too much waste by agreement with city waste management).

Redundancy—an expanded language function also known as a linguistic function that refers to the way that meaning overlaps increasing the cognitive meaning while limiting the structural redundancy of language.

Refer (referring function)—a language function that specifies ideas; the act of referring occurs at the language thinker's level of function.

Referent—that idea which is specified.

Referential clarity—the act of being able to use specific meaning of a referent that is shared or conventional in nature.

Rejecting (rejection)—the language function of not accepting what a person says, does, or offers; often developed in the first couple of years of language and can be demonstrated non-verbally or verbally.

Relational languages—those languages that contextually use a culture where the relationships among people, their actions, objects and locations are more important than the meaning of words.

Requesting—an early language function that is also a speech act; as an early function a child wants an object, an action, or an agent. Requests become more advanced and change from simple speech acts to performatives such as promise (see **performative**).

Restricted language—refers to limited linguistic function of language; typically, restricted function occurs in children up to seven years old or in pidgin language; restricted language utilizes limited grammatical complexity as well as limited meaning of concepts.

Retag—refers to the use of a synonym or similar meaning for another word. Dachshund retags dog.

Scaffold—an interactive process between a learner and another person who assigns meaning to verbal and non-verbal acts of the learner; in this way, the learning increases in a spiral process of overlapping meanings to more complex layers of meaning.

Semantic complexity—patterns, concepts, and language are comprised of meaningful features that increase over time. This increase in feature attainment refers to the complexity of the meaning or semantics of the pattern, concept, or language function.

Semantic correction—process of assigning a new meaning so as to refine or correct the meaning expressed; e.g., a parent says "that is a dog" to a child's use of "cat" for a four-legged animal in a friend's home.

Semantic features—these are the parts of the sensory input such as particular sounds or sights or pieces of a whole such as seeing the wings on an insect but not seeing the insect.

Semantic field—a collection of related terms such as cooking utensils is a type of semantic field.

Semantic relationships—cognitive development of the connections among the basic concepts of people (agents), their actions, and their objects within a context or setting; an understanding of these relationships may occur non-verbally such as with pointing or verbally by using words to indicate the meaning among these concepts such as "mommy juice." Semantic meaning also increases through expanded or linguistic functions to increase the complexity of relationships.

Semantic word errors—misuse of a word meaning such as saying the teacher gave us several "school" words for "skill" words which could also be an auditory misperception; misuse of conventional meaning of words such as "I lit the light" where light is used in place of candle.

Semanticity—an expanded language function also known as a linguistic function that refers to an increase of meaning for any concept; for example, a cat becomes more specified as a type of cat, Persian, which then becomes more specified as the "neighbor's Persian cat." The concept can continue to acquire meaning until it no longer refers to a tangible concept; for example, the lady is a cat means that she is spiteful, not a four-legged feline.

Semantics—the study of the meaning of language; at four levels; or as a study of the conceptual, thinking level of language.

Sensation—the first level of neuro-semantic meaning where sensory input is organized by the receptor organs (eyes, ears, mouth, skin, nose).

Sensori-motor cognition—the first stage of cognitive development typically between 0 and two years of age where the input is in sensory form and the output is in a motor form.

Sensory input—the first level of meaning from the physical forms of light, sound, touch, taste, and smell.

Shared referent—two or more people are able to understand the meaning of an idea through common context of agents, their actions, their objects within an event.

Signs—a verbal or non-verbal meaning that must be interpreted; for example, an octagonal shape with the letters "S-t-o-p" is a pattern that means something or the movement of the hands into a manual sign means something to another person who is able to interpret the sign.

Silent period—refers to the time when a speaker of a first language other than English is beginning to learn English but has not yet developed the English structures; so, the English language learner is listening and waiting to learn the structures to represent ideas and is therefore silent in English.

Social competence—the ability to initiate and maintain healthy relationships.

Social development—one of five developmental domains that defines the way a person is like others within a culture.

Social intentions—the purpose for communicating to another person, especially used to describe young children's utterances (see **intend**).

Social interactions—the way that a culture defines appropriate communication or spending time together.

Spatial development—a semantic field of ideas related to understanding the properties of space around a person; horizontal, vertical, and diagonal space represented by words such as up, down, on, in, between, for, over, and so forth.

Spatial words—these concepts refer to the movement across horizontal, vertical, and diagonal planes; languages can use spatial relationships among ideas to create context for communication, such as American Sign Language or Mandarin are both spatial languages.

Speaking—the use of acoustic-motor patterns to represent conceptual language as a literacy function.

Speech acts—the function of verbal and non-verbal acts in relationship to a hearer and a speaker as defined by semantic constituent rules; for example, assertions, statements of information, requests, and rule orders are all speech acts.

Spontaneous imitation—a language function that occurs around 18 to 24 months used to assign underlying conceptual meaning to language structures; the use of spontaneous imitation increases the child's cognitive development from sensory input recognition to more conceptual preoperational thinking.

Strategy learning—process by which a person acquires ways to access his or her learning system better for developing higher order thinking or more complex conceptualization.

Strong test of grammar—the language shows maximum semantic complexity through expanded and extended language functions of displacement, semanticity, flexibility, productivity, and limited structural redundancy.

Structures—parts like in building or the whole of the parts as the building; see language structures.

Subject-verb-object (S-V-O)—this is typically considered the way that words are put together for the syntax of English.

Symbolization—an advanced language function also known as a linguistic function that raises the meaning of a concept through the use of a complete grammar to form meaning that is greater than the parts; for example, symbolization of the words, "If you report him, then he will be arrested" symbolizes the "if-then" statement as conditional; one thing happens as a result of something else.

Symbols—advanced level of meaning for representing a concept; for example, a stop sign only indicates (see **indicates**) a pattern or rule to stop until a reader of the sign thinks about all of the relationships of what might happen if the driver of a car does not stop at the sign (see **signs**).

Syntax—the study of word order of a language.

Tag—the individual marker or specific lexicon that a person uses; for example, a child may use the word "pop" for a drink and therefore the child's tag is "pop" whereas another child says "soda" and so that child's tag for a drink is "soda" and so forth.

Tangential (tangentiality)—a semantic problem; redundancy of ideas where related concepts are discussed.

Telegraphic—ideas that are represented with one or two words; usually represents underlying cognitive semantic relationships.

Temporal words—these words refer to meanings about time such as before, during, while, when, so, also, day, afternoon, forever, whenever, and so forth.

Thinking—a literacy function that refers to the development of concepts created by the synergy of neuronal circuits of the brain; could be visual or auditory.

Time—a property of English represented by a variety of temporal words as well as by the structure of the language and the use of specific ways to assign meaning to referents (use of functors); time is multidirectional in that time can go through a speaker or a speaker can go through time resulting in properties of time allowing for multi-tasking in a culture; time-based languages use temporal properties.

Time-based—English is a language that marks time which makes the language very portable in that language can go into the future, past, or present in relationship to time.

Utterances—the spoken phrases or sentences of a speaker.

Viconic Language Methods™—the use of what is known about visual languages imposed upon auditory English so as to help a visual thinker translate visual cognition into auditory English.

Viewing—a language function of literacy; the ability to understand one's world in the way that concepts develop.

Visual languages—those languages that use field-sensitive contexts for specifying the relationship among people, their actions, objects, and locations, such as Mandarin and Hopi are both visual languages.

Visual patterns—vision provides sensory input in light and movement. These light and movement features form patterns from the points of light and edges or shapes of movement also known as visual patterns.

Visual thinking—the use of a visual meta-cognition; utilizes the same properties as a relational or visual language.

Vowels—the energy of speech is carried by the constriction of airflow in the oral cavity at the same time as producing a vibratory resonance within the trachea.

Weak test of grammar—the language is restricted to the interpretation of the listener; examples of restricted grammars are pidgins, texting, and chimpanzee language.

Words—the unit of English analysis typically consisting of consonant-vowel-consonant combinations; alphabetic in nature; word-based languages like English do not consider the context important in understanding the meaning of a word.

Writing—the ability to encode visual-motor patterns or sounds-letters into meaningful constructs that others read.

References

American Psychiatric Association (2000). *The diagnostic and statistical manual of mental disorders: Fourth edition text-revision* (DSMIV-TR). Washington, DC: Author.

Angus, G. (1977). Thinking with restricted language: A personal construct investigation of pre-lingually profoundly deaf apprentices. *British Journal of Psychology, 68*(2), 253–255.

Arwood, E. (1983). *Pragmaticism: Theory and application.* Gaithersberg, MD: Aspen.

Arwood, E. (1985). *APRICOT I Kit*. Portland, OR: APRICOT.

Arwood, E. (1991a). *Semantic and pragmatic language disorders* (2nd ed.). Gaithersberg, MD: Aspen.

Arwood, E. (1991b). *Video-tape of nine adults*. Unpublished manuscript, Portland, OR: APRICOT.

Arwood, E. (2003). *Video-tape of six adults*. Unpublished manuscript, Portland, OR: APRICOT.

Arwood, E. (2010). *Efficacy of VLMs*. Unpublished manuscript, University of Portland, Portland, OR.

Arwood, E., Bahls, G., & Crabtree, R. (1986). *Acoustic reflex, reading, writing, and oral language found in learning disabled adults matched with typical learning adults*. Unpublished manuscript, Lubbock, TX: Texas Tech University.

Arwood, E., & Beggs, M. (1989). *Temporal analysis of propositions (TEMPRO)* [Test]. Portland, OR: APRICOT.

Arwood, E., & Brown, M. (1999). *A guide to cartooning and flowcharting.* Portland, OR: APRICOT.

Arwood, E., & Brown, M. (2001). *A guide to visual strategies for young adults.* Portland, OR: APRICOT.

Arwood, E., & Brown, M. (2002). *Balanced literacy: Phonics, viconics, kinesics*. Portland, OR: APRICOT.

Arwood, E., Brown, M., & Robb, B. (2005). *Make it visual in the classroom*. Portland, OR: APRICOT.

Arwood, E., & Kaakinen, J. (2004). Visual language strategies for innovative teaching of science. *Journal of Science Education for Students with Disabilities, 10*, 27–36.

Arwood, E., & Kaakinen, J. (2008). Visual teaching in an auditory world [DVD]. *Advanced academy for teaching and learning.* Corvallis, OR: Center for Teaching and Learning, Oregon State University.

Arwood, E., & Kaakinen, J. (2009). SIMulation Based on Language and Learning (SIMBaLL): The model. *International Journal for Nursing Education Scholarship, 6*(1), article 9. Retrieved from: www.bepress.com/ijnes/vol6/issi/art9. Accessed September 6, 2010.

Arwood, E., Kaakinen, J., & Wynne, A. (2002). *Nurse educators: Using visual language*. Portland, OR: APRICOT.

Arwood, E., & Kaulitz, C. (2007). *Learning with a visual brain in an auditory world: Language strategies for individuals with autism spectrum disorders.* Shawnee Mission, KS: Autism Asperger Publishing Company.

Arwood, E., Kaulitz, C., & Brown, M. (2009). *Visual thinking strategies for individuals with autism spectrum disorders: The language of pictures.* Shawnee Mission, KS: Autism Asperger Publishing Company.

Arwood, E., & McInroy, J. (1995). *Introduction to pragmaticism: The workshop*. Portland, OR: APRICOT.

Arwood, E., & Robb, B. (2008). Language events in a classroom. *ESL Magazine, 61*. Chichester: Keyways Publishing.

Arwood, E., & Unruh, I. (1997). *Reading/writing: It's so easy to see (RISES II)*. Portland, OR: APRICOT.

Arwood, E., & Young, E. (2000). *The language of RESPECT: The right of each student to participate in an environment of communicative thoughtfulness*. Portland, OR: APRICOT.

Austin, J. L. (1962). *How to do things with words* [Lectures for Harvard]. London: Oxford University Press.

Ballenger, T. (2009, October 26). Multi-tangle. *The Boston Globe*. Boston, MA: Globe.

Barr, R. G., & Peters, R. (Eds.) (2005). *Encyclopedia on early childhood development*, 1–5 [Online]. Montreal, Quebec: Centre of Excellence for Early Childhood Development. Retrieved from: www.child-encyclopedia.com/documents/CleaveANGxp.pdf. Accessed January 28, 2010.

Basor, E. (2006). The theory of the whole-brain-work. *International Journal of Psychophysiology, 60*, 133–138.

Begley, S. (2007). *Train your mind: Change your brain*. New York: Ballantine.

Berenstain Bears (1962). *The big honey hunt: Beginner books*. New York: Random House.

Bloom, L., & Lahey, M. (1978). *Language development and language disorders*. Somerset, NJ: John Wiley & Sons.

Bookheimer, S. (2004). Overview on learning and memory: Insights from functional brain imaging. *Learning Brain Expo Conference Proceedings*. San Diego, CA: Brain Store.

Bradford, J. D., & National Research Council (2000). *Brain, mind, experience, and school*. Washington, DC: National Academy Press.

Breedlove, S. M., Rosenzweig, M., & Watson, N. V. (2007). *Biological psychology* (5th ed.). Sunderland, MA: Sinauer Associates.

Britten, R. J. (2002). Divergence between samples of chimpanzee and human DNA sequences is 5% counting indels. *Proceedings National Academy Science, 99*, 13,633–13,635.

Brown, M. (1979). *Speech act types in three-year-old children*. Unpublished thesis, Pullman, WA: Washington State University.

Brown, R. (1973). *A first language: The early stages*. Cambridge, MA: Harvard University Press.

Bruner, J. S. (1983). *Child's talk: Learning to use language*. New York: Norton.

Buccino, G., Vogt, S., Ritzl, A., Fink, G., Zilles, K., Freund, H., & Rizzolatti, G. (2009). Neural circuits underlying imitation learning of hand actions. An event-related FMRI study. *Neuron, 42*(2), 323–334.

Butler, A. B., & Hodos, W. (2008). *Comparative vertebrate neuroanatomy: Evolution and adaptation*. New York: John Wiley & Sons.

Caffarel, A., Martin, J. R., & Matthiessen, C. M. I. M. (Eds.) (2004). *Language typology: A functional perspective*. Philadelphia, PA: John Benjamins.

Calvert, G. A., Brammer, M. J., Bullmore, E. T., Campbell, R., Iversen, S. D., & David, A. S. (1999). Brain imaging: Response amplification in sensory-specific cortices during crossmodal binding. *NeuroReport, 10*(12), 2619–2623.

Calvin, W. H. (1996). *How brains think: Evolving intelligence then and now*. New York: Basic Books.

Carroll, J. B. (1956). *Language, thought, and reality: Selected writings by Benjamin Lee Whorf*. Cambridge, MA: MIT Press.

Carruthers, S. A. (1997). *Language, thought, and consciousness: An essay in philosophical psychology*. Cambridge: Cambridge University Press.

Chomsky, N. (2002). *Syntactic structures*. Berlin: Walter de Gruyter. (Original work published 1957)

Cleave, P. L. (2005, January 17). Services and programs supporting young children's language development: Comments on Girolametto, and Thiemann and Warren. *Encyclopedia on early childhood development* [Online]. Retrieved from: The neurobiology of www.enfant-encyclopedie.com/Pages/PDF/CleaveANGxp.pdf. Accessed November 18, 2009.

Coltman, P., Petyaeva, D., & Anghileri, J. (2002). Scaffolding learning through meaningful tasks and adult interaction. *Early Years: Journal of International Research and Development, 22*(1), 39–49.

Compagni, A., & Manderscheid, R. W. (2006). A neuroscientist–consumer alliance to transform mental health care. *Journal of Behavioral Health Services and Research, 23*(2), 265–274.

Cooper, J. D. (2006). *Literacy: Helping children construct meaning*. Burlington, MA: Houghton Mifflin.

Damasio, A. (1994). *Descartes' error: Emotion, reason, and the human brain*. New York: Putnam.

Damasio, A. (2003). *Looking for Spinoza: Joy, sorrow, and the feeling brain*. New York: Harcourt Brace.

Dana Foundation (2007). *Cerebrum*. New York: Dana Press.

Dance, F. E. X. (1985). The functions of human communication. In B. D. Ruben (Ed.) *Information and behavior* (Vol. 1). New Brunswick, NJ: Transaction.

Deacon, T. W. (1997). *The symbolic species: The co-evolution of language and the brain*. New York: Norton.

Decety, J., Grezes, J., Costes, N., Perani, D., Jeannerod, M., Procyk, E., Grassi, F., & Fazio, F. (1997). Brain activity during observation of actions: Influence of action content and subject's strategy. *Brain, 120*(10), 1763–1777.

Dore, J. (1975). Holophrases, speech acts, and language universals. *Journal of Child Language, 2*(1), 21–40.

Emmorey, K. (1993). Processing a dynamic visual–spatial language: Psycholinguistic studies of American Sign Language. *Journal of Psycholinguistic Research, 22*(2), 153–187.

Fletcher, P., & Garman, M. (1997). *Language acquisition* (2nd ed.). New York: Press Syndicate of the University of Cambridge.

Fouts, R. S., Jensvold, M. L. A., & Fouts, D. H. (2002). Chimpanzee signing: Darwinian realities and Cartesian delusions. In M. Bekoff, C. Allen & G. Burghardt (Eds.) *The cognitive animal: Empirical and theoretical perspectives in animal cognition* (pp. 285–291). Cambridge, MA: MIT Press.

Fouts, R. S., & Waters, G. (2001). Chimpanzee sign language and Darwinian continuity: Evidence for a neurology continuity of language. *Neurological Research, 23*, 787–794.

Franke, P., Leboyer, M.,Gänsicke, M., Weiffenbach, O., Biancalana, V., Cornillet-Lefebre, P., Croquette, M. F., *et al.* (1998). Genotype–phenotype relationship in female carriers of the premutation and full mutation of FMR-1. *Psychiatry Research, 80*(2), 113–127.

Fry, P. G., Phillips, K., Lobaugh, G., & Madole, S. (1996). Halliday's functions of language: A framework to integrate elementary-level social studies and language arts. *Social Studies, 87*, 76–78.

Gal, S., & Irvine, J. T. (1995). The boundaries of languages and disciplines: How ideologies construct difference. *Social Research, 62*, 967–1002.

Galaburda, A., & Livingstone, M. (1993). Evidence for a magnocellular defect in developmental dyslexia. *Annals New York Academy of Sciences, 682*, 70–82.

Gallese, V. (1999). From grasping to language: Mirror neurons and the origins of social communication. In S. R. Hameroff, A. W. Kaszniak, & D. J. Chalmers (Eds.) *Toward a science of consciousness III: The third Tucson discussions and debates* (MIT conference proceedings). New York: Bradford Books.

Gallese, V., & Lakoff, G. (2005). The brain's concepts: The role of the sensory-motor system in conceptual knowledge. *Cognitive Neuropsychology, 22*(3–4), 455–479.

García, O., & Otheguy, R. (1989). *English across cultures, cultures across English: A reader in cross-cultural communication.* Berlin: Walter de Gruyter.

Gazzaniga, M. S. (1999). *The new cognitive neurosciences* (2nd ed.). Cambridge, MA: MIT Press.

Gazzaniga, M. S. (2005). *The ethical brain.* New York: Dana Press.

Gil, D. (2004, January 8). Babel's children. *Economist, 370*, 69–70. Retrieved from: http://tinyurl.com/3zmbxq (www.economist.com/science). Accessed July 27, 2010.

Gill, H. (2008). *Thinking and learning through drawing in the primary classrooms.* Thousand Oaks, CA: Sage.

Givon, T. (2009). *The genesis of syntactic complexity.* Amsterdam: John Benjamins.

Gleason, J., Berko, J., & Weintraub, S. (1976). The acquisition of routines in child language. *Language in Society, 5*, 129–136.

Goldberg, E. (2001). *The executive brain: Frontal lobes and the civilized mind.* New York: Oxford University Press.

Goldblum, N. (2001). *The brain-shaped mind: What the brain can tell us about the mind.* Cambridge: Cambridge University Press.

Goodwin, C. (Ed.) (2003). *Conversation and brain damage.* New York: Oxford University Press.

Greenfield, S. A. (1997). *The human brain: A guided tour.* New York: Basic Books.

Greenough, W. T., Black, J. E., & Wallace, C. S. (1987). Experience and brain development. *Child Development, 58*, 539–559.

Grice, H. P. (1989). *Studies in the way of words.* Cambridge, MA: Harvard University Press.

Hall, C. J. (2005). *An introduction to language and linguistics.* New York: Continuum.

Halliday, M. A. K. (1975). *Learning how to mean: Explorations in the development of language.* New York: Elsevier North Holland.

Halpern, D. (1990). Teaching for critical thinking: Helping college students develop the skills and dispositions of a critical thinker. *New Directions for Teaching And Learning, 80*, 69–74.

Hampson, R. E., Pons, T. P., Stanford, T. R., & Deadwyler, S. A. (2004). Categorization in the monkey hippocampus: A possible mechanism for encoding information into memory. *Proceedings of the National Academy of Sciences (USA), 101*(9), 3184–3189.

Hart, B., & Risley, T. R. (1999). *The social world of children learning to talk.* Baltimore, MD: Paul H. Brookes.

Heilman, A. W. (2005). *Phonics in proper perspective* (10th ed.). Columbus, OH: Merrill-Prentice Hall. (Original work published 1964)

Hirsch, M. C., & Kramer, T. (1999). *Neuroanatomy: 3D-stereoscopic atlas of the human brain.* Heidelberg: Springer-Verlag.

Holm, A., & Dodd, B. (1996). The effect of first written language on the acquisition of English literacy. *Cognition, 59* (2), 119–147.

Holmes, A.,Murphy, D. L., & Crawley, J. N. (2003). Abnormal behavioral phenotypes of serotonin transporter knockout mice: Parallels with human anxiety and depression. *Biological Psychiatry, 54*(10), 953–959.

Honda, H. (2003). Competition between retinal ganglion axons for targets under the servomechanism model explains abnormal retinocollicular projection of eph receptor-overexpressing or ephrin-lacking mice. *Journal of Neuroscience, 23*(32), 10,368–10,377.

Hood, L. J. (1998). An overview of neural function and feedback control in human communication. *Journal of Communication Disorders, 31(6)*, 461–470.

Horner, R. H. (2000). Positive behavior supports. *Focus on Autism and Other Developmental Disabilities, 15*(2), 97–105.

Howard, P. J. (2006). *Owner's Manual of the Brain* (3rd ed.). Austin, TX: Bard Press.

Hubel, D. H. (1988). *Eye, brain, and vision*. New York: Scientific American Library and W. H. Freeman.

Hux, K., Morris-Friehe, M., & Sanger, D. D. (1993). Language sampling practices: A survey of nine states. *Speech Language Hearing Services in the Schools, 24*, 84–91.

Just, M. A., Carpenter, P. A., Keller, T. A., Eddy, W. F., & Thulborn, K. A. (1996). Brain activation modulated by sentence comprehension. *Science, 274*(5284), 114–116.

Kasher, A. S. A. (1998). *Pragmatics: Critical concepts*. London: Routledge.

Katz, J. J., & Fodor, J. A. (1963). The structure of a semantic theory. *Language, 39*(2), 170–210.

Kernan, K. T. (1970). Semantic relationships and the child's acquisition of language. *Anthropological Linguistics, 12*(5), 171–187.

Klima, E., & Bellugi, U. (1979). *The signs of language*. Cambridge, MA: President and Fellows of Harvard College.

Koruga, D., Ribar, S., Ratkaj, Z., Radonjic, M., & Matija, L. (2004). Synergy of classical and quantum communications channels in brain: Neuron-astrocyte network. *Neural Network Applications in Electrical Engineering: NEUREL, 23–25*, 177–182.

Kramsch, C. (2004). *Context and culture in language teaching* (6th ed.). Oxford: Oxford University Press.

Lakatos, P., Shah, A. S., Knuth, K. H., Ulbert, I., Karmos, G., & Schroeder, C. E. (2005). An oscillatory hierarchy controlling neuronal excitability and stimulus processing in the auditory cortex. *Journal of Neurophysiology, 94*, 1904–1911.

Launer, P. B., & Lahey, M. (1981). Passages: From the fifties to the eighties in language assessment. *Topics in Language Disorders, 1*(3), 11–30.

Lenneberg, E. H. (1967). *Biological foundations of language*. New York: John Wiley & Sons.

Leonard, W. M. (1988). *A sociological perspective of sport* (3rd ed.). New York: Macmillan.

Lou, H. C., Henriksen, L., Bruhn, P., Børner, H., & Bieber Nielsen, J. (1989). Striatal dysfunction in attention deficit and hyperkinetic disorder. *Archives of Neurology, 46*(1), 48–52.

Lucas, E. V. (1978). The feasibility of speech acts as a language approach for emotionally disturbed children. Doctoral dissertation, University of Georgia, 1977. *Dissertation Abstracts International, 38*, 3479B–3967B.

Lucas, E. V. (1980). *Semantic and pragmatic language disorders*. Rockville, MD: Aspen Systems Corporation.

Lund, N. J., & Duchan, J. F. (1983). *Assessing children's language in naturalistic contexts*. Englewood Cliffs, NJ: Prentice-Hall.

Lust, B., & Foley, C. (Eds.) (2004). *First language acquisition: The essential readings*. Malden, MA: Blackwell.

Malafouris, L. (2010). The brain–artefact interface (BAI): A challenge for archaeology and cultural neuroscience. *Social, Cognitive, Affective Neuroscience,* doi: 10.1093/scan/nsp057. First published online January 19, 2010; accessed March 30, 2010.

Manhart, K. (2004). The limits of multitasking. *Scientific American Mind*, December, 62–67.

Maurice, C., Green, G., & Luce, S. (1996). *Behavioral intervention for young children with autism: A manual for parents and professionals.* Austin, TX: Pro-Ed.

Maybin, J. (2003). *Language and literacy in social practice*. Tonawanda, NY: The Open University.

McCawley, J. D. (Ed.) (1976). *Papers on syntactic and semantic topics*. New York: Academic Press.

McCombs, J., Kirby, S., Barney, H., Darilek, H., & Magee, S. (2005). *Achieving state and national literacy goals: A long uphill road. A report to Carnegie Corporation of New York*. Santa Monica, CA: Rand Corporation.

McEwen, B. S. (2007). *The Dana Foundation's cerebrum*. New York: Dana Foundation.

McEwen, B. S. (2008). Central effects of stress hormones in health and disease: Understanding the protective and damaging effects of stress and stress mediators. *European Journal of Pharmacology,583*(2–3), 174–185.

McGuinness, D. (2005). *Language development and learning to read*. Cambridge, MA: MIT Press.

Merzenich, M. M., Saunders, G., Jenkins, W. M., Miller, S., Peterson, B., & Tallal, P. (1999). Pervasive developmental disorders: Listening training and language abilities. In S. H. Broman & J. M. Fletcher (Eds.) *The changing nervous system: Neurobehavioral consequences of early brain disorders* (pp. 365–385). New York: Oxford University Press.

Merzenich, M. M., Tallal, P., Peterson, B., Miller, S. L., & Jenkins, W. M. (1998). Some neurological principles relevant to the origins of—and the cortical plasticity based remediation of—language learning impairments. In J. Grafman & Y. Christen (Eds.) *Neuroplasticity: Building a bridge from the laboratory to the clinic* (pp. 169–187). Amsterdam: Elsevier.

Miller, C. A., Kail, R., & Tomblin, J. B. (2001). Speed of processing in children with specific language impairment. *Journal of Speech, Language, and Hearing Research, 44*, 416–433.

Miller, S. L., Linn, N., Tallal, P., Merzenich, M. M., & Jenkins, W. M. (1999). Acoustically modified speech and language training: A relationship between auditory word discrimination training and measures of language outcomes. *Reeducation Orthophonique, 197*, 159–182.

Mitchell, T. M., Shinkareva, S. V., Kai-Min Chang, A. C., Malave, V. L., Mason, R. A., & Just, M. A. (2008). Predicting human brain activity associated with the meanings of nouns. *Science, 30*(320), 1191–1195.

Monchi, O., Petrides, M., Petre, V., Worsley, K., & Dagher, A. (2001). Wisconsin card sorting revisited: Distinct neural circuits participating in different stages of the task identified by event-related functional magnetic resonance imaging. *Journal of Neuroscience, 21*(19), 7733–7741.

Moore, D., & Shepherd, R. (2008). The auditory brain—A tribute to Dexter R.F. Irvine. *Hearing Research,238*, 1–2.

Morgan, M., Greene, J. O., Gill, E. A., & McCullough, J. D. (2009). The creative character of talk: Individual differences in narrative production ability. *Communication Studies, 60*, 180–196.

Overath, T. (2009*). Representation of statistical sound properties in human auditory cortex.* Unpublished doctoral thesis, University College London.

Peirce, C. S. (2000). *Writings of Charles S. Peirce: Volume 1. 1857–1866*. Peirce Edition Project. Bloomington, IN: Indiana University Press and Association of American University Presses.

Piaget, J. (1952). *The origins of intelligence in children* (M. Cook, Trans.). New York: International Universities Press.

Pulvermueller, F. (2002). *The neuroscience of language*. Cambridge: Cambridge University Press.

Qi, C. H., Kaiser, A. P., Milan, S., & Hancock, T. (2006). Language performance of low-income African American and European American preschool children on the PPVT–III. *Language, Speech, and Hearing Services in Schools, 37,* 5–16.

Robb, B. (2010). *My approach to my classroom*. Unpublished manuscript, Portland, OR: Portland Public School District Teacher and Consultant.

Robinson, W. P. (2003). *Language in social worlds*. Malden, MA: Blackwell.

Rostamizadeh, A. (2009a). *My approach to teaching*. Unpublished manuscript, McMinnville, OR: McMinnville School District Teacher.

Rostamizadeh, A. (2009b). *Visual strategies for critical literacy: Assigning meaning to formal concepts in social justice texts*. Unpublished thesis, Western Oregon University, Monmouth, OR.

Rowe, B., & Levine, D. P. (2009). *Linguistics: A concise introduction* (2nd ed.). Boston, MA: Allyn & Bacon.

Sadato, N., Pascual-Leone, A., Grafman, J., Ibanez, V., Deiber, M., Dold, G., & Hallett, M. (1996). Activation of the primary visual cortex by Braille reading in blind subjects. *Nature, 380*(11), 526–528.

Sanda, P., & Marsalek, P. (2009). Sound encoding in auditory pathway, implications for cochlear implants. Eighteenth Annual Computational Neuroscience Meeting, Berlin, Germany. *Neuroscience, 10*(Suppl. 1), 104, 18–23.

Schmidt, M. F. (2008). Using both sides of your brain: The case for rapid interhemispheric switching. *PLoS Biology 6*(10): e269. doi:10.1371/journal.pbio.0060269.

Schumann, J. H. (2004). *The neurobiology of learning*. Mahwah, NJ: Lawrence Erlbaum.

Searle, J. (1969). *Speech acts: An essay in the philosophy of language*. Cambridge: Cambridge University Press.

Shanker, S. G., & King, B. J. (2002). The emergence of a new paradigm in ape language research. *Behavioral and Brain Sciences, 25*(5), 605–620.

Shaywitz, S., Shaywitz, B., Pugh, K., Fulbright, R., Constable, R. T., Mencl, W. E., Shankweiler, D., *et al.* (1998). Functional disruption in the organization of the brain for reading in dyslexia. *Proceedings of the National Academy of Sciences, 95*(5), 2636–2641.

Siegel, D. J. (2007). *The mindful brain.* New York: Norton.

Simmons, A. (2002). *The story factor: Inspiration, influence, and persuasion through the art of storytelling*. Cambridge, MA: Perseus.

Simos, P. G., Fletcher, J. M., Bergman, E., Breier, J. J., Foorman, B. R., Castillo, E. M., Davis, R. M., Fitzgerald, M., & Papanicolaou, A. C. (2002). Dyslexia-specific brain activation profile becomes normal following successful remedial training. *Neurology, 58*, 1203–1213.

Slobin, D. I. (2004). Cognitive prerequisites for the development of grammar. In B. C. Lust, & C. Foley (Eds.) *First language acquisition: The essential readings*. Malden, MA: Blackwell.

Smith, B. L. (1978). Temporal aspects of English speech production: A developmental perspective. *Journal of Phonetics, 6*(1), 37–67.

Smith, F. (1992). Learning to read: The never-ending debate. *The Phi Delta Kappan, 73*(6), 432–435, 438–441.

Smith, F. (2004). *Understanding reading: A psycholinguistic analysis of reading and learning to read.* Hillsdale, NJ: Lawrence Erlbaum.

Sparks, B. F., Friedman, S. D., Shaw, D. W., Aylward, E. H., Echelard, D., Artru, A. A., Maravilla, K. A., *et al.* (2002). Brain structural abnormalities in young children with autism spectrum disorder. *Neurology, 59*, 184–192.

Starr, M. D., Amlie, R., Martin, W. H., & Sanders, S. (1977). Development of auditory function in newborn infants revealed by auditory brainstem potentials. *Pediatrics, 60*(6), 831–839.

Stremming, N. (2009). *Creating a visual classroom: Strategies for developing meaning through visual teaching.* Unpublished capstone project, University of Portland, Portland, OR.

Stremming, N. (2010). *Visual teaching in the high school*. Unpublished manuscript, University of Portland, Portland, OR.

Sylwester, R. (1995). *A celebration of neurons*. Alexandria, VA: Association for Supervision and Curriculum Design.

Sylwester, R. (2003). *A biological brain in a cultural classroom: Enhancing cognitive and social development through collaborative classroom management*. Thousand Oaks, CA: Corwin Press.

Sylwester, R. (2005). *How to explain a brain: An educator's handbook of brain terms and cognitive processes.* Thousand Oaks, CA: Corwin Press.

Trask, R. L. (1992). *A dictionary of grammatical terms in linguistics.* London: Routledge.

Traugott, E. C. (1975). Spatial expressions of tense and temporal sequencing: A contribution to the study of semantic fields. *Semiotica, 15*(3), 207–230.

Trelfert, D. A., & Wallace, G. L. (2007). *Islands of the mind.* Mind Special Edition, *Scientific American.*

Verschueren, J. (1999). *Understanding pragmatics*. London: Arnold.

Villegas, M., Neugebauer, R., & Venegas, K. R. (Eds.) (2008). *Indigenous Knowledge and Education.* Cambridge, MA: Harvard Educational Review.

Vygotsky, L. S. (1962). *Thought and language*. Cambridge, MA: MIT Press. (Original work published 1934)

Walker, D., Greenwood, C., Hart, B., & Carta, J. (1994). Prediction of school outcomes based on early language prediction and socio-economic factors. *Child Development, 65*, 606–621.

Walker, H. M., Kavanagh, K., Stiller, B., Golly, A., Severson, H. H., & Feil, E. G. (1998). First step to success: An early intervention approach for preventing school antisocial behavior. *Journal of Emotional and Behavioral Disorders, 6*(2), 66–80.

Walker, I., & Hulme, C. (1999). Concrete words are easier to recall than abstract words: Evidence for a semantic contribution to short-term serial recall. *Journal of Experimental Psychology: Learning, Memory, and Cognition, 25*(5), 1256–1271.

Webster, D. B. (1999). *Neuroscience of communication*. San Diego, CA: Singular.

Webster, J. J. (Ed.) (2008). *Meaning in context*. New York: Continuum.

Wheeler, S. C. (1978). Quantification in English. *Philosophia, 8*(1), 31–42.

Winkler, E. G. (2007). *Understanding language*. New York: Continuum.

Wittgenstein, L. (2001). *Philosophical investigations: The German text, with a revised English translation.* Malden, MA: Blackwell. (Original work published 1953)

Subject Index

Author Index

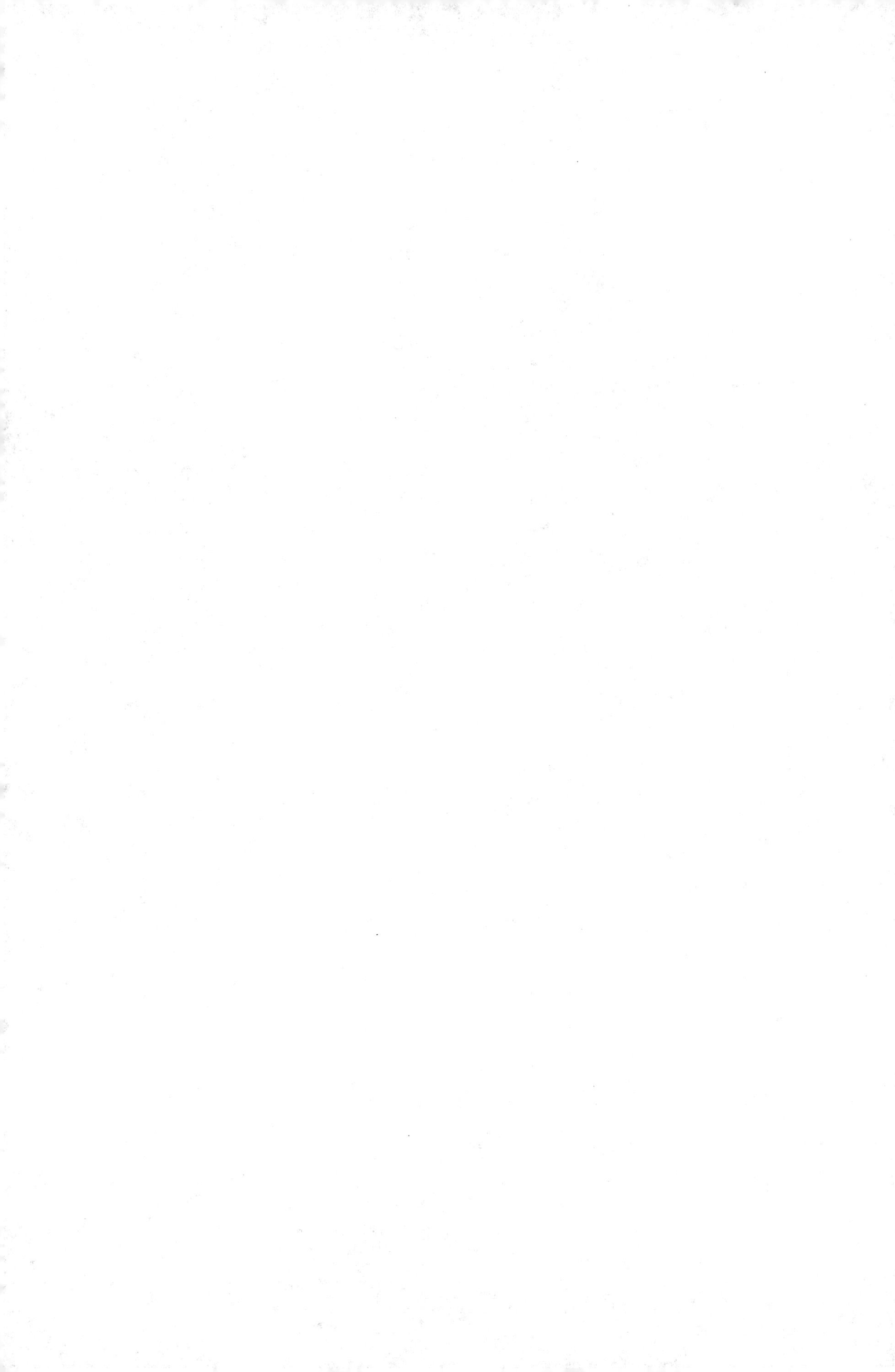